Chalk Talks in Internal Medicine

Somnath Mookherjee • Lauren A. Beste
Jared W. Klein • Jennifer Wright
Editors

Chalk Talks in Internal Medicine

Scripts for Clinical Teaching

Springer

Editors
Somnath Mookherjee
University of Washington Medical Center
Department of Medicine
Division of General Internal Medicine
University of Washington
Seattle, WA
USA

Lauren A. Beste
VA Puget Sound Health Care System
Department of Medicine
Division of General Internal Medicine
University of Washington
Seattle, WA
USA

Jared W. Klein
Harborview Medical Center
Department of Medicine
Division of General Internal Medicine
University of Washington
Seattle, WA
USA

Jennifer Wright
University of Washington Medical Center
Department of Medicine
Division of General Internal Medicine
University of Washington
Seattle, WA
USA

ISBN 978-3-030-34813-7 ISBN 978-3-030-34814-4 (eBook)
https://doi.org/10.1007/978-3-030-34814-4

This Springer imprint is published by the registered company Springer Nature Switzerland AG
The registered company address is: Gewerbestrasse 11, 6330 Cham, Switzerland

SM dedicates this book to his parents: anything I have accomplished as a physician and a scholar I owe to them.

LAB dedicates this book to all who spend their lives in the service of learning, teaching, and healing and to the families who support us on that journey.

JWK dedicates this book to his family for their boundless support.

JW dedicates this book to Patrick: for your love and support.

Preface

Chalk talks immerse high yield, and relevant teaching in the clinical setting – immediately linking clinical experiences with the skills of physicianship. Chalk talks not only enhance the learning of students and trainees but also enable fun, satisfying, and meaningful teaching. We hope this book positively contributes to the experience of teaching and learning medicine for all readers

This book is the result of a unique endeavor by the Division of General Internal Medicine, University of Washington. We recruited ninety-six faculty members from our Division to create teaching scripts for commonly encountered inpatient and outpatient clinical scenarios. In addition to creating the teaching scripts, we encouraged co-authors to engage in peer mentorship around career development and satisfaction. Thus, faculty not only used their expertise and experience to create these teaching scripts, many developed partnerships supporting their career development.

This is a guide for teaching clinical medicine and not a manual for clinical practice. Readers should be vigilant for advances in medical science and changes in clinical practice that supersede the details of this book. While we did our utmost to avoid errors and omissions, the responsibility for verifying the accuracy of the content lies with the reader.

We hope that you will find Chalk Talks in Internal Medicine to be useful and engaging. We wish you the best in your teaching career.

Seattle, WA, USA
July 8, 2019

Somnath Mookherjee
Lauren A. Beste
Jared W. Klein
Jennifer Wright

Contents

Contributors

Albert Ackil, MD University of Colorado Hospital, Department of Medicine, Division of Hospital Medicine, University of Colorado, Denver, CO, USA

Nicole Chow Ahrenholz, MD Harborview Medical Center, Department of Medicine, Division of General Internal Medicine, University of Washington, Seattle, WA, USA

Tyler Albert, MD VA Puget Sound Health Care System, Department of Medicine, Division of General Internal Medicine, University of Washington, Seattle, WA, USA

Bradley D. Anawalt, MD University of Washington Medical Center, Department of Medicine, Division of General Internal Medicine, University of Washington, Seattle, WA, USA

Neil Argyle, MD, MPH Boise VA Medical Center, Department of Medicine, Division of General Internal Medicine, University of Washington, Seattle, WA, USA

Pallavi R. Arora, MBBS, MD, MPH Harborview Medical Center, Department of Medicine, Division of General Internal Medicine, University of Washington, Seattle, WA, USA

Amy Baernstein, MD University of Washington Medical Center, Department of Medicine, Division of General Internal Medicine, University of Washington, Seattle, WA, USA

Maralyssa Bann, MD Harborview Medical Center, Department of Medicine, Division of General Internal Medicine, University of Washington, Seattle, WA, USA

Gabrielle Berger, MD University of Washington Medical Center, Department of Medicine, Division of General Internal Medicine, University of Washington, Seattle, WA, USA

Lauren A. Beste, MD, MS VA Puget Sound Health Care System, Department of Medicine, Division of General Internal Medicine, University of Washington, Seattle, WA, USA

Daniel Cabrera, MD Harborview Medical Center, Department of Medicine, Division of General Internal Medicine, University of Washington, Seattle, WA, USA

Tiffany Chen, MD University of Washington Medical Center, Department of Medicine, Division of General Internal Medicine, University of Washington, Seattle, WA, USA

John H. Choe, MD, MPH Harborview Medical Center, Department of Medicine, Division of General Internal Medicine, University of Washington, Seattle, WA, USA

Andrea S. Christopher, MD, MPH, FACP Boise VA Medical Center, Department of Medicine, Division of General Internal Medicine, University of Washington, Seattle, WA, USA

Paul Cornia, MD VA Puget Sound Health Care System, Department of Medicine, Division of General Internal Medicine, University of Washington, Seattle, WA, USA

James Darnton, MD Harborview Medical Center, Department of Medicine, Division of General Internal Medicine, University of Washington, Seattle, WA, USA

Stefanie A. Deeds, MD VA Puget Sound Health Care System, Department of Medicine, Division of General Internal Medicine, University of Washington, Seattle, WA, USA

Neha S. Deshpande, MD University of Washington Medical Center, Department of Medicine, Division of General Internal Medicine, University of Washington, Seattle, WA, USA

Anne Eacker, MD Kaiser Permanente Bernard J. Tyson School of Medicine, Pasadena, CA, USA

Leslie Enzian, MD Harborview Medical Center, Department of Medicine, Division of General Internal Medicine, University of Washington, Seattle, WA, USA

Ginger Evans, MD VA Puget Sound Health Care System, Department of Medicine, Division of General Internal Medicine, University of Washington, Seattle, WA, USA

Brandon Fainstad, MD Veterans Affairs, Rocky Mountain Regional Medical Center, Aurora, CO, USA

Tyra Fainstad, MD University of Washington Medical Center, Department of Medicine, Division of General Internal Medicine, University of Washington, Seattle, WA, USA

Joana Lima Ferreira, MD University of Washington Medical Center, Department of Medicine, Division of General Internal Medicine, University of Washington, Seattle, WA, USA

Stephanie A. Field, MD Harborview Medical Center, Department of Medicine, Division of General Internal Medicine, University of Washington, Seattle, WA, USA

Barak Gaster, MD University of Washington Medical Center, Department of Medicine, Division of General Internal Medicine, University of Washington, Seattle, WA, USA

Lindsay Gibbon, MD Harborview Medical Center, Department of Medicine, Division of General Internal Medicine, University of Washington, Seattle, WA, USA

Mellena Giday, MD Harborview Medical Center, Department of Medicine, Division of General Internal Medicine, University of Washington, Seattle, WA, USA

Divya Gollapudi, MD Harborview Medical Center, Department of Medicine, Division of General Internal Medicine, University of Washington, Seattle, WA, USA

Anna L. Golob, MD VA Puget Sound Health Care System, Department of Medicine, Division of General Internal Medicine, University of Washington, Seattle, WA, USA

Deborah Greenberg, MD University of Washington Medical Center, Department of Medicine, Division of General Internal Medicine, University of Washington, Seattle, WA, USA

Anna Hagan, MD Harborview Medical Center, Department of Medicine, Division of General Internal Medicine, University of Washington, Seattle, WA, USA

Scott Hagan, MD VA Puget Sound Health Care System, Department of Medicine, Division of General Internal Medicine, University of Washington, Seattle, WA, USA

Melissa M. Hagman, MD, FACP Boise VA Medical Center, Department of Medicine, Division of General Internal Medicine, University of Washington, Seattle, WA, USA

Mahri Haider, MD, MPH Harborview Medical Center, Department of Medicine, Division of General Internal Medicine, University of Washington, Seattle, WA, USA

Meghaan Hawes, MD Harborview Medical Center, Department of Medicine, Division of General Internal Medicine, University of Washington, Seattle, WA, USA

Ken He, MD VA Pittsburgh Health Care System, Pittsburgh, PA, USA

Allison Himmel, MD Harborview Medical Center, Department of Medicine, Division of General Internal Medicine, University of Washington, Seattle, WA, USA

Ronald Huang, MD, MPH University of Washington Medical Center, Department of Medicine, Division of General Internal Medicine, University of Washington, Seattle, WA, USA

Sara L. Jackson, MD, MPH Harborview Medical Center, Department of Medicine, Division of General Internal Medicine, University of Washington, Seattle, WA, USA

Kamala B. Jain, MD VA Puget Sound Health Care System, Department of Medicine, Division of General Internal Medicine, University of Washington, Seattle, WA, USA

Jocelyn James, MD Harborview Medical Center, Department of Medicine, Division of General Internal Medicine, University of Washington, Seattle, WA, USA

Kay M. Johnson, MD, MPH VA Puget Sound Health Care System, Department of Medicine, Division of General Internal Medicine, University of Washington, Seattle, WA, USA

Catherine P. Kaminetzky, MD, MPH VA Puget Sound Health Care System, Department of Medicine, Division of General Internal Medicine, University of Washington, Seattle, WA, USA

Mehraneh Khalighi, MD VA Puget Sound Health Care System, Department of Medicine, Division of General Internal Medicine, University of Washington, Seattle, WA, USA

Jared W. Klein, MD, MPH Harborview Medical Center, Department of Medicine, Division of General Internal Medicine, University of Washington, Seattle, WA, USA

Christopher Knight, MD University of Washington Medical Center, Department of Medicine, Division of General Internal Medicine, University of Washington, Seattle, WA, USA

Eve Lake, MD Harborview Medical Center, Department of Medicine, Division of General Internal Medicine, University of Washington, Seattle, WA, USA

David S. Levitt, MD Harborview Medical Center, Department of Medicine, Division of General Internal Medicine, University of Washington, Seattle, WA, USA

Yuree Lin, MD Kaiser Permanente Moanalua Medical Center, Honolulu, HI, USA

Adelaide McClintock, MD University of Washington Medical Center, Department of Medicine, Division of General Internal Medicine, University of Washington, Seattle, WA, USA

Karen A. McDonough, MD University of Washington Medical Center, Department of Medicine, Division of General Internal Medicine, University of Washington, Seattle, WA, USA

Susan Merel, MD University of Washington Medical Center, Department of Medicine, Division of General Internal Medicine, University of Washington, Seattle, WA, USA

Joseph Merrill, MD, MPH Harborview Medical Center, Department of Medicine, Division of General Internal Medicine, University of Washington, Seattle, WA, USA

Kara Mitchell, MD University of Washington Medical Center, Department of Medicine, Division of General Internal Medicine, University of Washington, Seattle, WA, USA

Sylvia Mollerstrom, MD Harborview Medical Center, Department of Medicine, Division of General Internal Medicine, University of Washington, Seattle, WA, USA

Alexandra Molnar, MD Harborview Medical Center, Department of Medicine, Division of General Internal Medicine, University of Washington, Seattle, WA, USA

Somnath Mookherjee, MD University of Washington Medical Center, Department of Medicine, Division of General Internal Medicine, University of Washington, Seattle, WA, USA

Alexandra Moretti Morrison, MD Harborview Medical Center, Department of Medicine, Division of General Internal Medicine, University of Washington, Seattle, WA, USA

Kelly Nakamura, MD Harborview Medical Center, Department of Medicine, Division of General Internal Medicine, University of Washington, Seattle, WA, USA

Maya Narayanan, MD, MPH University of Washington Medical Center, Department of Medicine, Division of General Internal Medicine, University of Washington, Seattle, WA, USA

Kari M. Nelson, MD, MSHS VA Puget Sound Health Care System, Department of Medicine, Division of General Internal Medicine, University of Washington, Seattle, WA, USA

Michael Northrop, MD VA Puget Sound Health Care System, Department of Medicine, Division of General Internal Medicine, University of Washington, Seattle, WA, USA

Kim O'Connor, MD University of Washington Medical Center, Department of Medicine, Division of General Internal Medicine, University of Washington, Seattle, WA, USA

Maryann K. Overland, MD VA Puget Sound Health Care System, Department of Medicine, Division of General Internal Medicine, University of Washington, Seattle, WA, USA

Doug Paauw, MD University of Washington Medical Center, Department of Medicine, Division of General Internal Medicine, University of Washington, Seattle, WA, USA

Grady Paden, MD VA Puget Sound Health Care System, Department of Medicine, Division of General Internal Medicine, University of Washington, Seattle, WA, USA

Genevieve L. Pagalilauan, MD, FACP University of Washington Medical Center, Department of Medicine, Division of General Internal Medicine, University of Washington, Seattle, WA, USA

Thomas Payne, MD University of Washington Medical Center, Department of Medicine, Division of General Internal Medicine, University of Washington, Seattle, WA, USA

Heidi Powell, MD University of Washington Medical Center, Department of Medicine, Division of General Internal Medicine, University of Washington, Seattle, WA, USA

Alexander Pratt, MD Harborview Medical Center, Department of Medicine, Division of General Internal Medicine, University of Washington, Seattle, WA, USA

Thomas Rea, MD, MPH Harborview Medical Center, Department of Medicine, Division of General Internal Medicine, University of Washington, Seattle, WA, USA

Jeffrey Redinger, MD VA Puget Sound Health Care System, Department of Medicine, Division of General Internal Medicine, University of Washington, Seattle, WA, USA

Caroline Rhoads, MD Harborview Medical Center, Department of Medicine, Division of General Internal Medicine, University of Washington, Seattle, WA, USA

Daniel Santovasi, MD VA Puget Sound Health Care System, Department of Medicine, Division of General Internal Medicine, University of Washington, Seattle, WA, USA

Sabeena Setia, MD, MPH Landmark Health, Seattle, WA, USA

John Sheffield, MD Harborview Medical Center, Department of Medicine, Division of General Internal Medicine, University of Washington, Seattle, WA, USA

Naomi Shike, MD, MSc Harborview Medical Center, Department of Medicine, Division of General Internal Medicine, University of Washington, Seattle, WA, USA

Toby Sinton, MD VA Puget Sound Health Care System, Department of Medicine, Division of General Internal Medicine, University of Washington, Seattle, WA, USA

Shobha W. Stack, MD, PhD University of Washington Medical Center, Department of Medicine, Division of General Internal Medicine, University of Washington, Seattle, WA, USA

Lindee M. Strizich, MD, MSc University of Washington Medical Center, Department of Medicine, Division of General Internal Medicine, University of Washington, Seattle, WA, USA

Nancy Sugg, MD, MPH Harborview Medical Center, Department of Medicine, Division of General Internal Medicine, University of Washington, Seattle, WA, USA

Paul R. Sutton, MD, PhD University of Washington Medical Center, Department of Medicine, Division of General Internal Medicine, University of Washington, Seattle, WA, USA

Traci Takahashi, MD, MPH VA Puget Sound Health Care System, Department of Medicine, Division of General Internal Medicine, University of Washington, Seattle, WA, USA

Genji S. Terasaki, MD Harborview Medical Center, Department of Medicine, Division of General Internal Medicine, University of Washington, Seattle, WA, USA

Jill Watanabe, MD, MPH Harborview Medical Center, Department of Medicine, Division of General Internal Medicine, University of Washington, Seattle, WA, USA

William Weppner, MD, MPH Boise VA Medical Center, Department of Medicine, Division of General Internal Medicine, University of Washington, Seattle, WA, USA

Stephanie Wheeler, MD VA Puget Sound Health Care System, Department of Medicine, Division of General Internal Medicine, University of Washington, Seattle, WA, USA

Andrew White, MD University of Washington Medical Center, Department of Medicine, Division of General Internal Medicine, University of Washington, Seattle, WA, USA

Joyce Wipf, MD VA Puget Sound Health Care System, Department of Medicine, Division of General Internal Medicine, University of Washington, Seattle, WA, USA

Jessica Woan, MD VA Puget Sound Health Care System, Department of Medicine, Division of General Internal Medicine, University of Washington, Seattle, WA, USA

Christopher Wong, MD University of Washington Medical Center, Department of Medicine, Division of General Internal Medicine, University of Washington, Seattle, WA, USA

Jennifer Wright, MD University of Washington Medical Center, Department of Medicine, Division of General Internal Medicine, University of Washington, Seattle, WA, USA

Yilin Zhang, MD University of Washington Medical Center, Department of Medicine, Division of General Internal Medicine, University of Washington, Seattle, WA, USA

Diana Zhong, MD University of Washington Medical Center, Department of Medicine, Division of General Internal Medicine, University of Washington, Seattle, WA, USA

Chapter 1
Introduction

Somnath Mookherjee, Lauren A. Beste, Jared W. Klein, and Jennifer Wright

Why We Created This Book

Every year, thousands of teaching physicians are asked to train the next generation of learners in a growing body of knowledge. Formal teaching time has become increasingly limited because of rising clinical workload, medical documentation requirements, duty hour restrictions, and other time pressures. In addition, today's learners expect teaching sessions that deliver focused content integrated into their clinical workflow. One classic teaching method that is ideally suited to meet these needs is the "chalk talk," a focused teaching session typically delivered with just a white board for drawing visual aids and extensive audience participation.

We have all observed master teachers deliver riveting chalk talks off the cuff. However, most of us would benefit from structured content and guidance on how to deliver this content-also known as a teaching script. A good teaching script anticipates learners' misconceptions, highlights a select number of teaching points, uses strategies to engage the learners, and provides a cognitive scaffold for teaching the topic that the teacher can refine over time.

S. Mookherjee (✉) · J. Wright
University of Washington Medical Center, Department of Medicine, Division of General Internal Medicine, University of Washington, Seattle, WA, USA
e-mail: smookh@u.washington.edu

L. A. Beste
VA Puget Sound Health Care System, Department of Medicine, Division of General Internal Medicine, University of Washington, Seattle, WA, USA

J. W. Klein
Harborview Medical Center, Department of Medicine, Division of General Internal Medicine, University of Washington, Seattle, WA, USA

S. Mookherjee et al. (eds.), *Chalk Talks in Internal Medicine*,
https://doi.org/10.1007/978-3-030-34814-4_1

Intended Audience

The primary target audience for this book are trainees in internal medicine and attending physicians who teach in inpatient or outpatient clinical settings. In addition, physician's assistants, nurse practitioners, and others who teach general medicine will be interested in this book. Finally, we anticipate that learners throughout the continuum of medical education, from first-year medical students to experienced attending physicians, will deepen their comfort with these important concepts by practicing to teach them.

Guiding Principles

All teaching scripts share the same overall goal: to help teachers plan and execute effective teaching sessions. The structure and content of a script depend on the teaching setting, audience, experience of the teacher, and many other factors. For our teaching scripts, we determined the following guiding principles to facilitate the structure and content:

- While teaching based on clinical trials and prominent studies is important, this collection focuses on important principles of diagnosis and care without relying on extensive references to the literature.
- Well-designed learning objectives are critical for each teaching script: limited in scope and number, realistic for the teaching session, and behaviorally anchored.
- The content should be explicitly engaging to the learner.
- Visual representations (drawings, tables, and diagrams) are essential, both for maximizing ease of use for the teacher and for aiding in knowledge retention by the learners.
- The visual elements of the teaching scripts should be easily reproducible by hand.
- Salient parts of the teaching script should be able to be taught in about 10 min with content provided to give lengthier or more in-depth chalk talks.

Finally, we wish to emphasize key internal medicine concepts that an early clinician (students and residents) should know, and acknowledge that this is not meant to be a comprehensive textbook of internal medicine.

Structure

After reading the chapter and practicing the teaching script, the reader should be able to give a chalk talk on the topic. Each teaching script is anchored by a brief clinical scenario and structured around questions the teacher may ask of the learners. Each step in the teaching scripts is explicitly linked with a portion of the diagram for the teacher to use as they teach the content. Figure 1.1 outlines the structure of the teaching scripts provided in this book.

Description of teaching script component	Examples from Chapter 38: Approach to microscopic hematuria
Objectives: these were designed to complete the sentence: "After this talk, the learner will be able to…"	1. Use a systematic approach to evaluation of microscopic hematuria 2. Describe common causes of microscopic hematuria 3. Distinguish between "glomerular" and "non-glomerular" sources of microscopic hematuria 4. Identify risk factors for genitourinary (GU) malignancy
Clinical vignette: a brief description of a clinical scenario that anchors the teaching script. As with all aspects of the teaching scripts offered, the teacher can modify this based on their own experiences or points which they wish to emphasize.	A 62-year-old man comes to see you because he received notification that his insurance examination urine dipstick had shown "blood". He is confused by these results as he has never seen blood in his urine
Questions for the learner: these questions link to the visually represented content. In this example, the letter "A" refers to the point in diagram that the teacher should be writing on the white board.	**A. How do we define hematuria - do we know that he really has it?**
Brief directions to the teacher: these questions are included to clarify the steps of the teaching script for the teacher.	Write the definition as shown in the Figure.

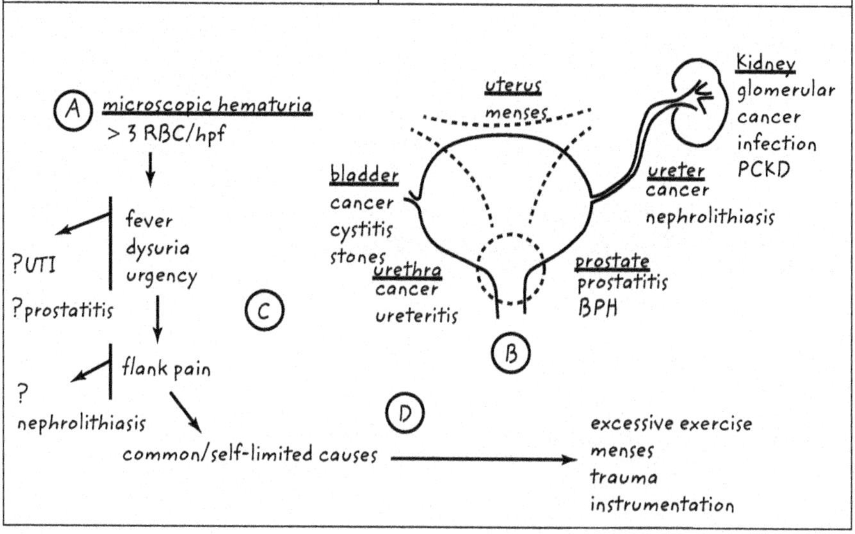

Fig. 1.1 Structure of the teaching scripts in this book

Teaching points: these are the key points to answer the questions to the learner and comprise the bulk of the content. We endeavored to minimize the overlap between the teaching points listed in the script and in the visual representations.	• The term "gross hematuria" is used to describe visible blood in the urine. The term "microscopic hematuria" is used when blood is not visible to the naked eye, only noted upon microscopic examination. • Positive blood on urine dipstick is not sufficient to diagnose microscopic hematuria, as this is a very sensitive test with frequent false positives. ... continued in Chapter 38.
Return to objectives and emphasize key points: this section was included at the end of each teaching script to reinforce the importance of repeating the key points. The content provided intentionally overlaps with the teaching points and objectives previously provided.	1. Recognize common causes of microscopic hematuria – circle these in the figure • Cancer • Infection (e.g., bladder, kidney, prostate) • Stones • IgA nephropathy • Post streptococcal • Benign (e.g., menses, exercise) ... continued in Chapter 38.
Resources: for each teaching script, we included for a list of key resources that support the content and provide further reading. This not meant to be a comprehensive list of references supporting the content of the teaching script.	1. Nielsen M, Quaseem A. Hematuria as a Marker of Occult Urinary Tract Cancer: Advice for High-Value Care from the American College of Physicians. Ann Intern Med 2016;164(7):488-497. ... continued in Chapter 38.

Fig. 1.1 (continued)

Based on our own clinical teaching experiences and in consultation with our colleagues, we selected topics that often arise in the inpatient and outpatient contexts. The scope of each topic is deliberately narrow enough that a key portion can be taught in 10 min, but each chapter contains enough content such that the length of the teaching script can be adjusted, as needed (see Chap. 2).

Using Teaching Scripts

Our goal is to encourage clinical teachers to deliver these and other chalk talks. Teaching "on the fly" can be challenging, but we hope that these scripts provide valuable support and content to meet this challenge. In addition, we provide guidance on creating your own teaching scripts (Chap. 2) and detailed advice on delivering a chalk talk using a teaching script (Chap. 3). Figure 1.1 outlines how to use the teaching scripts in this book.

Chapter 2
How to Create a Teaching Script for a Chalk Talk

Diana Zhong and Somnath Mookherjee

Introduction

This book provides teaching scripts for 48 chalk talks on a variety of inpatient and outpatient internal medicine topics. We hope that the teaching scripts will be exceedingly useful, but ultimately, we aspire to encourage readers to create their own teaching scripts to use and share. Creating a teaching script can seem like an intimidating proposition. In this chapter, we provide guidance to clinical teachers on how to create their own teaching scripts.

Choosing the Topic

Uncertainty over your own level of content mastery is a common barrier to clinical teaching. Lack of confidence in recalling the names of salient clinical trials, the mechanism of action of drugs, or the pathophysiology once learned in medical school (but long forgotten) can discourage clinicians from taking on important teaching topics. In reality, you know much more than you think you do, and in the realm of practical knowledge, you will have much more to share with the learners than you anticipate. It takes less work than you might expect to fill in any knowledge gaps in order to create an effective teaching script, and taking the additional step of creating a teaching script will push you to better understand the topic.

D. Zhong (✉) · S. Mookherjee
University of Washington Medical Center, Department of Medicine, Division of General Internal Medicine, University of Washington, Seattle, WA, USA
e-mail: zhongd@uw.edu

S. Mookherjee et al. (eds.), *Chalk Talks in Internal Medicine*,
https://doi.org/10.1007/978-3-030-34814-4_2

When creating a teaching script (or selecting one to use from this book), consider the following questions:

- What are some common scenarios that you encounter in your clinical work?
- What are recurring clinical decision points that you consider on a regular basis?
- Are there high-risk scenarios that are important to emphasize in your teaching?
- Are there situations that are commonly confusing to learners or may have been previously confusing to you?
- What are common misconceptions that you have encountered in your interactions with learners?

In addition, consider what clinical experiences your learners may have been exposed to and may be interested in learning more about. If on an inpatient or outpatient teaching service, teaching about medical conditions for patients recently seen together is often a great source of teaching topics.

Get Started by Creating a "Hook" and Defining Learning Objectives

Once you have a general idea for a chalk talk, start the script with an interesting opener—our recommendation is a brief clinical vignette. Think about classic presentations for your clinical topic. Rare variations may seem more interesting, but they may be less helpful to early learners who are starting to build their own "illness scripts" based on your teaching. Once you have established the patient presentation, formulate the two or three most important learning objectives that you want learners to take away from the talk. The SMART framework [1, 2] can help you create effective learning objectives:

- Specific: describes what the learner will be able to do as a result of your talk.
- Measurable: the objectives are tangible—they can be observed or counted.
- Action-oriented: behavior change or acquisition of knowledge, skills, or attitudes (in contrast to passive words such as "learn," "know," or "understand").
- Reasonable: realistic expectations for the learner in terms of the scope of the talk and the stage of the learner.
- Time-bound: achievable within the time allotted to teach.

Well-crafted learning objectives can help frame your learners' thinking before your talk and provide context for your learners to apply their knowledge. Table 2.1 provides some examples of good and suboptimal learning objectives.

Table 2.1 Good and suboptimal learning objectives

Examples of good learning objectives	Examples of suboptimal learning objectives
By the end of this talk, learners should be able to: 1. Define sepsis by SIRS and qSOFA criteria 2. Risk stratify patients with sepsis 3. Describe the initial treatment strategies for sepsis	1. Learn about sepsis (*too passive*) 2. Take care of patients with sepsis (*too broad, unreasonable, and unlikely to be achieved in the scope of a chalk talk*)

Table 2.2 Strategies for delivering content in a chalk-talk [3]

Discuss clinical reasoning	Explain complex physiologic principles	Prepare to discuss calculations or methods	Compare and contrast
Do you have a specific patient case that you'd like to discuss? You can go through the case like a morning report. Even with a simple structural organizer like a list, you can number the list (e.g., diagnostic criteria), or rank the list (e.g., sorting from most common to least common, or ranking a differential diagnosis from most likely to least likely). If you want to focus on clinical reasoning, consider emphasizing methods and approaches over facts.	Physiologic principles often work well with frameworks, drawings, and visual organizers. You can use chalk talks to discuss feedback loops and interactions. It can be helpful to evolve your concepts, such as explaining normal physiology and then transitioning to explaining abnormal pathophysiology.	Chalk talks are a great way to demonstrate specific calculations or methods, such as analyzing an arterial blood gas. Even if you're an expert at the calculations, create sample problems and prepare all the math and analyses in advance. This will ensure that your talk is accurate and fluent, and will allow you to focus on teaching the concepts and answering learner questions during the talk.	You can use charts or lists to compare and contrast clinical syndromes (e.g., Crohn disease vs ulcerative colitis) or management strategies (e.g., different antibiotic regimens). You can also compare and contrast old guidelines and new guidelines.

Determine the Most Salient Content and Start Organizing the Flow of the Talk

Once you have established your learning objectives, you are ready to create the content of your chalk talk. There are many ways to present your content, including the suggestions below. Use whichever strategies are most appropriate for your topic and your audience. While creating content, try to keep your information concise and high-yield, always considering how it relates to the learning objectives. Resist the urge to stray too far from your learning objectives or to provide excessive detail. For interested learners, you can always provide supplemental information with a handout, or send them journal articles with the evidence basis. Table 2.2 provides four important strategies to help guide and effectively deliver your content. Other key points to remember are as follows:

Consider your audience If teaching learners of different levels, earmark certain concepts depending on the level of training (e.g., ask one type of question to the medical student and another to the senior resident).

Use frameworks and visual organizers Create frameworks to help improve your learners' recall. Does your topic lend itself to any visual organizers like diagrams, tables, graphs, or flowcharts? Whenever possible, find ways to order, sort, and enumerate information. The more visually clear and appealing your information, the more you will take advantage of the chalk talk format.

Create take-home points These are not the same as your learning objectives, but rather one or two "must knows" or "don't forgets." Ask yourself, "What are the crucial things that I want them to remember from this talk?"

Map Out the Chalk Talk

Now that you have considered the key content needed to accomplish the learning objectives, start to draw out the talk, using your clinical vignette as the starting point. At this stage it is normal to go through several iterations. The rest of this book provides many examples of potential ways to organize a chalk talk. Again, always link the content to your learning objectives.

Create your beginning template Create a rough outline, including placeholders for what you can draw before the talk starts and what you will populate during the talk [3]. What content should already be on the board before you begin speaking? It can be very helpful to write your learning objectives on the board in a corner to help structure your learners' thinking throughout the talk. You can even create placeholders and pre-draw parts of your talk before you begin. Do you have any graphs or tables? You can draw blank *x* and *y* graph axes, or you can label an empty table. You should aim to structure your board, not clutter it. What will you explain verbally? What will you write down? Try your best to have your highest yield points written out.

Decide when to ask questions As you've laid out your content, you can pinpoint specific places where you'll want to elicit learner participation (e.g., a learner-generated differential). Are there specific questions you want to ask? Should you designate certain questions for specific learner levels? Again, consider that you can discuss some ideas verbally, while others you will also write down. Don't rely exclusively on asking questions to populate the chalk talk—some of the content can be directly provided by you.

Get creative Consider using color to emphasize points (e.g., underline) or create contrast (e.g., draw different plots on a graph, or comparing and contrasting normal and abnormal feedback loops). This can improve the visual interest and clarity of your talk.

Evaluate your talk visually Step back and imagine what your talk would look like on an actual whiteboard (or chalkboard, or projected screen). Is it legible? Is it cluttered? Do you need to reassess?

Narrow the Scope of Your Talk as Appropriate for the Time Frame and the Audience

Teaching scripts will inevitably start out lengthier than intended. Fortunately, the script can easily be tailored for the amount of time available. One practical way to do this is by providing more information (such as in the opening clinical vignette) and narrowing the learning objectives.

For example, the learning objectives for a chalk talk on microscopic hematuria with a vignette describing a 62-year-old man presenting with a urine dipstick positive for blood may be:

1. Demonstrate an approach to microscopic hematuria.
2. Distinguish between glomerular and nonglomerular hematuria.
3. List risk factors for bladder cancer.

The teaching script for these objectives would be rather lengthy, as shown in Fig. 2.1. You can narrow the scope of the talk by deciding to emphasize a limited aspect of the case and by listing just two learning objectives:

1. Demonstrate an approach to microscopic hematuria.
2. List risk factors for bladder cancer.

Figure 2.2 shows this abbreviated teaching script, which could practically be accomplished in less than 10 min. To further narrow the teaching script, you can give more information in the clinical vignette and create a more discrete teaching point that you want to emphasize. For example:

Learning Objective

1. Suspect cancer if a man has blood in his urine.

Vignette: A 62-year-old man is presenting with a urine dipstick positive for blood. He has no other symptoms. He has smoked 1 pack of cigarettes per day for 40 years.

The teaching script for this highly condensed chalk talk is shown in Fig. 2.3.

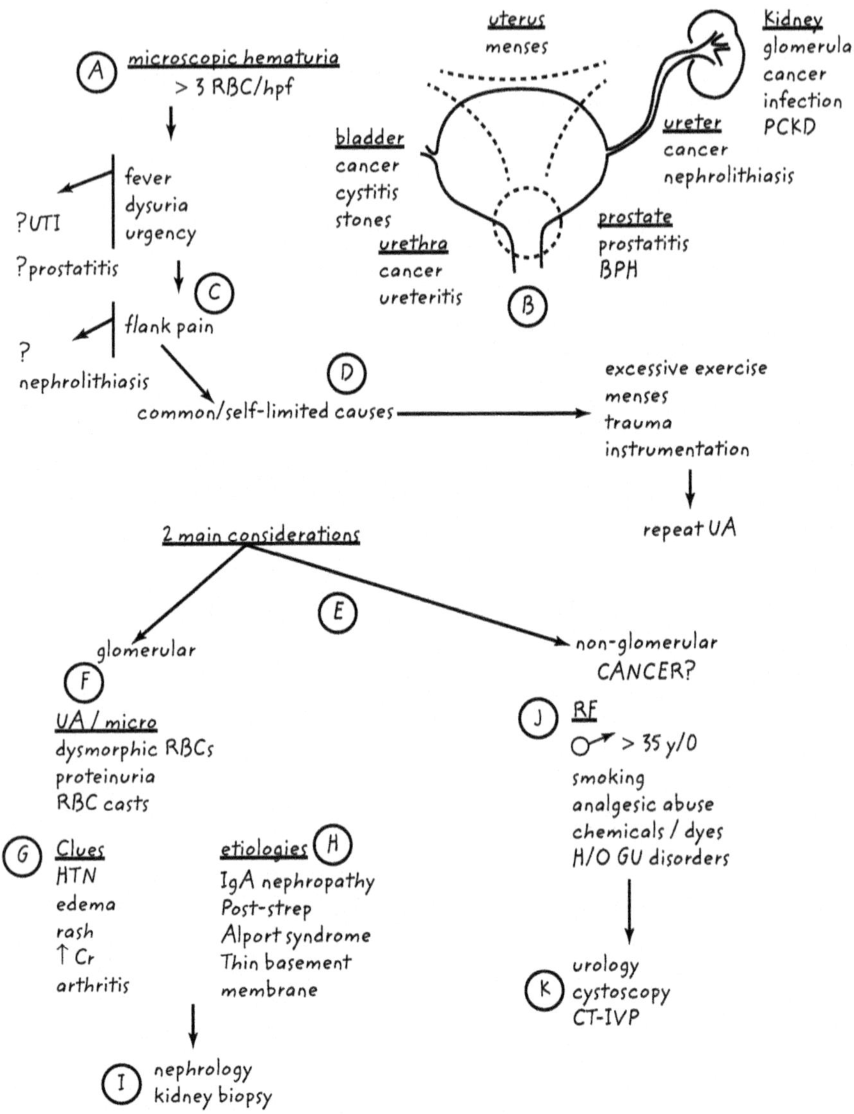

Fig. 2.1 Full-length chalk talk example for microscopic hematuria

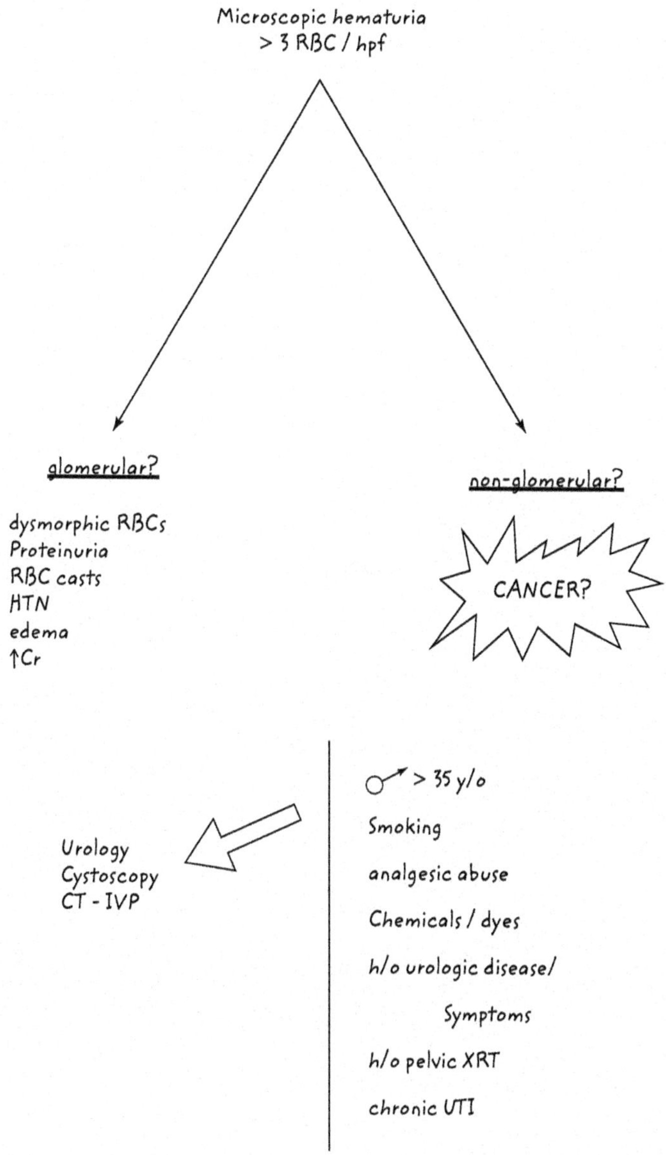

Fig. 2.2 Chalk talk trimmed to emphasize two objectives

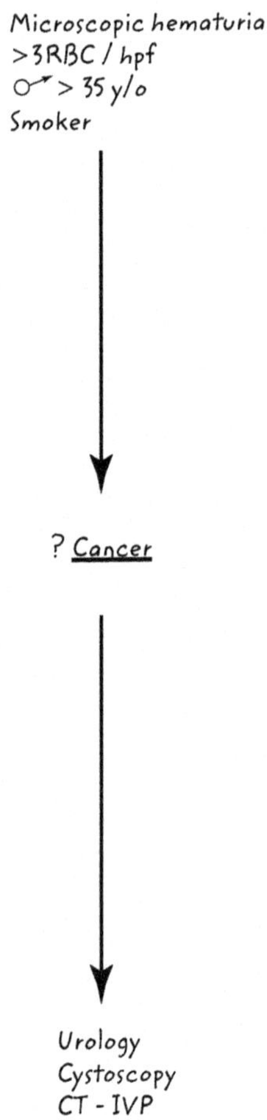

Fig. 2.3 Minimal chalk talk for one key point about microscopic hematuria

Practice!

If possible, run through your whole talk aloud. At a minimum, draw and redraw the script on a piece of paper or a whiteboard. While practicing, take the time to write legibly and leave pauses for eliciting learner questions. Time how long it takes and then trim the content as needed.

Resources

1. I-TECH. Writing good learning objectives. I-TECH technical implementation Guide #4. 2010.
2. Doran GT. There's a SMART way to write management's goals and objectives. Manag Rev. 1981;70(11):35–6.
3. Berger GN, Kritek PA. How to give a great "chalk talk". In: Mookherjee S, Cosgrove EM, editors. Handbook of clinical teaching. Cham: Springer; 2016. p. 77–84.

Chapter 3
How to Use a Teaching Script to Deliver a Chalk Talk

Diana Zhong and Somnath Mookherjee

Introduction

The previous chapter provided tips on creating teaching scripts. This chapter describes best practices in using these teaching scripts to provide excellent clinical teaching. Many of the principles provided here are applicable to any teaching scenario, but we have provided examples to illustrate how they are applicable to chalk talks in particular.

Prepare Your Room and Materials

Create a physical environment conducive for learning. This can be as simple as ensuring there is enough room for all attendees and that all will be able to see the board.

Bring necessary materials. Bring your own markers, especially if you need specific colors.

Draw your template in advance, including your learning objectives. If possible, thoroughly erase any existing content on the board and give yourself as much empty space as possible.

D. Zhong (✉) · S. Mookherjee
University of Washington Medical Center, Department of Medicine, Division of General Internal Medicine, University of Washington, Seattle, WA, USA
e-mail: zhongd@uw.edu

S. Mookherjee et al. (eds.), *Chalk Talks in Internal Medicine*,
https://doi.org/10.1007/978-3-030-34814-4_3

Establish a Positive Learning Environment

The learning climate is the tone or atmosphere of a teaching setting [1]. There are many strategies to promote effective learning that can be implemented far in advance of your chalk talk through the creation of a safe and positive learning climate. Many of these strategies may seem intuitive, but their importance cannot be overstated.

Be respectful The learning climate begins the moment you meet your learners. You can create a culture of respect and caring through simple but important interactions like remembering your learners' names, getting to know them, and asking how they're doing. Be positive and affirm good work, and be considerate when providing constructive feedback.

Make teaching a priority You can stimulate learners through your own enthusiasm to teach. Show that teaching is a priority for you by deliberately setting aside time for it in advance, and hold yourself and your learners to it. Also demonstrate that you embrace the humility of medicine and the principle of lifelong learning by admitting your own limitations. Don't be afraid of saying "I don't know"—use these occasions as teaching opportunities to role model your own curiosity and demonstrate how you find answers.

Introducing Your Talk

Before diving into your content, get your learners' attention, set the agenda, and state the learning objectives.

Get your learners' attention! Consider in advance how you are going to emphasize the importance of your topic.

- Why did you choose your topic?
- Do you have a personal story or patient case that's relevant?
- Have you seen a medical error occur because of the lack of understanding?
- Will learners be seeing a lot of patients with the disease you're teaching about?
- Is it something you've struggled with?
- If you have a clinical vignette, you can introduce it at this point.

Set the agenda Just as you would during a patient encounter, set an agenda for the teaching session. Let your learners know how many minutes your talk will take, and then complete your talk in that timeframe. This prepares learners to be engaged for the duration of the talk and shows that you are mindful of their time. If the learning environment allows, request the learners to devote maximal attention to learning for the specified period of time. For example, in an inpatient setting, you can ask your learners to minimize responses to nonurgent pages or have the senior resident cover students' and interns' pages.

State the learning objectives See Chap. 2 for guidance on crafting learning objectives. It is optimal to both state them out loud and have them written on the board. This will hold you accountable for the content that is to follow and provide signposts to the learners for what they are expected to accomplish.

Delivering Your Talk

Write and speak clearly Take your time—speak clearly and audibly, and write legibly. If your tendency is to talk fast, this is your opportunity to slow down! Avoid talking and writing at the same time, so that you avoid talking to the board instead of to your learners—the time you spend writing is time that your learners can spend thinking. Avoid writing on areas of the board that have minimal visibility.

Position yourself Be mindful of your physical presence and try not to block the learners' view of the board. Sitting down with the learners will engage them and emphasize that you are part of a discussion rather than "performing" or "teaching *at* them."

Be excited! Allow your knowledge and your passion about your topic to show through. This will stimulate enthusiasm in your learners as well.

Ask questions Consider a mix of asking questions to the group at large as well as to specific learners. This is your opportunity to ask any questions you've earmarked for certain learner levels. Having established a positive learning climate is critical to being able to ask learners' questions without them feeling uncomfortable or pressured. Depending on available time and physical space, you can have learners come up and write on the board themselves.

Utilize peer-to-peer teaching [1] Utilize your learners to teach each other. This is especially effective if the learners are at different levels of training—giving senior learners the opportunity to teach can be highly satisfying for them. For example, if a learner asks a question, you can open the floor and allow your other learners to answer questions before you answer. This can also allow you to gauge the understanding of your other learners.

Emphasize important points For the most important points, explicitly call attention to them (e.g., "this is really important" or "this is the biggest take-home point"). Similarly, you can explicitly de-emphasize details that are not your take-home points ("It's okay if you don't remember all of these details"). Draw attention to specific audience members or to learner levels, by explicitly stating what is most applicable (e.g., "as a third-year resident, it is important to understand ___").

Gauge understanding At key stopping points, ask questions not only to achieve your learning objectives, but also to gauge how well learners are understanding the content. Pay attention to facial expressions and nonverbal cues. When learners answer questions, ask them to discuss their thought process.

Adapt your talk for a large group If you are in a larger space, ensure your writing is legible to all audience members. Repeat questions and answers from the audience to ensure that everyone can hear. Pause at key points to encourage small group discussions or pair-share activities, then solicit responses from the small groups. In a large group or more formal setting, you may want to answer questions directly rather than asking for input from other learners. This will allow the discussion to remain audible and stay on track [1].

Concluding Your Talk

Emphasize take-home points Be sure to emphasize the take-home point; if there is adequate time, you can solicit take-home points from the audience as well (e.g., "everyone state one thing they learned").

Reflect and make plans to improve Take a picture of your board right after the talk—was everything legible? Was the board crowded or sparse? Would the talk have benefited from more visual organization? What went well? What could you do better next time? Was the flow of information logical? Were you able to engage sufficiently with your learners? Did you finish on time? You can take notes and even annotate on the board directly before taking a picture for future reference. Some teachers catalogue their talks, and those of their colleagues, to build a library of talks. Ask learners or any colleagues who attended for feedback.

Resource

1. Berger GN, Kritek PA. How to give a great "chalk talk". In: Mookherjee S, Cosgrove EM, editors. Handbook of clinical teaching. Cham: Springer; 2016. p. 77–84.

Chapter 4
Management of Acute Coronary Syndromes

Stephanie A. Field and Jared W. Klein

Learning Objectives

1. Recognize the presentation of acute coronary syndrome (ACS).
2. Manage initial interventions for ACS.
3. Differentiate among ST-elevation myocardial infarction (STEMI), high-risk unstable angina or non-ST-elevation myocardial infarction (UA/NSTEMI), and low-intermediate risk UA/NSTEMI.

Clinical Vignette: A 65-year-old man with a history of hypertension and ongoing tobacco use presents to the emergency department, reporting a 1-day history of worsening chest pressure.

You may personalize this by using a patient you or your team has cared for. Consider making the patient a woman, given underdiagnosis of this syndrome in women.

A. **What are the risk factors for coronary artery disease (CAD)?**

Write the risk factors on Fig. 4.1 *as learners name them, filling in the list as needed.*

Teaching points

- Risk factors for CAD can be divided into modifiable and nonmodifiable risk factors.
- Nonmodifiable risk factors include older age, male sex, and family history.

S. A. Field (✉) · J. W. Klein
Harborview Medical Center, Department of Medicine, Division of General Internal Medicine, University of Washington, Seattle, WA, USA
e-mail: safield@uw.edu

S. Mookherjee et al. (eds.), *Chalk Talks in Internal Medicine*,
https://doi.org/10.1007/978-3-030-34814-4_4

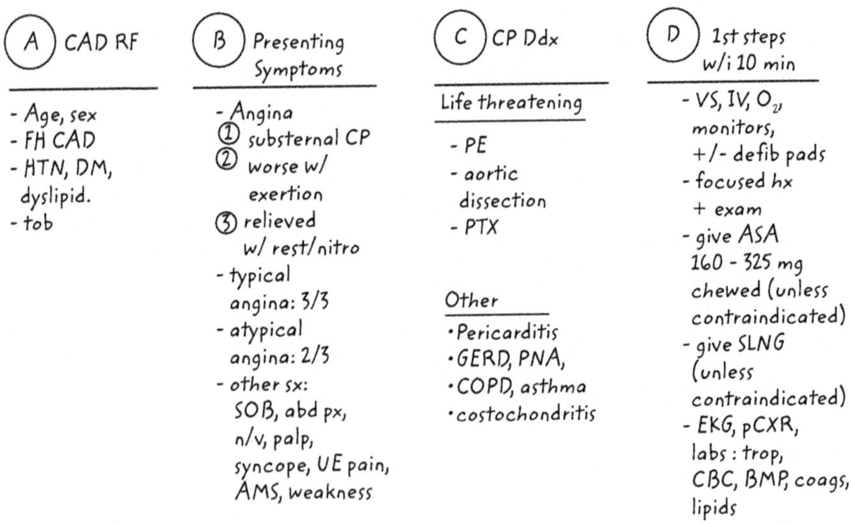

Fig. 4.1 Management of acute coronary syndromes, A–D

- Family history of cardiovascular disease is particularly significant when it is in first-degree relatives, diagnosed in males younger than 55 years or females younger than 65 years.
- Modifiable risk factors include hypertension, diabetes mellitus, dyslipidemia, and tobacco use.

B. **What are the various ways ACS can present?**

Write the presenting symptoms on Fig. 4.1 *as learners name them, filling in the list as needed.*

Teaching points

- Acute coronary syndrome classically presents with angina.
- Typical angina has the following three components:

  1. substernal chest pain (often described as pressure or discomfort rather than pain)
  2. exacerbated by exertion/stress
  3. alleviated by rest or nitroglycerin

- Atypical angina has only two of these components.
- Noncardiac chest pain has only one component.
- However, patients who are women, older, and/or have diabetes are more likely to present with atypical or "noncardiac" symptoms.
- ACS can also present with dyspnea, abdominal pain, nausea and vomiting, palpitations, syncope, upper extremity pain, altered mental status, or generalized weakness.

C. **As you do your initial evaluation, what other causes of chest pain are you considering in our patient?**

Write Differential Diagnosis on Fig. 4.1 *as learners name them, filling in the list as needed.*

D. **Let's think about our patient (*repeat the 1-liner*). You have identified that he has CAD risk factors (*circle them*) and symptoms concerning for ACS (*circle chest pressure).* What are the first steps in managing this patient?**

Write first steps on Fig. 4.1 *as learners name them filling in the list as needed.*

Teaching points for the first steps

- If aortic dissection is a strong contender on the differential, consider ruling out dissection before giving aspirin and other antiplatelets or anticoagulants.
- Oxygen should not be given if O_2 saturation >90%, in the absence of a separate indication.

E. **The electrocardiogram (ECG) helps classify the type of ACS underway and determines the next steps in management.**

Draw out the depictions of ST depression, T-wave inversion, and ST elevation. Prompt learners to tell you how to fill out the pain pattern, extent of coronary thrombosis, and troponin level for UA, NSTEMI, and STEMI. This is a great place to personalize the talk by sharing an ECG from a real patient.

Teaching points for ECGs

- The initial ECG may NOT have any changes. The initial ECG is nondiagnostic in about 45% and normal in about 20% of patients subsequently found to have an acute myocardial infarction (MI). If you have clinical concern for acute MI and the initial ECG is nondiagnostic, repeat it every 20–30 minutes if patient is having ongoing pain.
- Serial ECGs (every 20 minutes for average of 2 hours) are more sensitive than a single initial ECG for detecting acute MI while specificity remains the same at about 95%.

F. **What if our patient's ECG has ST elevations?**

Draw an arrow from the STEMI column in Fig. 4.2 *and ask the learners to tell you what they would do if they were handed that ECG in the ED. Fill out answers on the board. Tailor this section to local protocols—general rules are given in the figure.*

G. **What if our patient's ECG has ST depressions or T-wave inversions (this is also known as NSTE-ACS)?**

Draw an arrow from the "UA/NSTEMI" columns in Fig. 4.2 *and fill in management principles as learners name them. Emphasize the importance of risk stratification.*

Teaching points on medical management of ACS

- Nitroglycerin should be avoided if patient is hypotensive, has right ventricular infarct or aortic stenosis, or has taken a phosphodiesterase inhibitor within 24 hours.
- Beta-blockers should be given within 24 hours to patients without (1) signs of heart failure, (2) evidence of low-output cardiac state, (3) increased risk for cardiogenic shock, or (4) other contraindications to beta-blockade (e.g., PR interval > 0.24 seconds, second- or third-degree heart block without a cardiac pacemaker, active asthma, or reactive airway disease). If the patient has a contraindication to beta-blocker initially, reevaluate periodically and start when the contraindication resolves.
- Intravenous morphine has been associated with increased risk of death, so should be used as a last resort for patients with intractable pain.
- Most patients do not need a GPIIb/IIIa inhibitor such as eptifibatide or abciximab, consult with cardiology before starting one.

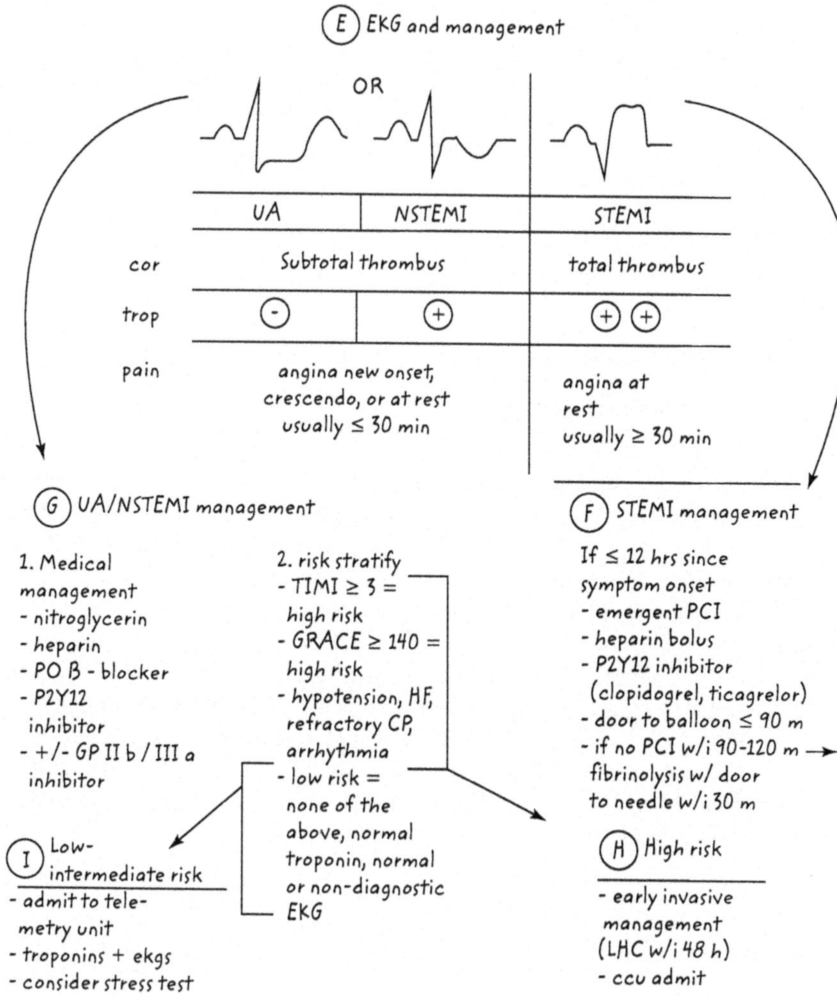

Fig. 4.2 Management of acute coronary syndromes, E–I

Teaching points on risk stratification

- Risk stratification should be performed for all patients with ACS. Thrombolysis in Myocardial Infarction (TIMI) and Global Registry of Acute Coronary Events (GRACE) score calculators are available through online medical calculators and apps.
- Patients with high risk for mortality based on risk-stratification scores should undergo left heart catheterization within 24–48 hours.
- Very high-risk patients should undergo immediate cardiac catheterization similar to those with STEMI. "Very high-risk" includes those with hypotension, heart failure, refractory chest pain, ventricular arrhythmias, dynamic ST-segment and T-wave changes on ECG, mechanical dysfunction such as acute mitral regurgitation, or ventricular septal defect.

H. **If our patient is high risk, what is your next step?**

Write "High risk" on Fig. 4.2 *and fill in management principles as learners name them.*

I. **If our patient is low-intermediate risk, what is your next step?**

Write "Low-Intermediate Risk" on Fig. 4.2 *and fill in management principles as learners name them.*

Return to objectives and emphasize key points

1. Recognize the presentation of ACS. It is important to consider both clinical risk factors (older age, male sex, family history of CAD, hypertension, diabetes, hyperlipidemia, or smoking history) as well as clinical symptoms (triad of substernal chest pain/pressure, worse with exertion, and relieved by rest or nitroglycerin).
2. Provide initial interventions for ACS. In the absence of contraindications, these include aspirin, sublingual nitroglycerin, oxygen (if hypoxic), and additional relevant diagnostic testing (ECG, CXR, cardiac biomarkers and other labs).
3. Differentiate between STEMI, high-risk UA/NSTEMI, and low-intermediate risk UA/NSTEMI. This can be accomplished by a combination of clinical history, ECG findings, and biomarkers.

Resources

1. Thygesen K, Alpert JS, Jaffe AS, Simoons ML, Chaitman BR, White HD, et al. Third universal definition of myocardial infarction. Circulation. 2012;126(16):2020–35.
2. Hofmann R, James SK, Jernberg T, Lindahl B, Erlinge D, Witt N, et al. Oxygen therapy in suspected acute myocardial infarction. N Engl J Med. 2017;377(13):1240–9.
3. Fesmire FM, Percy RF, Bardoner JB, Wharton DR, Calhoun FB. Usefulness of automated serial 12-lead ECG monitoring during the initial emergency department evaluation of patients with chest pain. Ann Emerg Med. 1998;31(1):3–11.
4. O'Gara PT, Kushner FG, Ascheim DD, Casey DE Jr, Chung MK, de Lemos JA, et al. ACCF/AHA guideline for the management of ST-elevation myocardial infarction: a report of the

American College of Cardiology Foundation/American Heart Association Task Force on Practice Guidelines. Circulation. 2013;127(4):e362–425.
5. Amsterdam EA, Wenger NK, Brindis RG, Casey DE Jr, Ganiats TG, Holmes DR Jr, et al. 2014 AHA/ACC guideline for the management of patients with non-ST-elevation acute coronary syndromes: executive summary: a report of the American College of Cardiology/American Heart Association Task Force on Practice Guidelines. Circulation. 2014;130(25):2354–94.
6. Antman EM, Cohen M, Bernink PJ, McCabe CH, Horacek T, Papuchis G, et al. The TIMI risk score for unstable angina/non-ST elevation MI: a method for prognostication and therapeutic decision making. JAMA. 2000;284(7):835–42.
7. Granger CB, Goldberg RJ, Dabbous O, Pieper KS, Eagle KA, Cannon CP, et al. Predictors of hospital mortality in the global registry of acute coronary events. Arch Intern Med. 2003;163(19):2345–53.
8. Gibbons RJ, Balady GJ, Bricker JT, Chaitman BR, Fletcher GF, Froelicher VF, et al. ACC/AHA 2002 guideline update for exercise testing: summary article: a report of the American College of Cardiology/American Heart Association Task Force on Practice Guidelines (Committee to update the 1997 exercise testing guidelines). Circulation. 2002;106(14):1883–92.
9. Mukherjee D, Fang J, Chetcuti S, Moscucci M, Kline-Rogers E, Eagle KA. Impact of combination evidence-based medical therapy on mortality in patients with acute coronary syndromes. Circulation. 2004;109(6):745–9.

Chapter 5
Management of Acute Decompensated Heart Failure

Pallavi R. Arora and Genji S. Terasaki

Learning Objectives
1. Define heart failure (HF).
2. Correlate pathophysiology of HF to management.
3. Triage acute decompensated heart failure (ADHF) patients to the appropriate clinical setting

Clinical Vignette: A 66 year old gentleman with 'past medical' history of myocardial infarction 2 years ago, hypertension, hyperlipidemia, and heart failure (HF), has been on a stable medical regimen of aspirin, atorvastatin, carvedilol, lisinopril, and furosemide for months. He presents to the emergency department with progressively worsening shortness of breath. He noticed 'onset of symptoms' a few days ago while he was out of town at a wedding and forgot to take his medications as prescribed. The dyspnea is worse at night, requiring him to sleep propped up on three pillows. He has also noticed weight gain with worsening swelling of both legs.

His heart rate is 110 beats per minute and regular. Respiratory rate is 26 per minute, blood pressure is 145/96 mm of Hg, and oxygen saturation is 86% on ambient air. He is breathing using accessory muscles, has bibasilar crackles on lung exam, and pitting edema on bilateral lower extremities. His skin is warm and he is mentating normally. Chest x-ray reveals bilateral pulmonary edema. His kidney function is normal (creatinine 1.0 mg/dL). You are called to admit the patient for a HF exacerbation.

P. R. Arora (✉) · G. S. Terasaki
Harborview Medical Center, Department of Medicine, Division of General Internal Medicine, University of Washington, Seattle, WA, USA
e-mail: parora@uw.edu

S. Mookherjee et al. (eds.), *Chalk Talks in Internal Medicine*,
https://doi.org/10.1007/978-3-030-34814-4_5

A. **What is heart failure (HF)? Heat failure is defined as failure of the heart to pump blood forward sufficiently to meet the metabolic demands the body, or the ability to do so only at abnormally high cardiac filling pressures.**

Write out the definition and two major categories of HF in Fig. 5.1.

Teaching points for heart failure with reduced ejection fraction (HFrEF) and heart failure with preserved ejection fraction (HFpEF)

- Heart failure with reduced ejection fraction (HFrEF) is also known as systolic heart failure or pump failure. It is defined by the presence of cardiac ejection fraction <40%.
- Heart failure with preserved ejection fraction (HFpEF) is also known as diastolic heart failure. It occurs when the left ventricle fails to relax and fill normally, leading to elevated pressures. In HFrEF, cardiac ejection fraction exceeds >50%.
- Epidemiologic studies have shown that HFpEF is as prevalent as HFrEF

B. **In a normal heart, cardiac output increases as preload increases. However, beyond a certain point, further increase in volume (sarcomere length) leads to decreased contractility/pump function and cardiac output.**

Draw the "cardiac output" and "preload" axes and draw the normal Frank–Starling curve.

Teaching points

- The Frank–Starling curve illustrates the relationship between cardiac preload (volume) on the x-axis and cardiac output (perfusion) on the y-axis.
- The sympathetic nervous system and the renin angiotensin aldosterone system modulate the Frank–Starling curve.
- At times of stress or exercise, the sympathetic nervous system response will shift this curve upward, followed by activation of the renin-angiotensin-aldosterone system (RAS).

C. **How does a person move from having a normal heart to having HF?** Heart failure is initiated by an index event that causes damage to the heart muscle and disrupts the ability of the myocardium to generate force.

Ask the learners to list examples of index events, fill in the examples as they are named. Draw the lower line on the Frank–Starling curve and the arrow in between the two curves indicating the activation of the sympathetic nervous system and the renin-angiotensin-aldosterone system.

Teaching points

- Following an index event, the Frank–Starling curve shifts downward. Compensatory mechanisms are activated to restore cardiac function to the normal range (these include the sympathetic nervous system and renin-angiotensin-aldosterone system).

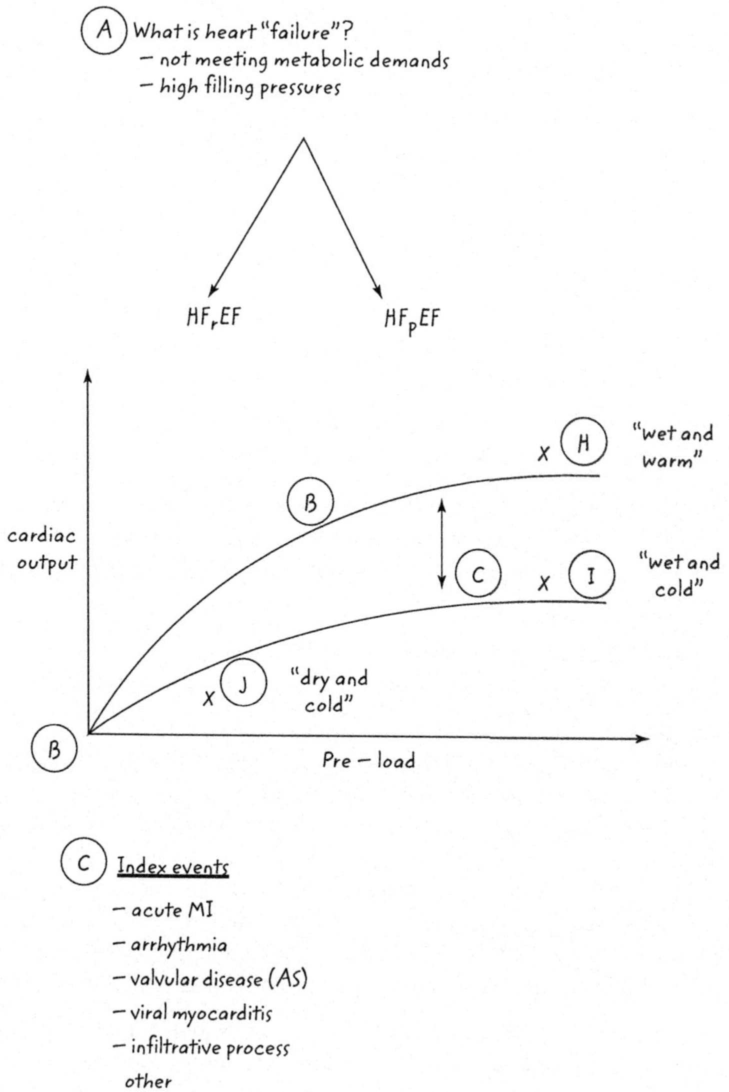

Fig. 5.1 Management of acute decompensated heart failure, A–C, H–J

- In the short term, the patient remains at the top of the Frank–Starling curve. However, sustained activation of these compensatory mechanisms results in cardiac remodeling, with damage to the ventricle and subsequent cardiac decompensation.

D. **You can think about the clinical presentation and management of acute decompensated heart failure (ADHF) in terms of the patient's volume status and peripheral perfusion**

On Fig. 5.2, *draw the "volume" and "perfusion" axes, and write out "dry," "wet," "warm," and "cold" in the appropriate places.*

Teaching points
- "Wet" means increasing volume, high filling pressure, cardiac congestion.
- "Cold" means inability to pump blood forward, not meeting perfusion demands.

E. **ADHF can be thought of symptoms due to increased congestion and decreased perfusion. What are some common symptoms of each?**

List major signs and symptoms at the end of the appropriate arrows on Fig. 5.2 *for "increased congestion" and "decreased perfusion."*

F. **Return to the case. Our patient had an index event of an MI 2 years ago, was medically managed, and was in compensated HF prior to the recent events. What box would he fit in when he was compensated? What are the key elements of maintenance management?**

Draw the "plus sign" in the middle of the axes, and write out the key characteristics of compensated HF ("dry and warm") with outpatient management.

Teaching points
- Our patient started out with compensated HF. Patients like him are managed in the outpatient setting (primary care, heart failure clinic).
- The goal for management of compensated HF is to prevent deleterious cardiac remodeling.
- Evidence-based interventions include beta-blockers to block the sympathetic system and angiotensin converting enzyme inhibitors (ACE-I)/angiotensin receptor blockers (ARB) to block the renin-angiotensin-aldosterone system. Patients with compensated HF are also sometimes on an oral diuretic regimen.

G. **As a patient moves from a well-perfused (or "warm") and euvolemic (or "dry") state to any of the other boxes, it signals the development of ADHF. There is usually a precipitant that shifts a patient from compensated to decompensated HF. What are common precipitants of HF? What might have precipitated ADHF in our patient?**

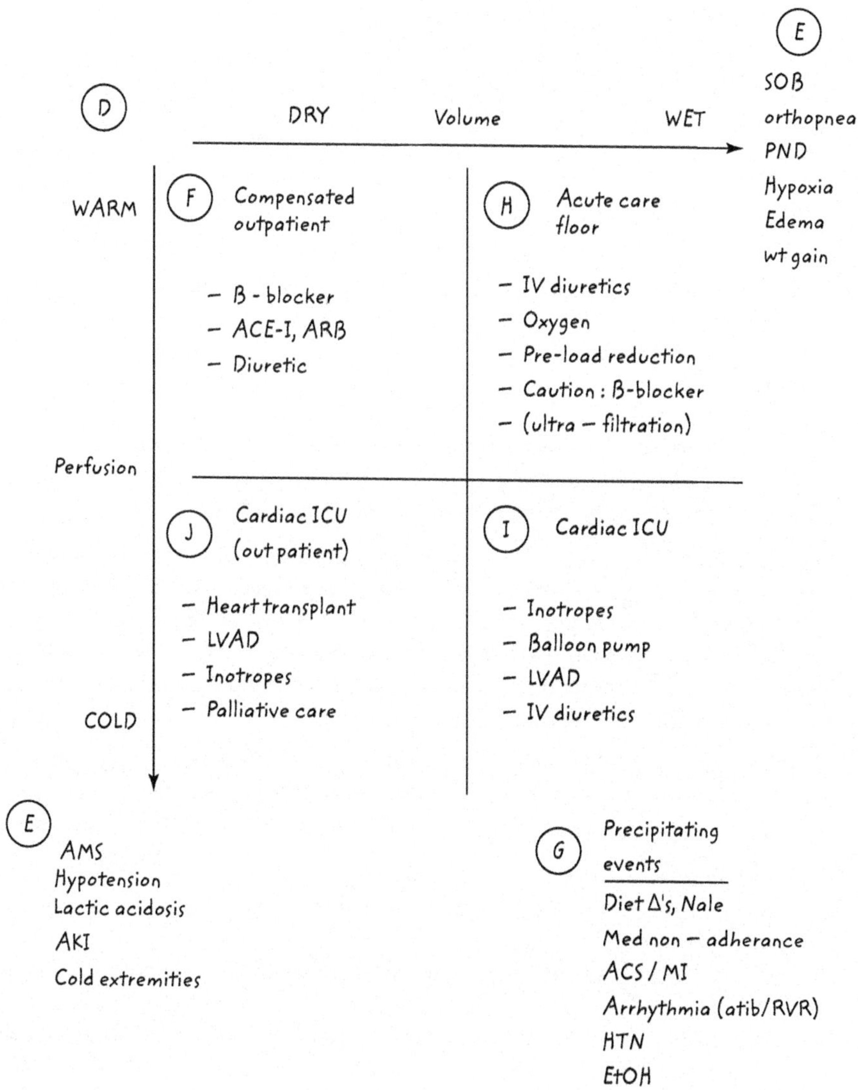

Fig. 5.2 Management of acute decompensated heart failure, D–J

Write down some of the precipitants for heart failure.

H. **Returning to the case, in which box would our patient fit when he presented to the ED? A compensated patient can become hypervolemic ("wet") to the point of becoming symptomatic, but still have adequate cardiac output. How would you manage this patient?**

Fill out the key characteristics of the "wet and warm" patient in Fig. 5.2. *In* Fig. 5.1, *indicate with an "X" where he would be represented on the Frank–Starling curve.*

Teaching points

ADHF can sometimes be managed in the outpatient setting if symptoms are mild, but it is primarily managed on acute care floors. Typical interventions include:

- Intravenous diuresis (more reliably bioavailable than oral diuretics in the setting of gut edema).
- Supplemental oxygen.
- Preload reduction with transdermal nitroglycerin as an adjunct to diuresis, or if poor response to diuresis.
- Rarely, ultrafiltration is used in patients who do not respond to diuretics.
- Use beta-blockers cautiously in ADHF patients due to negative inotropic effects. There is a risk of precipitating cardiogenic shock.

I. **Imagine that our patient fails to respond to diuresis. He begins to clinically deteriorate with decreasing blood pressure, cool extremities, increasing creatinine, and poor urine output. Our patient has moved from the "wet and warm" box to the "wet and cold" box. In addition to the volume overload, there is now inadequate perfusion. What should we do for patients who are in the "cold and wet" box?**

Indicate with an "X" where he would be represented on the Frank–Starling curve. Fill out the location of care and key management steps in the "wet and cold" box.

Teaching points

- Our patient is in cardiogenic shock and should be managed in a cardiac critical care unit.
- Pulmonary artery catheter placement for hemodynamic monitoring can be considered.
- These patients need improvement in cardiac output in order to move from the "cold" to "warm" box.
- Inotropic support with dobutamine, dopamine, or milrinone
- Mechanical pump support (intra-aortic balloon pump, temporary, or destination left ventricular assist devices)
- Continue intravenous diuresis for volume management to move them from a "wet" to "dry" state.

J. **The final box is the "dry and cold" box. These patients have advanced pump dysfunction independent of their volume status. Patients present with low blood pressure, cool extremities, fatigue, and poor exercise tolerance.**

Indicate with an "X" where he would be represented on the Frank–Starling curve. Fill out the "location of care" and key management steps in the "dry and cold" box.

Teaching points

- Decompensations are managed in cardiac critical care units.
- Palliative care/hospice should be considered for goals of care planning and symptom management.
- Management involves pump support.
- Heart transplant. This is the gold standard of management (5-year survival is greater than 70%). However, not all patients are eligible for transplantation, and it has limited availability due to scarcity of donors.
- Mechanical circulatory support. Left ventricular assist devices can be used as a bridge to transplant or as a destination device in patients not eligible for transplant (2-year survival with newer devices is 46%).
- Chronic inotropic support can be considered in patients who are not candidates for transplant or mechanical circulatory support. This can improve symptoms but at the cost of increased mortality.

Return to objectives and emphasize key points

1. Define heart failure

   - Failure of the heart to pump blood forward at a rate sufficient to meet metabolic demands of vital organs, or the ability to do so only at abnormally high cardiac filling pressures.
   - An index event causes damage to the heart muscle leading to the sustained activation of compensatory mechanisms driven by the RAS and the sympathetic nervous system.

2. Correlate pathophysiology of HF to management

   - HF can remain compensated, that is, well-perfused (warm) and euvolemic (dry).
   - Precipitating events lead to decompensation of HF.
   - Symptoms of decompensated HF come from volume overload and hypoperfusion.

3. Triage acute decompensated heart failure (ADHF) patients to the appropriate clinical setting based on clinical presentation in terms of volume status and perfusion.

Resources

1. Braunwald's heart disease, 10th ed. 2014.
2. Forrester, et al. Correlative classification of clinical and hemodynamic function after acute myocardial infarction. Am J Cardiol. 1977;39:137.
3. Stehlik J, Edwards LB, Kucheryavaya AY, et al. The registry of the International Society for Heart and Lung Transplantation: twenty-eighth adult heart transplant report–2011. J Heart Lung Transplant. 2011;30:1078–94.
4. McMurray JJ, et al. Systolic heart failure. N Engl J Med. 2010;362(3):228–38.
5. Yancy CW, Jessup M, Bozkurt B, Butler J, Casey DE, Drazner MH, Fonarow GC, Geraci SA, Horwich T, Januzzi JL, Johnson MR. 2013 ACCF/AHA guideline for the management of heart failure. J Am Coll Cardiol. 2013;62(16):e147–239. https://doi.org/10.1016/j.jacc.2013.05.019.

Chapter 6
Interpretation of Pacemaker Settings

Divya Gollapudi and Thomas Rea

Learning Objectives
1. Describe the indications for pacemaker placement.
2. Recognize the various pacemaker types and settings.
3. Identify complications of pacemakers.

Clinical Vignette: An 89-year-old man presents to the emergency department after an episode of syncope. His evaluation is negative for abnormalities in troponin, blood counts, and electrolytes. His electrocardiogram (ECG) does not demonstrate ST- or T-wave changes consistent with acute ischemia, but does reveal third-degree atrioventricular block. *Consider bringing an example of an ECG with third-degree atrioventricular block for added learning.*

A. **What is the indication for a pacemaker in this patient? What are other indications for pacemaker placement?**

Draw the schematic of the conduction system. Write down indications for pacemaker placement in a list as they are mentioned. Relate the indications to the location of the lesion in the conduction system.

Teaching points
- Major indications for pacemaker placement include conduction abnormalities, arrhythmias, structural heart disease, and neurocardiogenic syncope.
- Cardiac synchronization therapy is indicated in selected patients with heart failure.

D. Gollapudi (✉) · T. Rea
Harborview Medical Center, Department of Medicine, Division of General Internal Medicine, University of Washington, Seattle, WA, USA
e-mail: gollapud@uw.edu

S. Mookherjee et al. (eds.), *Chalk Talks in Internal Medicine*,
https://doi.org/10.1007/978-3-030-34814-4_6

B. **How does pacing look on an ECG?**

Draw an ECG tracing on the board. Ask a volunteer to show you where the atrial and ventricular spikes would show up. Alternatively, this would be another great place to bring in an ECG example from a real patient with a pacemaker.

C. **Where do pacemaker leads go? Name the basic components of pacemakers.**

Draw the pulse generator (battery), each of the leads, and the sensing and pacing arrows.

Teaching points

- Single-chamber pacemaker: one lead only—paces a single heart chamber (either atria or ventricle).
- Dual-chamber pacemaker: two leads—one lead is placed in the atria and the other in the ventricle.
- Biventricular: three leads—one lead is placed in the right atrium, one in the right ventricle, and one in the left ventricle (via the coronary sinus).

D. **The electrophysiologist says that the patient needs a DDD pacemaker. What does that mean?**

Fill in NBG pacemaker code table in Fig. 6.1.

Teaching points for pacer nomenclature

- Pacemakers are classified by the nature of their pacing mode using the NBG code, a series of up to five letters.
- NBG is the acronym for the North American Society of Pacing and Electrophysiology (NASPE)/British Pacing and Electrophysiology Group (BPEG) (2002) Generic Pacemaker Code.
- Each of the five letters in the NBG taxonomy describes a different pacemaker characteristic, depending on the position of the letter.
  - Position I—chamber paced (A = atria, V = ventricles, D = dual-chamber).
  - Position II—chamber sensed (A = atria, V = ventricles, D = dual-chamber, 0 = none).
  - Position III—response to sensed event (T = triggered, I = inhibited, D = dual—T and I, R = reverse).
  - Pacemakers are commonly described with the first three letters, so the fourth (rate modulation) and fifth (multisite pacing) positions are not discussed here.
- Synchronous/demand pacing signals the pacemaker to discharge only when the patient's heart rate fails to reach a predetermined rate. Synchronous/demand settings include AAI and VVI.
- Dual-chamber AV sequential pacing means that the atrium is stimulated to contract, followed by the ventricle. Dual-chamber AV sequential settings include VDD, DVI, and DDD.

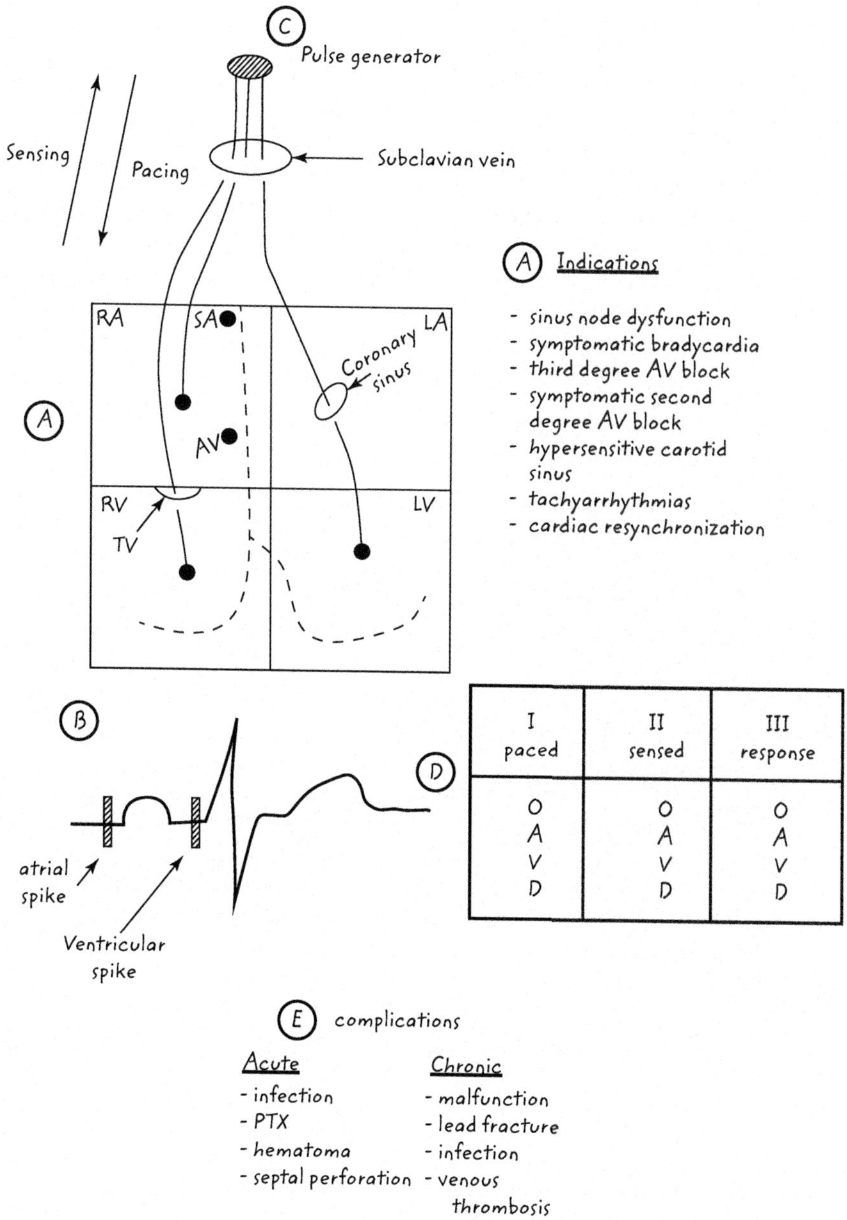

Fig. 6.1 Interpretation of pacemaker settings, A–E

E. **The patient has severe shortness of breath the day after his pacemaker is placed. What are examples of acute complications of pacemaker implantation? What might cause shortness of breath months or years after pacemaker implantation?**

Write down complications as they are mentioned, categorized by acute and chronic.

Teaching points
- Complications can also be characterized by procedure-related versus device-related.
- Acute complications are mainly procedure-related. These include infection, pneumothorax, hematoma, and septal perforation.
- Chronic complications include pacemaker malfunction, lead fracture, infection, and venous thrombosis.
- Patients with pacemakers require additional consideration before undergoing magnetic resonance imaging (MRI), anesthesia, and surgeries.

Return to objectives and emphasize key points
1. Describe the indications for pacemaker placement
   - Indications for pacemaker placement include conduction abnormalities, arrhythmias, structural heart disease, and neurocardiogenic syncope.
2. Recognize the various pacemaker types and settings
   - Pacemakers can have single, dual, or biventricular leads and pace in a fixed rate or demand fashion.
   - Pacemakers are classified by the nature of their pacing mode using the five-letter NBG coding system.
3. Identify complications of pacemakers
   - Acute complications include infection, pneumothorax, and septal perforation.
   - Chronic complications include pacemaker malfunction and infection.
   - Patients with pacemakers require additional consideration before undergoing MRI and anesthesia.

Resources

1. Gregoratos G, Cheitlin MD, Conill A, et al. ACC/AHA guidelines for implantation of cardiac pacemakers and antiarrhythmia devices: a report of the American College of Cardiology/American Heart Association Task Force on Practice Guidelines (Committee on Pacemaker Implantation). J Am Coll Cardiol. 1998;31:1175–209.
2. Mulpuru SK, et al. Cardiac pacemakers: function, troubleshooting, and management. J AM Coll Cardiol. 2017;69(2):189–210.
3. Rapsang AG, Bhattacharyya P. Pacemakers and implantable cardioverter defibrillators – general and anesthetic considerations. Braz J Anesthesiol. 2014;64(3):205–14.
4. Kusumoto FM, Goldschlager N. Cardiac pacing. New Engl J Med. 1996;334(2):89–97.

Chapter 7
Secondary Hypertension

Yuree Lin and Anne Eacker

Learning Objectives
1. Recognize when it is appropriate to screen for diseases that cause secondary hypertension.
2. Describe common causes of secondary hypertension and the pathophysiology of each of these diseases.
3. Determine the next appropriate diagnostic test(s) to identify a cause for secondary hypertension.

Clinical Vignette: A 38-year-old man sees you in primary care clinic for management of hypertension. Despite adequate compliance with maximally dosed amlodipine, hydrochlorothiazide, and lisinopril, his blood pressure remains persistently elevated at 165/100 mm Hg.

A. **When is it appropriate to screen for secondary hypertension? What features of our patient's presentation raise concern for a secondary cause of hypertension?**

Write the mnemonic "MARCY" on the board and write the first word of each sentence below.

Teaching points for when to screen
- **M**alignant hypertension: defined as severe hypertension with signs or symptoms of end-organ damage
- **A**brupt worsening: sudden worsening of hypertension in a previously well-controlled patient

Y. Lin (✉)
Kaiser Permanente Moanalua Medical Center, Honolulu, HI, USA

A. Eacker
Kaiser Permanente Bernard J. Tyson School of Medicine, Pasadena, CA, USA

S. Mookherjee et al. (eds.), *Chalk Talks in Internal Medicine*,
https://doi.org/10.1007/978-3-030-34814-4_7

- Resistant hypertension: defined as inadequate blood pressure control despite adequate doses of ≥3 antihypertensive agents from different classes, including one diuretic
- Clinical features: look for features of an underlying disorder associated with hypertension
- Young age of onset: defined as hypertension in a patient <30 years old, in the absence of obesity or family history of hypertension

B. **This patient has resistant hypertension. It would be appropriate to initiate a workup for causes of secondary hypertension. What are some common causes of secondary hypertension?**

Have learners list common causes and fill out the "AABBCCCDE" mnemonic as causes are mentioned. You may also use the graphic depictions to add visual interest or as a prompt for learners. If learners have ideas that don't fit in the mnemonic, list them under "Other" or explain why they are not a cause.

C. **Our patient is obese, snores loudly, and dozes off during the clinic visit. What secondary cause of hypertension is he at risk for? What are some common symptoms or findings for causes of secondary hypertension?**

Write down the risk factors for sleep apnea for your patient. Add other common symptoms as listed by learners—Fig. 7.1 *lists some of them.* Table 7.1 *provides further information.*

D. **What tests would you order if our patient did have any of the clinical features associated with a cause of secondary hypertension?**

Have learners list next diagnostic steps and write these next to the cause you would be testing for on the board.

Teaching points for diagnostic tests

- A detailed history and physical exam should be used to focus the diagnostic testing.
- Note that there may be no specific symptoms or exam findings for acute or chronic kidney disease, including renovascular disease.
- In the absence of an obvious cause, it is reasonable to screen all patients with resistant hypertension for kidney disease and renovascular disease.
- The table provides expanded information on physical exam findings and diagnostic testing is provided as a convenient reference for the teacher. It is not necessary to copy the entire Supplemental Table onto the board.

(A) Screen?

Malignant hypertension
Abrupt worsening
Resistant hypertension
Clinical features of underlying disorder
Young age of onset

(C) Symptom/findings

- obesity
- snoring
- moon facies
- hirsutism
- cold intolerance
- muscle weakness
- delayed femoral pulse
- tachycardia
- headache
- ↓K ↑Na
- bruit

(B) Causes

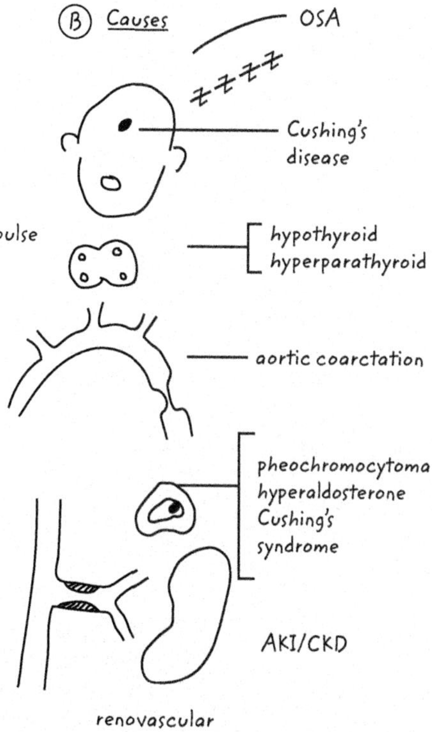

(B) Causes

(D) Tests

Apnea	- sleep study
Aldosteronism	- plasma aldo/renin, CT adrenal glands
Bruits (renovascular)	- renal artery duplex, MRA, CTA
Bad kidneys	- renal function tests
Catecholamines (pheo)	- 24 h urine metaneph, plasma free metaneph
Cushing's	- dexamethasone suppression test, 24 h urine free cortisol
Coarctation	- CTA
Drugs	
Endocrine	
- hypothyroid	- TSH
- hyperparathyroid	- Serum calcium

Fig. 7.1 Secondary hypertension (**a**–**d**)

Table 7.1 Expanded AABBCCCCDE mnemonic for secondary hypertension

	Causes	Key signs/symptoms, physical exam	Diagnostic testing
A	Apnea	Excessive daytime sleepiness, snoring, witnessed apnea, obesity, increased neck circumference	Sleep study
	Aldosteronism	Hypernatremia, hypokalemia	Plasma aldosterone to plasma renin ratio CT adrenal glands
B	Bruits (renovascular disease)	Abdominal bruit (low sensitivity), young patient (especially women—suspect fibromuscular dysplasia), recurrent episodes of flash pulmonary edema	Renal artery duplex MR or CT angiogram (to confirm diagnosis)
	Bad kidneys (acute or chronic kidney disease)		Renal function tests
C	Catecholamines (pheochromocytoma)	Paroxysmal hypertension, tachycardia, headaches, diaphoresis	24-h urine metanephrines and catecholamines (fewer false positives than plasma metanephrines; use if low pretest probability) Plasma free metanephrines (high sensitivity (96–100%), moderate specificity (85–89%); use if high pretest probability)
	Cushing syndrome	Weight gain, truncal obesity, moon facies, dorsal hump, fatigue, weakness, hirsutism, amenorrhea, and purple striae	Overnight dexamethasone suppression test or 24-h urine free cortisol
	Coarctation of the aorta	Hypertension in arms, decreased or delayed femoral pulses, rib notching on CXR	CT angiogram
D	Drugs	Oral contraceptives, NSAIDs, stimulants (cocaine, methylphenidate), calcineurin inhibitors, and antidepressants such as MAO inhibitors, TCAs, and venlafaxine	
E	Endocrine Hypothyroidism	Weight gain/loss, heat/cold intolerance, palpitations, exophthalmos, tremor, bradycardia/tachycardia, hair loss	TSH
	Hyperparathyroidism	Muscle weakness, lethargy, osteoporosis, kidney stones	Serum calcium

Return to objectives and emphasize key points

1. Recognize when it is appropriate to screen for diseases that cause secondary hypertension—*circle these in the figure ("MARCY").*
2. Describe common causes of secondary hypertension and the pathophysiology of each of these diseases—*asterisk each cause within the "AABBCCCDE" mnemonic and its corresponding pathophysiology in the anatomical figure.*
3. Determine the next appropriate diagnostic test(s) to identify a cause for secondary hypertension—*circle the list of diagnostic tests in the figure.*

Resources

1. Charles L, Triscott J, Dobbs B. Secondary hypertension: discovering the underlying cause. Am Fam Phys. 2017;96(7):453–61.
2. Vongpatanasin W. Resistant hypertension: a review of diagnosis and management. JAMA. 2014;311(21):2216–24.

Chapter 8
Approach to Hypertension

Stefanie A. Deeds and Kari M. Nelson

Learning Objectives

1. Diagnose essential hypertension in the adult patient and describe an approach to further evaluation.
2. Recognize complications of essential hypertension.
3. Identify and describe the impact of lifestyle changes and review the classes of antihypertensive medication used in the initial management of hypertension.
4. Distinguish blood pressure goals based on patient characteristics and select a treatment plan for a patient with essential hypertension.

Clinical Vignette: A 55-year-old African-American man returns to primary care clinic for his annual exam. You note his vitals 2 months ago during an acute care visit: blood pressure (BP) was 155/82 mmHg. Today it is 152/84 mmHg. He has a personal history of diabetes that is well controlled on metformin. Both of his parents have hypertension (HTN) and his father had a myocardial infarction at age 50 years. He is a former smoker. He is asymptomatic.

A. **How is essential hypertension (HTN) defined?**

Fill out the definition and pearls for accurate measurement in Fig. 8.1.

Teaching points for BP measurement

- Essential HTN is diagnosed when BP is >140/90 mmHg with proper measurement at least two times.
- Accurate measurement: Sit for 5 minutes, use the correct size cuff, support the arm, and take >1 measurement at separate visits.

S. A. Deeds (✉) · K. M. Nelson
VA Puget Sound Health Care System, Department of Medicine, Division of General Internal Medicine, University of Washington, Seattle, WA, USA
e-mail: sdeeds@uw.edu

S. Mookherjee et al. (eds.), *Chalk Talks in Internal Medicine*,
https://doi.org/10.1007/978-3-030-34814-4_8

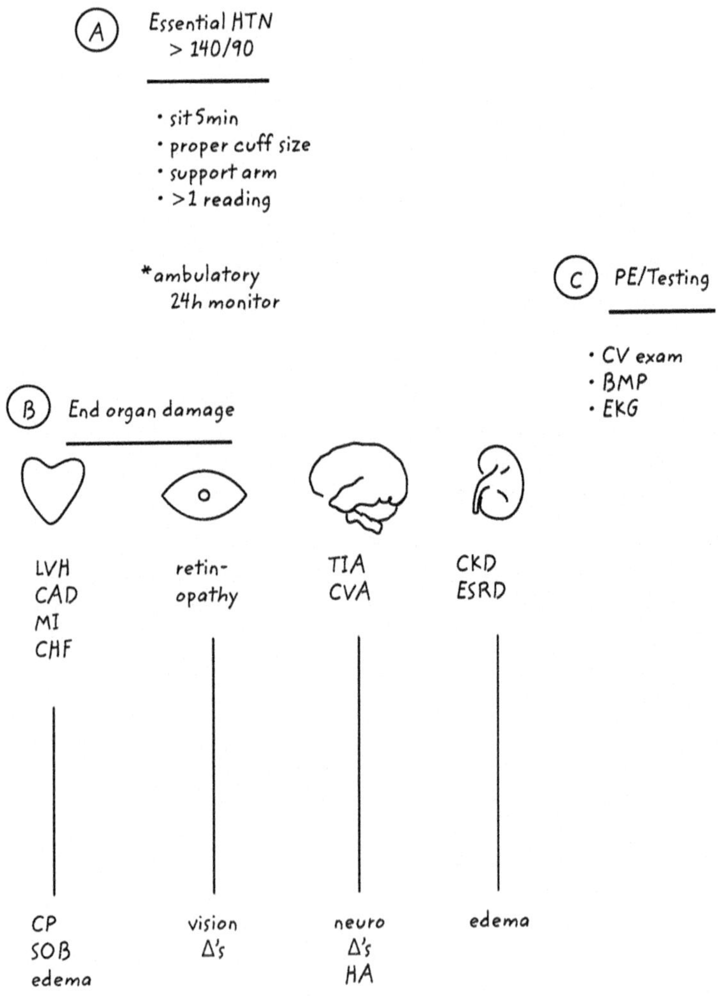

Fig. 8.1 Approach to hypertension, A–C

- If you want to confirm the diagnosis (and exclude white coat hypertension), you may consider 24-hour ambulatory BP monitoring.

B. **What organs are damaged by HTN? What are some signs and symptoms of end organ damage?**

Write down diseases on Fig. 8.1 *as they are mentioned and add any diseases that are missed and discuss any corollary signs and symptoms, if relevant.*

Teaching points
- Most patients with elevated BP have no symptoms unless organ damage is present.
- End organs damaged by HTN include the heart and vessels of the eyes, brain, and kidneys.

C. **Our patient is overweight but otherwise has a normal cardiovascular exam. He is diagnosed with essential hypertension. After performing a focused exam, what labs or other studies should be ordered?**

Teaching points
- At the diagnosis of HTN, check a basic metabolic panel (BMP) for renal damage and an electrocardiogram (ECG) for evidence of left ventricular hypertrophy.

D. **What are modifiable risk factors of HTN? Lifestyle changes of modifiable risk factors are recommended for all patients newly diagnosed with HTN.**

Draw the arrow depicting increasing effectiveness of lifestyle modification shown in Fig. 8.2. *Ask for examples and list them in the appropriate location by effectiveness.*

Teaching points
- Modifiable risk factors for HTN include tobacco use, alcohol, drug use, and obesity.
- Nonmodifiable risk factors include increased age, male sex, cardiovascular disease (CVD), diabetes, and family history of HTN and CVD.
- Weight loss is the most potent lifestyle intervention for improving BP.

E. **After 6 months of making lifestyle changes, he returns to the clinic and his BP is 148/88 mmHg. You decide it is time to start an antihypertensive medication. What are the classes of antihypertensive medications?**

List the major classes of antihypertensive medications, using the mnemonic ABCD, adding any that are missed. Add brief information about the major indications for each class of medications.

Teaching points
- Calcium channel blocker and diuretics tend to be more effective for African-American patients.
- Beta-blockers and diuretics tend to be lower cost than the other classes.

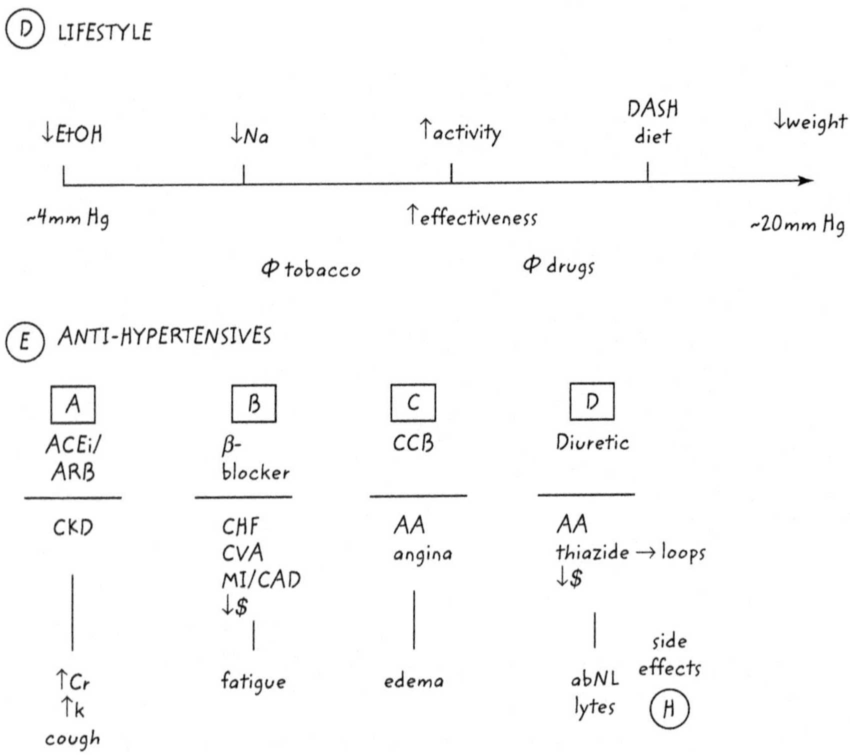

Fig. 8.2 Approach to hypertension, D–E

F. **Goals for BP are different for different patients. The main patient characteristics that determine BP goals are age, presence of diabetes mellitus, or chronic kidney disease. What is the blood pressure goal for most patients?**

Fill the appropriate goals based on patient characteristics and complete Fig. 8.3.

Teaching points

- The recommended BP targets come from guidelines included in the reference section.
- Note: Some recent trials, such as the SPRINT trial, have argued for lower BP goals, but most practitioners still follow the JNC-8 recommendations (see references).

G. **Our patient is 55 years old, is African-American, and has diabetes mellitus, so his target is <140/90 mmHg. Which antihypertensive would you recommend to this patient?**

- The recommended medical management based on patient characteristics and targets comes from guidelines in the references.
- Based on his age, presence of diabetes, and race, a calcium channel blocker or thiazide should be selected.

H. **It is important to monitor for side effects after starting any new antihypertensive medication.**

Return to Fig. 8.2 *to list the major side effects for the different classes of antihypertensive medications.*

Return to objectives and emphasize key points

1. Diagnose hypertension in the adult patient and describe an approach to further evaluation—circle or place an asterisk by each of these points in Fig. 8.1.
   - Measurement of BP > 140/90 mmHg.
   - Perform a focused exam.
   - Obtain a BMP and an ECG.
2. Recognize the complications of essential hypertension—circle or place an asterisk by each of these points in Fig. 8.1.
   - Patients are at risk for end organ damage if HTN goes untreated.
   - Major systems include the heart, eye, brain, and kidneys.
3. Identify and describe the impact of lifestyle changes and review the classes of antihypertensive medication used in the initial management of hypertension.
   - Lifestyle modifications of major risk factors should be recommended to all patients. Weight loss is most impactful in controlling BP.
   - The major classes of antihypertensives can be remembered by "ABCD."

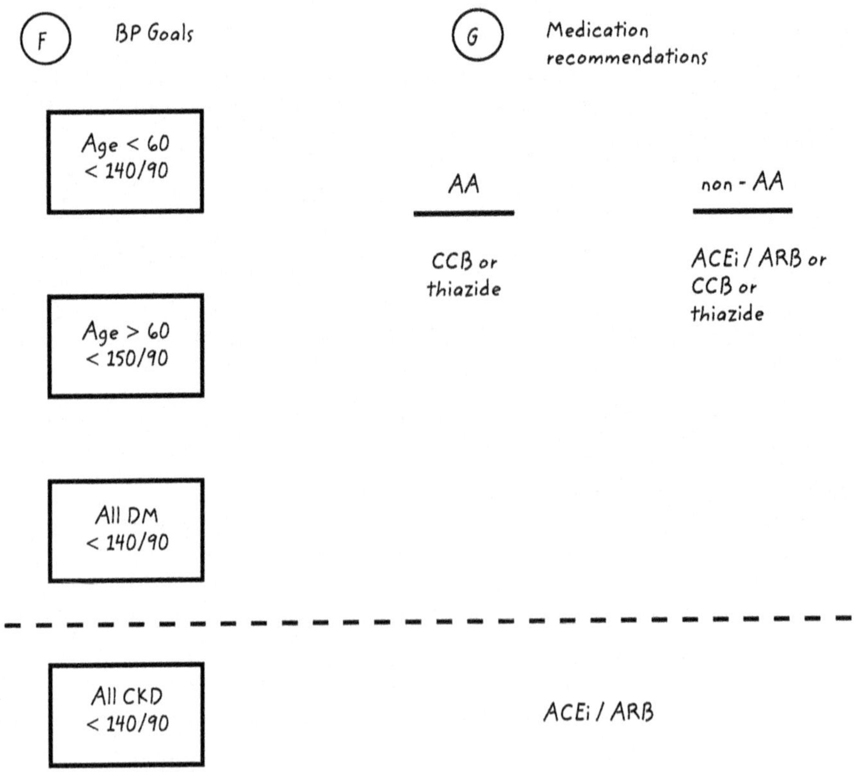

Fig. 8.3 Approach to hypertension, F–G

4. Distinguish blood pressure goals based on patient characteristics and select a treatment plan for a patient with essential hypertension.

- For most patients, the goal is BP < 140/90 mmHg.
- For patients aged >60 years, the goal is more lenient at <150/90 mmHg.
- Presence of comorbid diseases, such as CKD, and race can impact the selection of the initial antihypertensive medication.

Resources

1. James PA, Oparil S, Carter BL, Cushman WC, Dennison-Himmelfarb C, Handler J, et al. 2014 Evidence-based guidelines for the management of high blood pressure in adults. Report from the panel members appointed to the eighth Joint National Committee (JNC 8). JAMA. 2013;311(5):507–20.
2. Weir MR. Hypertension. Ann Intern Med. 2014;161(11):ITC1.
3. The SPRINT Research Group. A randomized trial of intensive versus standard blood-pressure control. N Engl J Med. 2015;373:2103–16.
4. Chobanian AV. Hypertension in 2017. JAMA. 2017;317(6):579–80.
5. Qaseem A, Wilt TJ, Rich R, Humphrey LL, Frost J, Forciea MA, et al. Pharmacologic treatment of hypertension in adults aged 60 years or older to higher versus lower blood pressure targets: a clinical practice guideline from the American College of Physicians and the American Academy of Family Physicians. Ann Intern Med. 2017;166:430–7.

Chapter 9
Stroke Prophylaxis in Atrial Fibrillation

Maya Narayanan and Paul R. Sutton

Learning Objectives

1. Evaluate a patient's stroke and bleeding risk by calculating the CHA_2DS_2-VASc and HAS-BLED scores.
2. Select an appropriate anticoagulant for stroke prophylaxis in patients with atrial fibrillation.
3. Identify treatments that are inferior to anticoagulation for stroke prophylaxis.

Clinical Vignette: A 70-year-old man with poorly controlled hypertension is admitted to the hospital with pneumonia and acute kidney injury. On physical exam, he is noted to have a temperature of 38.2 °C and blood pressure of 164/86 mmHg. He has an irregularly irregular heart rhythm and decreased breath sounds in the right lower lung fields. His creatinine is 2.3 mg/dL. Electrocardiogram shows new atrial fibrillation (AF) at 150 beats per minute.

A. **How can we assess this patient's risk of stroke related to atrial fibrillation?**

Ask for factors that increase risk of stroke and fill out the components of the CHA_2DS_2-VASc score in Fig. 9.1. *Explain that each variable equals one point except for age and stroke history.*

Teaching points

- The CHA_2DS_2-VASc score is used to predict risk of stroke in patients with atrial fibrillation. CHA_2DS_2-VASc calculators are widely available online and on medical calculator apps (reference below).
- Congestive heart failure history (clinical and objective evidence of systolic or diastolic dysfunction) = 1 point

M. Narayanan (✉) · P. R. Sutton
University of Washington Medical Center, Department of Medicine, Division of General Internal Medicine, University of Washington, Seattle, WA, USA
e-mail: mnarayan@uw.edu

S. Mookherjee et al. (eds.), *Chalk Talks in Internal Medicine*,
https://doi.org/10.1007/978-3-030-34814-4_9

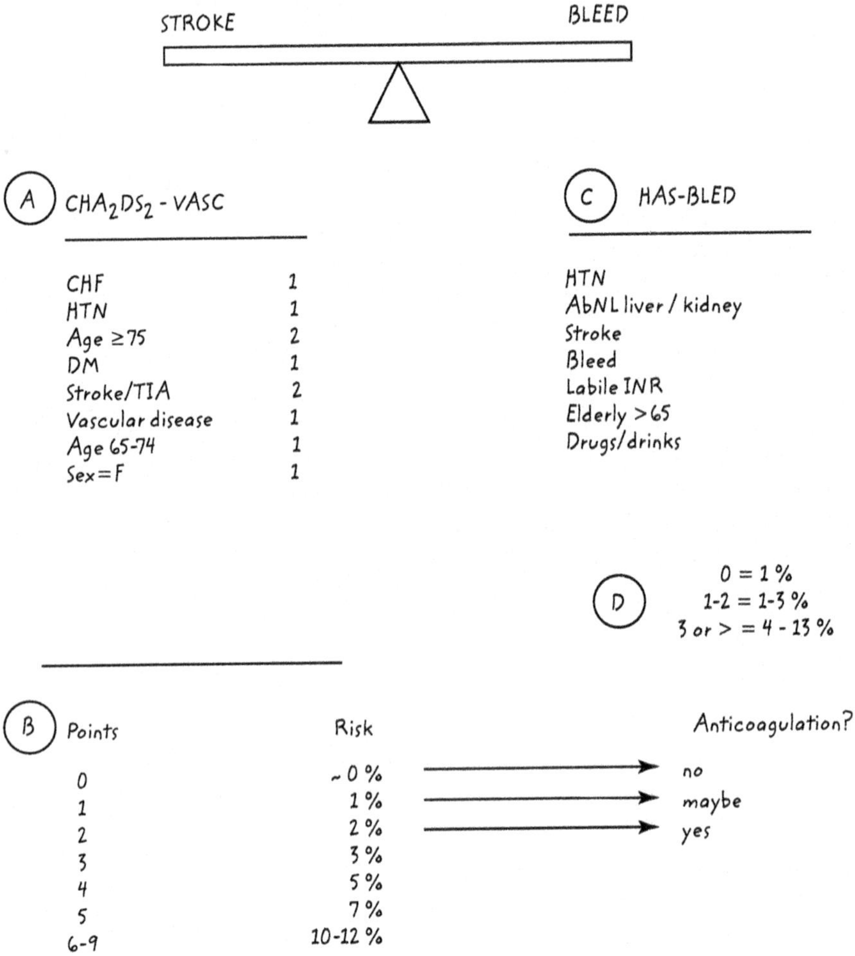

Fig. 9.1 Stroke prophylaxis in atrial fibrillation, A–D

- Hypertension history (or blood pressure controlled by medications) = 1 point
- Age >65 = 1 point, Age ≥75 = 2 points
- Diabetes mellitus history = 1 point
- Stroke or transient ischemic attack history = 2 points
- Vascular disease history (includes prior myocardial infarction, coronary interventions, other vascular interventions, symptoms of peripheral arterial disease (PAD), aortic plaque) = 1 point
- Female sex = 1 point

B. **Our patient has two stroke risk factors (hypertension and age >65 years), for a CHA_2DS_2-VASc score of 2. Would you offer anticoagulation for stroke prevention for a CHA_2DS_2-VASc score of 2?**

Write down the "points" column in Fig. 9.1. *Ask for estimated stroke risk for the number of points and fill out the "risk" column.*

Teaching points

- The number of CHA_2DS_2-VASc points corresponds to an approximate annual stroke risk.
- For CHA_2DS_2-VASc score of 0, the risk of stroke is so low that anticoagulation is not typically offered.
- For CHA_2DS_2-VASc score of 1, the decision to anticoagulate is variable and typically based on a discussion between the patient and the provider. These patients commonly receive aspirin rather than full anticoagulation.
- For CHA_2DS_2-VASc score of 2 or more (like our patient), anticoagulation is indicated in the absence of contraindications.
- Anticoagulation reduces stroke risk to about 1–2% a year (the fact that it is not zero may indicate treatment failure/inadequate anticoagulation or baseline stroke risk).

C. **On further interview, the patient reports an episode of AF during a past admission that converted back to sinus rhythm without intervention. He was prescribed aspirin 81 mg daily. The patient is worried about the risk of bleeding with anticoagulation. How can we assess his bleeding risk?**

Write out the HAS-BLED components under the "bleed" side of the scale in Fig. 9.1. *Ask learners to identify components that are potentially modifiable.*

Teaching points

- The HAS-BLED calculator is a useful tool to predict risk of major bleeding events in patients on anticoagulation (reference below).
- Note that the scoring system has only been validated for patients taking warfarin.
- Each HAS-BLED variable equals one point. Note that the score can change over time if the variables are modified:
  - Uncontrolled **H**ypertension ≥160 mmHg systolic (modifiable with medication)

- **A**bnormal renal function including dialysis, renal transplant, or creatinine >2.26 mg/dL or **A**bnormal liver function including cirrhosis or bilirubin >2× normal with AST/ALT/AP >3× normal (potentially modifiable)
- **S**troke history
- Prior major **B**leeding or predisposition to bleeding
- **L**abile INR or time in therapeutic range (TTR) <60% (potentially modifiable)
- **E**lderly >65 years old
- **D**rugs that predispose to bleeding like aspirin or ≥8 alcohol drinks/week (potentially modifiable)

D. **What is our patient's estimated bleeding risk? Should he be put on anticoagulation?**

Write down the annual risk of major bleeding with specific HAS-BLED scores in Fig. 9.1.

Teaching points

- His HAS-BLED risk factors include poorly controlled hypertension, abnormal kidney function, age greater than 65 years, and drugs (aspirin). Our patient's HAS-BLED score is 4.
- A HAS-BLED score of 3 or greater (conferring a 4–13% annual risk of bleed) is the generally accepted threshold above which the risk of major bleeding event exceeds the potential benefit of anticoagulation.
- Our patient's HAS-BLED score of 4 would typically preclude anticoagulation

E. **Given our patient's CHA2DS2-VASc score of 2, most providers would favor anticoagulation (and patients generally favor reducing stroke risk), yet the patient is at high risk for bleeding. Can any of our patient's HAS-BLED risk factors be modified to reduce his bleeding risk?**

Draw out a scale with greater weight on "BLEED" as shown in Fig. 9.2. *Indicate that if the bleeding risk cannot be modified, then anticoagulation probably shouldn't be started. Ask learners to consider how this patient's bleeding risk might be decreased.*

Teaching points

- His blood pressure can be modified with medication.
- His creatinine may improve with fluids.
- His aspirin can be stopped.
- If these interventions were successful, his HAS-BLED score would drop to 1 (or <4% annual risk of major bleeding risk).

F. **Having reduced our patient's bleeding risk, how would we choose the appropriate treatment to reduce his stroke risk?**

In Fig. 9.2, *write down "DOACs" as the preferred anticoagulant and list reasons NOT to give DOACs.*

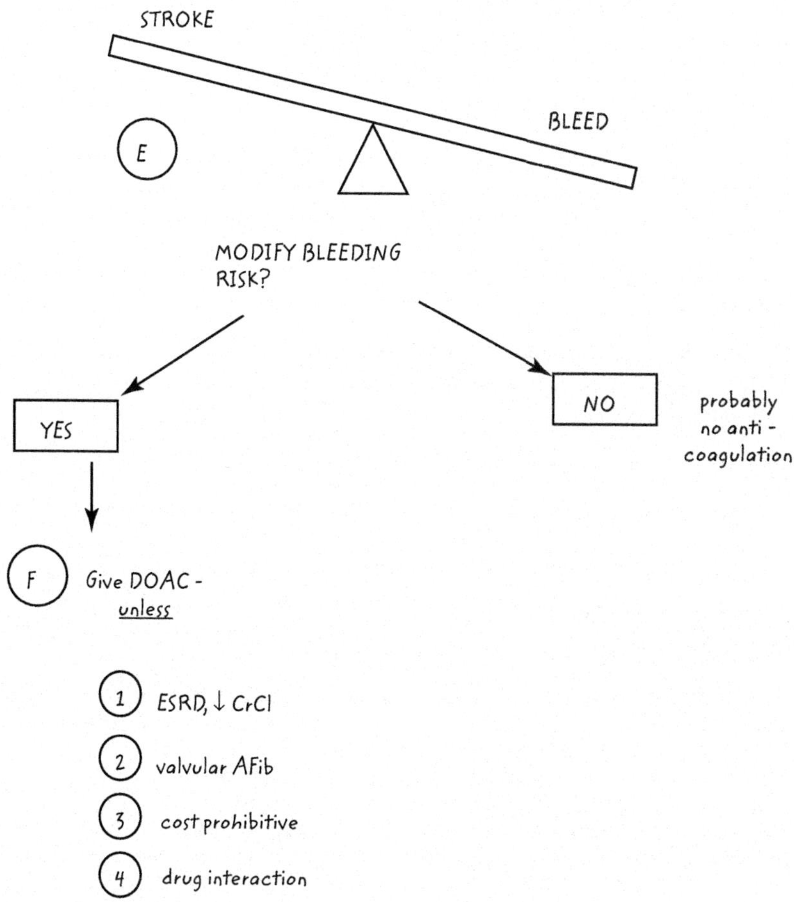

Fig. 9.2 Stroke prophylaxis in atrial fibrillation, E and F

Teaching points

- Direct oral anticoagulants (DOACs) like rivaroxaban or apixaban do not require monitoring with blood tests.
- DOACs are at least as effective as warfarin in reducing stroke risk and are associated with a lower risk for hemorrhagic stroke than warfarin.
- Warfarin is preferable to a DOAC in the listed select circumstances (see Fig. 9.2).
- Antiplatelets are inferior to therapeutic anticoagulation for stroke prevention.
- Risk of stroke is similar whether AF is paroxysmal or continuous.

Return to Objects and Emphasize Key Points

1. Stroke and bleeding risk among patients with AF can be calculated using the CHA_2DS_2-VASc and HAS-BLED scores.
    - Consider anticoagulation for CHA_2DS_2-VASc scores of 2 or greater.
    - Consider avoiding anticoagulation for HAS-BLED scores of 3 or greater.
    - Identify and address modifiable HAS-BLED variables.
2. Select an appropriate anticoagulant for stroke prophylaxis in patients with atrial fibrillation.
    - There are four main circumstances when warfarin is preferable to a DOAC.
    - Direct oral anticoagulants are effective and do not require blood test monitoring.
3. Identify treatments that are inferior to anticoagulation for stroke prophylaxis.
    - Antiplatelet therapy is inferior to anticoagulation for stroke prophylaxis.

Resources

1. Aguilar MI, Hart R, Pearce LA. Oral anticoagulants versus antiplatelet therapy for preventing stroke in patients with non-valvular atrial fibrillation and no history of stroke or transient ischemic attacks. Cochrane Database Syst Rev. 2007(3): CD006186.
2. Dogliotti A, Paolasso E, Giugliano RP. Novel oral anticoagulants in atrial fibrillation: a meta-analysis of large, randomized, controlled trials vs warfarin. Clin Cardiol. 2013;36:61–7.
3. Hart RG, Pearce LA, Rothbart RM, et al. Stroke with intermittent atrial fibrillation: incidence and predictors during aspirin therapy. Stroke Prevention in Atrial Fibrillation Investigators. J Am Coll Cardiol. 2000;35:183–7.
4. Lip GY, Nieuwlaat R, Pisters R, et al. Refining clinical risk stratification for predicting stroke and thromboembolism in atrial fibrillation using a novel risk factor based approach: the euro heart survey on atrial fibrillation. Chest. 2010;137:263–72.
5. Pisters R, Lane DA, Nieuwlaat R, et al. A novel user friendly score (has-bled) to assess one year risk of major bleeding in atrial fibrillation patients: the Euro Heart Survey. Chest. 2010;138:1093–100.
6. January CT, Wann LS, Calkins H, Chen LY, Cigarroa JE, Cleveland JC, Ellinor PT, Ezekowitz MD, Field ME, Furie KL, Heidenreich PA. 2019 AHA/ACC/HRS focused update of the 2014 AHA/ACC/HRS guideline for the management of patients with atrial fibrillation: a report of the American College of Cardiology/American Heart Association Task Force on Clinical Practice Guidelines and the Heart Rhythm Society. J Am Coll Cardiol. 2019;74(1):104–32.

Chapter 10
Workup for Chest Pain in the Clinic

Maryann K. Overland and Joseph Merrill

Learning Objectives
1. Generate a differential diagnosis of chest pain in clinic.
2. Explain key features of cardiac versus noncardiac chest pain.
3. Describe evidence-based physical exam and diagnostic testing in the evaluation of chest pain.
4. Recognize patients at high risk for cardiac events and justify indications for emergency or inpatient management of chest pain.

Clinical Vignette: A 66-year-old man presents to clinic for a routine checkup. He has a history of well-controlled type 2 diabetes mellitus on metformin, hypertension on lisinopril, gastroesophageal reflux disease on ranitidine as needed, and chronic knee and low back pain for which he uses occasional naproxen. His vital signs are within goal ranges and a brief exam is unremarkable. As you are wrapping up the visit, he says, "Oh, by the way my wife wanted me to mention this chest pain I've been having."

A. **What is the broad differential diagnosis of our patient's chest pain?**

As learners generate a differential diagnosis, draw and label the anatomic structures on the board as shown in Fig. 10.1. *Next to each structure, list the differential that your learners suggest. Fill in any gaps in the differential.*

B. **What key features on history are helpful in differentiating cardiac versus noncardiac chest pain?**

M. K. Overland (✉)
VA Puget Sound Health Care System, Department of Medicine, Division of General Internal Medicine, University of Washington, Seattle, WA, USA
e-mail: mko76@uw.edu

J. Merrill
Harborview Medical Center, Department of Medicine, Division of General Internal Medicine, University of Washington, Seattle, WA, USA

S. Mookherjee et al. (eds.), *Chalk Talks in Internal Medicine*,
https://doi.org/10.1007/978-3-030-34814-4_10

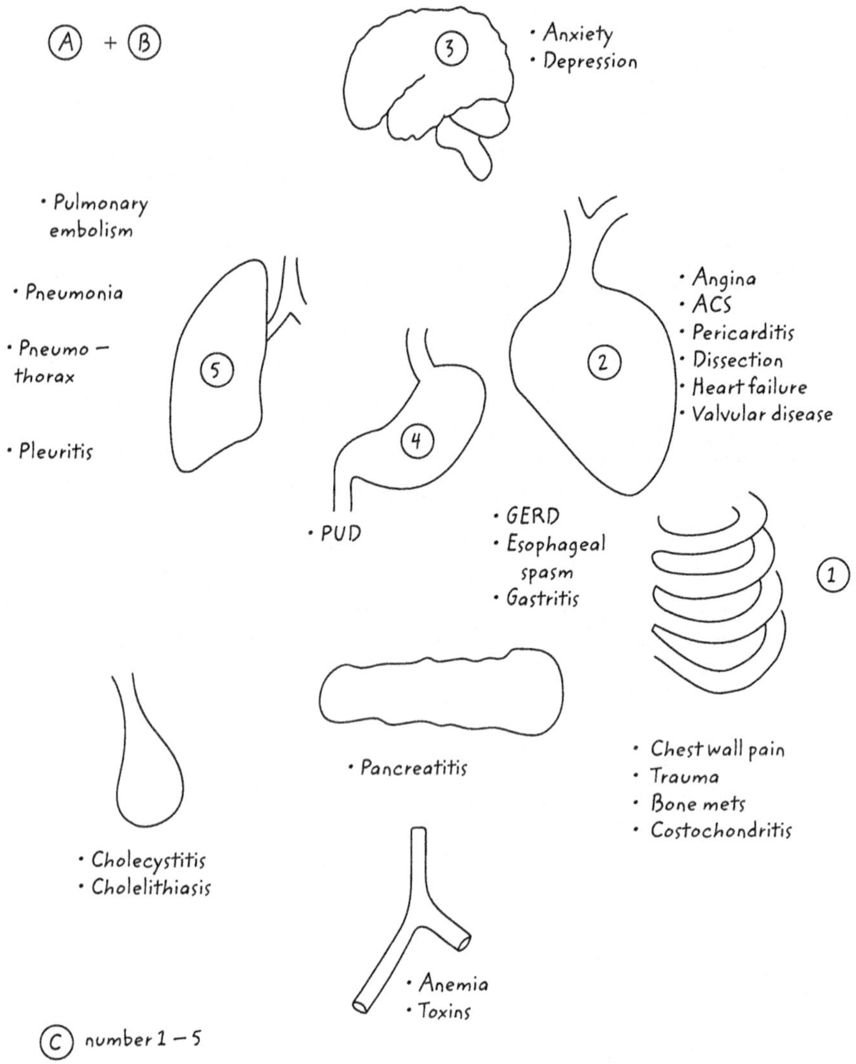

Fig. 10.1 Workup for chest pain in the clinic, A–C

Refer to Fig. 10.1 *as you discuss the typical characteristics of different sources of chest pain.*

Teaching points

- Cardiac ischemia pain tends to be retrosternal or epigastric, crushing or tight in quality, and can radiate to arms, shoulders, jaw, or neck.
- Chest pain or dyspnea caused by exertion or stress suggests stable angina.
- Aortic dissection is described as tearing/ripping pain radiating to the back.
- Gastroesophageal reflux disease (GERD) tends to be burning, postprandial, worse when supine.
- Cholecystitis/cholelithiasis typically presents as continuous epigastric or right upper quadrant pain, nausea, or vomiting. It is commonly triggered by fatty food.
- Pleural/pericardial pain tends to worsen with inspiration.
- Musculoskeletal chest pain is usually reproducible with palpation.
- Panic attacks are typically associated with anxiety, nonexertional dyspnea, or a history of panic disorder.

C. **How likely is each of these diagnoses to present in the clinic setting?**

Number the various causes in order of prevalence next to anatomic/category names in Fig. 10.1, *beginning with chest wall pain* (1) *through lung-related chest pain* (5).

D. **What questions should you ask the patient to characterize the chest pain?**

Elicit the pain characteristics listed in the acronym "SOCRATES" in Fig. 10.2.

E. **The patient reports dull, 5/10 substernal pain, that comes on with exertion, and dissipates after about 10 min of rest. What should your next steps be clinic?**

Start leading learners through the outpatient chest pain triaging algorithm in Fig. 10.2. *The very first step should be to verify clinical stability—if the patient is clinically unstable or has abnormal vital signs they should be sent to the emergency department (ED). If the patient is stable, they should be examined and an electrocardiogram (ECG) should be obtained.*

Teaching points

- Typical angina has the following three features: precipitated by exertion/stress, improved by rest or nitroglycerin, and lasts less than 10 min.
- Atypical angina has one or two features of typical angina.
- Nonanginal pain lacks all features of typical angina.
- Cardiac chest pain is more likely if there is diaphoresis, pain radiating to arm, jaw, or neck.
- Cardiac chest pain is less likely if pain worsens with inspiration, can be reproduced by palpation, or is triggered by food.

(D) **SOCRATES**

Site
Onset
Character
Radiation
Associations
Timing
Exacerbating / relieving factors
Severity

(E) OUTPATIENT TRIAGING OF CHEST PAIN

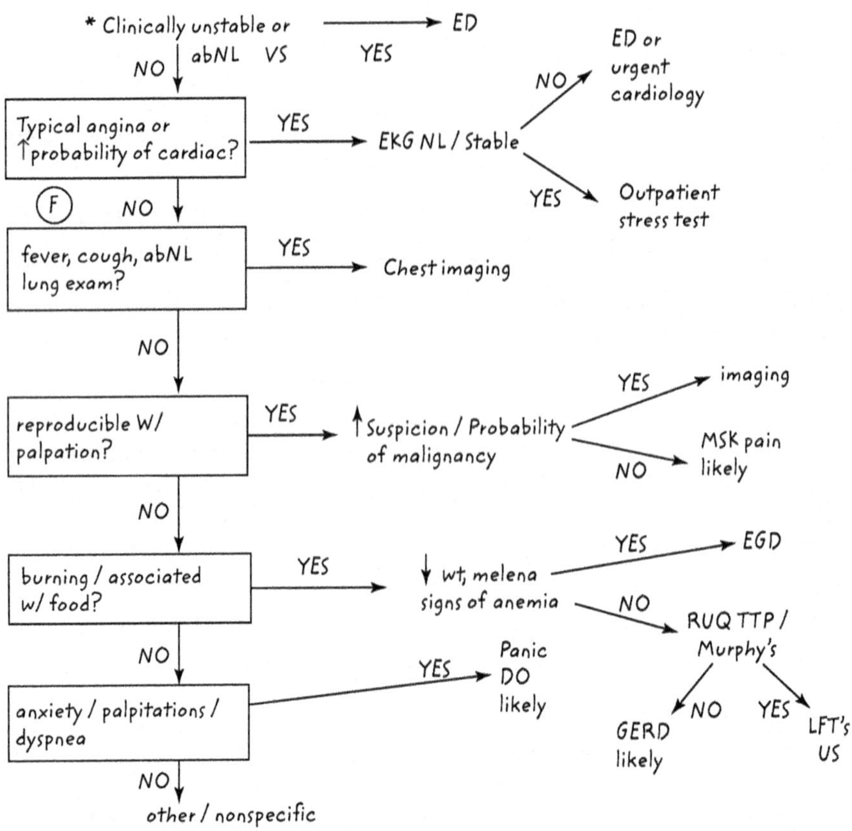

Fig. 10.2 Workup for chest pain in the clinic, D–F

- Historical features that increase the likelihood of coronary artery disease (CAD): typical angina description, age >70 years, prior myocardial infarction.
- Factors decreasing the likelihood of CAD: nonanginal description, pain >30 min duration, associated with dysphagia, young age.

Teaching points for the physical exam in evaluation of chest pain
- Patients with CAD often have no abnormal physical exam findings!
- Always assess heart rate, rhythm, and blood pressure.
- Cardiac auscultation—a pericardial rub suggests pericarditis.
- Rubs are best appreciated with patient leaning forward and holding his or her breath in deep expiration.
- Assess volume status to look for signs of heart failure.
- Palpate chest wall to evaluate for tenderness.
- Palpate abdomen to evaluate for tenderness, which might suggest of peptic ulcer disease or biliary colic.
- Auscultate lungs for pleural rubs or focal signs of pneumonia.
- Patient hand gestures are associated with probability of cardiac chest pain.
  - Levine sign—clenched fist against sternum increases probability.
  - Palm sign—open palm against sternum increases probability.
  - Arm sign—gripping left arm increases probability.
  - Pointing sign—pointing to a single spot reduces probability.

F. **Imagine the patient did NOT describe typical anginal pain. What would the next steps be?**

Lead learners through the rest of the algorithm in Fig. 10.2.

Return to objectives and emphasize key points
1. Generate a differential diagnosis of chest pain in clinic.
   - Cardiac: ischemia, pericarditis, aortic dissection
   - Pulmonary: pneumonia, pleuritis
   - GI: GERD, biliary colic, pancreatitis, gastritis
   - Musculoskeletal
   - Psych: panic/anxiety
2. Explain key patient history features in cardiac versus noncardiac chest pain.
   - Cardiac ischemia pain: retrosternal or epigastric, crushing/ tight in quality, can radiate to arms, shoulders, jaw, or neck. Typically brought on by exertion/ stress and relieved by rest/relaxation.
   - GERD: burning, postprandial, worse when supine.
   - Biliary colic: continuous epigastric or right upper quadrant pain, nausea, vomiting, often triggered by fatty food.

- Pleural/pericardial: worse with inspiration.
- Aortic dissection: tearing/ripping, radiates to back.
- Musculoskeletal: reproducible with palpation or movement.
- Panic: associated with anxiety, nonexertional dyspnea, history of panic disorder.

3. Describe evidence-based physical exam and diagnostic testing in the evaluation of chest pain.

   - Vital signs
   - Cardiopulmonary auscultation
   - Chest wall and abdominal palpation
   - Volume status
   - ECG

4. Recognize patients at high risk for cardiac events and justify indications for emergency or inpatient management of chest pain.

   - Factors increasing likelihood of CAD: typical angina description, age >70 years, prior myocardial infarction, ECG changes
   - Factors decreasing likelihood of CAD: Nonanginal description, triggered by food, associated dysphagia, worsened by inspiration, reproducible by palpation, pain >30 min duration, young age

Resources

1. Antman EM, et al. The TIMI risk score for unstable angina/non-ST elevation MI: a method for prognostication and therapeutic decision making. JAMA. 2000;284(7):835–42.
2. Cayley W. Diagnosing the cause of chest pain. Am Fam Physician. 2005;72(10):2012–21.
3. McGee S. Evidence-based physical diagnosis. 3rd ed. Philadelphia: Elsevier; 2012.
4. Scheuermeyer FX, et al. Development and validation of a prediction rule for early discharge of low-risk emergency department patients with potential ischemic chest pain. CJEM. 2014;16(2):106–19.
5. Six AJ, et al. Chest pain in the emergency room: value of the HEART score. Neth Heart J. 2008;16(6):191–6.
6. Than M, et al. Development and validation of the emergency department assessment of chest pain score and 2 h accelerated diagnostic protocol. Emerg Med Australas. 2014;26(1):34–44.

Chapter 11
Management of Hyperosmotic Hyperglycemia

Shobha W. Stack and Karen A. McDonough

Learning Objectives

1. Distinguish between diabetic ketoacidosis (DKA) and hyperosmotic hyperglycemic state (HHS).
2. Describe the management of HHS.
3. Identify the causes of HHS.

Clinical Vignette: A 58-year-old woman was found obtunded in a park, appearing profoundly dehydrated. A blood glucose check in the field was 1200 mg/dL. She was transported to the emergency department where her vital signs were: temperature 37.6 °C, BP 70/30 mmHg, HR 120 bpm, RR 18, O_2Sat 100% on RA.

A. **She clearly has a problem with elevated blood glucose—what are the two major hyperglycemic syndromes?**

Draw two overlapping circles in Fig. 11.1*; label the intersecting area "hyperglycemia," and label each circle "DKA" and "HHS."*

Teaching points

- Diabetic ketoacidosis (DKA) is an acute complication of diabetes mellitus type 1 (DM1). Deficiency of insulin prohibits muscle and liver cell glucose uptake. Insulin deficiency causes a shift from the normal carbohydrate metabolism to a state of fasting fat metabolism—lipolysis, which leads to ketoacidosis.
- Hyperosmolar hyperglycemic state (HHS) is associated with diabetes mellitus type 2 (DM2). Pancreatic production of insulin is sufficient to prevent ketoacidosis, but not adequate to cause glucose utilization.
- It takes one-tenth as much insulin to suppress ketoacidosis as it does to stimulate glucose uptake.

S. W. Stack (✉) · K. A. McDonough
University of Washington Medical Center, Department of Medicine, Division of General Internal Medicine, University of Washington, Seattle, WA, USA
e-mail: shobhaws@uw.edu

S. Mookherjee et al. (eds.), *Chalk Talks in Internal Medicine*,
https://doi.org/10.1007/978-3-030-34814-4_11

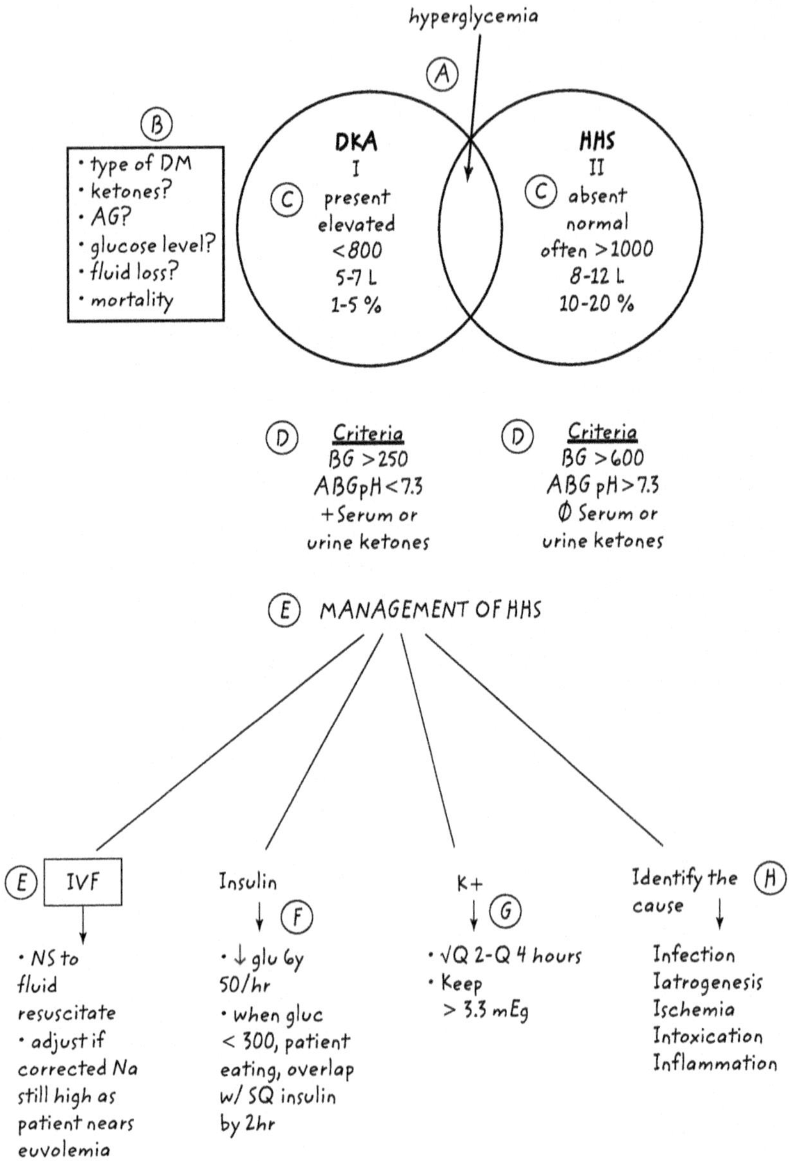

Fig. 11.1 Management of hyperosmotic hyperglycemia: A–H

B. **DKA and HHS have hyperglycemia in common, but the syndromes are different in several respects—what are some ways in which these syndromes are different?**

Write down the key distinguishing features in a column alongside the circles, making sure to include any not mentioned.

C. **For each of these variables, how do DKA and HHS typically present?**

Query learners about each of the characteristics and fill out the information for DKA and HHS as in Fig. 11.1.

Teaching points

- Although both DKA and HHS involve hyperglycemia, the ketones in DKA create an anion gap.
- Because HHS has no ketoacidosis, there is no anion gap (unless the precipitant of HHS also causes a gap acidosis).
- Ketosis-prone DM2 is uncommon but tends to occur in patients who are Hispanic or African American (nearly 50%). The etiology of this acute, transient β-cell failure is not currently known.
- HHS develops over days to weeks compared to hours for DKA. Therefore, HHS has a greater hyperglycemia and concurrent fluid loss compared to DKA.
- Lack of insulin leads to hyperglycemia through two mechanisms: loss of cellular glucose uptake and inhibited hepatic gluconeogenesis. This leads to osmotic diuresis and subsequent dehydration.

D. **Your patient had a blood gas sent. Her pH was 7.4, and urine did not have ketones. Does she have DKA or HHS?**

Write down the DKA and HHS criteria below the circles to reinforce the key distinguishing factors. This patient has HHS.

E. **After determining that circulation, airway, and breathing (CAB) are stable, what is the most important first step in the management of this patient?**

Write out IVF, insulin, K+ and "Identify the cause" under management of HHS in Fig. 11.1. *Put a box around "IVF"—the most important initial treatment for this patient.*

Teaching points

- Three of these cornerstones (fluids, insulin, and potassium) need constant monitoring.
- Fluids are critical to restore intravascular volume and concurrently decreasing plasma osmolarity.
- The initial fluid should be normal saline (NS) even if patients are initially hypernatremic. This is because normal saline is hypo-osmotic (285 mOsm/L) relative to the hyperosmotic patient (>320 mOsm/L).

- The initial serum sodium in HHS may be low, normal, or high. High plasma osmolality pulls water out of cells, diluting serum sodium and causing hyperosmolar hyponatremia. Osmotic diuresis with loss of free water eventually leads to hypernatremia, often made worse by poor oral intake due to altered mental status.
- The "corrected" serum sodium is an estimate of what the serum sodium level will be once blood glucose comes down to the normal range.
- As the patient approaches euvolemia and if the "corrected" sodium still appears to be high, ½ NS may be used to avoid ongoing hypernatremia.
- A rule of thumb for fluid resuscitation is to correct one-half of the fluid deficit in the first 8–12 h and the rest in the following 12–36 h.

F. **How quickly should the blood glucose be brought down?**

Fill out the second column under "Insulin."

Teaching points

- A rule of thumb for intravenous insulin infusion is to decrease blood glucose by 50 mg/dL per hour.
- When serum glucose reaches 250–300 mg/dL, a long-acting SQ insulin may be administered 30 min before a meal (the patient must be able to eat) and 2 h before discontinuing the infusion. The overlap accounts for the time to onset for the long-acting insulin, which is approximately 2 h.
- HHS is resolved when osmolarity reaches <320 mOsm/kg and mental status returns to baseline.

G. **What will happen to the potassium level as you give insulin and fluid to this patient?**

Fill out the third column under "K^+"

Teaching points

- The initial serum potassium may be high, normal, or low. Hyperosmolarity and insulin deficiency cause potassium to shift out of cells. However, total body potassium is typically very low due to urinary losses from osmotic diuresis.
- Serum potassium will fall rapidly with correction of hyperosmolality and administration of insulin. Itshould be monitored every 2–4 h.
- Delay potassium replacement until the serum level falls <5 mEq/L. If potassium is <3.3 mEq/L, pause the insulin until it reaches 3.3 mEq/L.
- There is usually no indication for bicarbonate or phosphate repletion as these levels are typically normal and self-limited, respectively. However, you should carefully replete phosphate if there is cardiac dysfunction, anemia, respiratory depression, or a serum phosphate level <1.0 mg/dL.

H. **What could have precipitated our patient's HHS?**

Fill out the fourth column under "Identify the cause."

Teaching points

- Infection (~45%)—leukocytosis is common in HHS, even without an infection. Nevertheless, the source of infection should be investigated in all cases.
- Iatrogenesis—inadequate insulin therapy (~30%), dehydration, medication side effects (e.g., glucocorticoids, thiazide diuretics, sympathomimetic drugs, antipsychotics).
- Ischemia—myocardial infarction, stroke.
- Intoxication—illicit drugs (particularly cocaine), alcohol.
- Inflammation—pancreatitis, appendicitis, pregnancy, trauma.

Return to objectives and emphasize key points

1. Distinguish between diabetic ketoacidosis (DKA) and hyperosmotic hyperglycemic syndrome (HSS)
   - HHS is more typical in type 2 diabetic patients.
   - HHS is diagnosed by a blood glucose >600 mg/dL, arterial pH > 7.30, and absent serum and urine ketones.
2. Describe the management of HHS: asterisk columns 1–3 below "Management of HHS"
   - Start with fluid resuscitation.
   - Correct blood glucose and potassium abnormalities.
   - Remember to concurrently find and treat the precipitating factor.
   - HHS is resolved when osmolarity reaches <320 mOsm/kg and mental status returns to baseline.
3. Identify the causes of HHS: asterisk column 4 below "Management of HHS"
   - Infection
   - Iatrogenesis
   - Ischemia
   - Intoxication
   - Inflammation

Resources

1. Van Ness-Otunnu R, Hack JB. Hyperglycemic crisis. J Emerg Med. 2013;45(5):797–805. https://doi.org/10.1016/j.jemermed.2013.03.040.
2. Wilson JF. In the clinic. Diabetic ketoacidosis. Ann Intern Med. 2010;152:ITC1–ITC15. PMID: 20048266
3. Maletkovic J, Drexler A. Diabetic ketoacidosis and hyperglycemic hyperosmolar state. Endocrinol Metab Clin North Am. 2013;42(4):677–95. https://doi.org/10.1016/j.ecl.2013.07.001.

4. Corwell B, Knight B, Olivieri L, Willis GC. Current diagnosis and treatment of hyperglycemic emergencies. Emerg Med Clin North Am. 2014;32(2):437–52. https://doi.org/10.1016/j.emc.2014.01.004.
5. Kitabchi AE, Umpierrez GE, Murphy MB, et al. American Diabetes Association. Hyperglycemic crises in diabetes. Diabetes Care. 2004;27(Suppl 1):S94–S102. PMID: 14693938
6. Gosmanov AR, Gosmanova EO, Kitabchi AE. Hyperglycemic crises: diabetic ketoacidosis (DKA), and hyperglycemic hyperosmolar state(HHS). In: De Groot LJ, et al., editors. Endotext [Internet]. South Dartmouth: MDText.com, Inc.; 2000.

Chapter 12
Management of Symptomatic Hypercalcemia

Yilin Zhang and John Sheffield

Learning Objectives

1. Identify patients who require urgent or emergent inpatient treatment of hypercalcemia.
2. Recognize symptoms of hypercalcemia.
3. Identify the main treatments for inpatient management hypercalcemia and limitations of their use.

Clinical Vignette: A 66-year-old woman with a history of squamous cell lung cancer presents to the emergency department with a 2-week history of abdominal pain, nausea, and vomiting. Initial labs are notable for serum creatinine of 5.52 mg/dL (from a baseline 0.8), serum calcium (Ca) of 12.8 mg/dL, and albumin of 3.0. On review of systems, she reports fatigue, constipation, and generalized weakness.

A. **How severe is her hypercalcemia?**

Starting with Fig. 12.1, *note the need to correct for albumin level; write out levels of serum and ionized calcium for mild, moderate, and severe hypercalcemia.*

Teaching points

- About 45% of our body's Ca is bound to albumin, so the total measured Ca should be corrected for albumin.
- Corrected serum Ca = (4 − serum albumin) × 0.8 + measured serum Ca.
- Our patient has a corrected Ca of (4 − 3) × 0.8 + 12.8 = 13.6.

Y. Zhang (✉)
University of Washington Medical Center, Department of Medicine, Division of General Internal Medicine, University of Washington, Seattle, WA, USA
e-mail: yilin2@uw.edu

J. Sheffield
Harborview Medical Center, Department of Medicine, Division of General Internal Medicine, University of Washington, Seattle, WA, USA

S. Mookherjee et al. (eds.), *Chalk Talks in Internal Medicine*,
https://doi.org/10.1007/978-3-030-34814-4_12

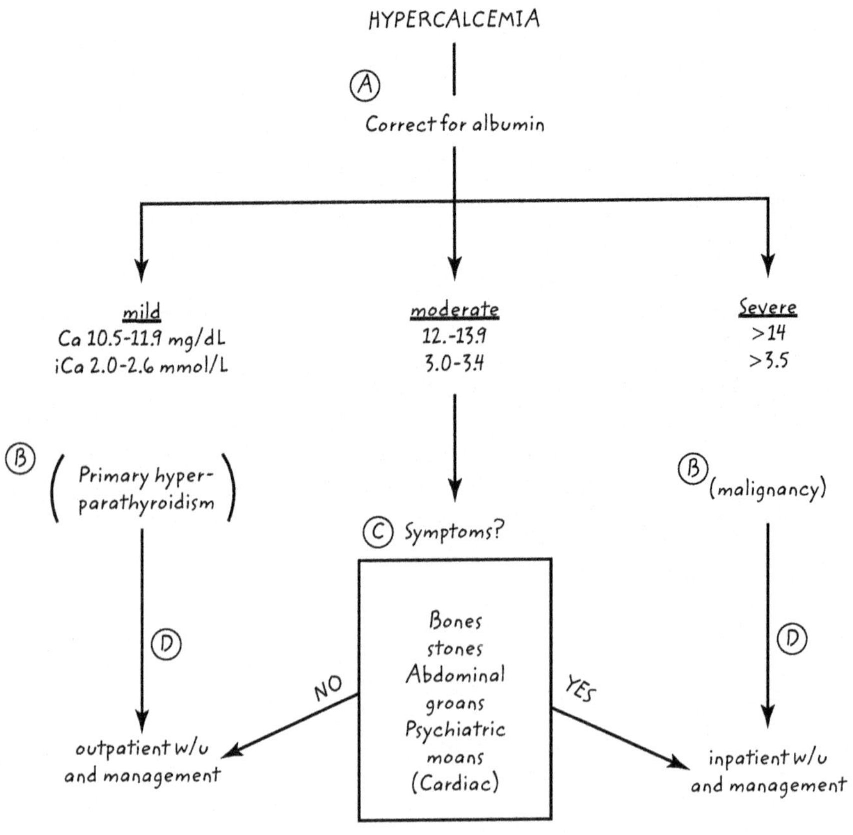

Fig. 12.1 Management of symptomatic hypercalcemia, A–D

B. **Our patient has moderate hypercalcemia. What are the most common causes of hypercalcemia?**

Write primary hyperparathyroidism and malignancy below mild and severe hypercalcemia respectively.

Teaching points

- The most common causes of hypercalcemia are primary hyperparathyroidism and hypercalcemia of malignancy, accounting for 90% of diagnoses.
- Primary hyperparathyroidism typically results in mild hypercalcemia, whereas hypercalcemia of malignancy can result in severe hypercalcemia.
- Our patient's underlying cancer diagnosis and her moderate hypercalcemia make hypercalcemia of malignancy the most likely diagnosis.

C. **What are some common symptoms of hypercalcemia?**

Fill out the box of symptoms below "moderate" hypercalcemia.

Teaching points

- The classic mnemonic is "stones, bones, psychiatric moans, and abdominal groans," which illustrates the multiorgan effects of hypercalcemia.
- "Stones"—renal symptoms.
  - Hypercalcemia has a diuretic effect and provokes nephrogenic diabetes insipidus, which leads to dehydration and acute kidney injury.
  - Nephrocalcinosis, kidney stones.
- "Bones"—musculoskeletal symptoms include muscle weakness and bone pain.
- "Psychiatric moans"—neuropsychiatric symptoms.
  - Fatigue, memory loss, and poor concentration.
  - Delirium, coma.
  - Psychosis, hallucination.
- "Abdominal groans"—gastrointestinal symptoms include constipation, nausea, vomiting, and pancreatitis.
- Not included in this mnemonic are the cardiac effects of hypercalcemia, which include shortened QTc interval and heart block.

D. **What are the indications for urgent or emergent treatment of hypercalcemia?**

Complete Fig. 12.1, *showing inpatient and outpatient follow-up needed.*

Teaching points

- Urgency of treatment is determined by symptoms and the severity of hypercalcemia.
  - Long-standing hypercalcemia may result only in mild symptoms (e.g., constipation, fatigue).
  - Acute rise in Ca levels can lead to more severe symptoms (e.g., acute kidney injury, altered mental status).
- All patients with severe hypercalcemia require hospital admission and urgent treatment.
- Mild hypercalcemia rarely requires hospitalization and can be evaluated in the outpatient setting.
- Urgency of treatment for moderate hypercalcemia depends on symptom severity and chronicity.

E. **Our patient has severe symptoms (acute kidney injury) and moderate hypercalcemia, which should prompt inpatient admission. Let's walk through some of the basic principles of inpatient management. What are some therapies for hypercalcemia in this situation?**

Start Fig. 12.2, *drawing an arrow indicating the onset of action from hours to weeks, and ask learners to suggest treatments for hypercalcemia; insert the treatments at the appropriate place and fill in any not mentioned.*

F. **Aggressive intravenous (IV) fluid resuscitation is a cornerstone of therapy for hypercalcemia. What are the mechanisms and limitations of fluid administration?**

Add to Fig. 12.2.

Teaching points

- Mechanism: reverses dehydration caused by hypercalcemia-induced nephrogenic diabetes insipidus and diuresis.
- Limitations: risk of volume overload.
- Intravenous fluids should be administered between 200 and 300 mL/hour with a target of ~2 L urine output per day.
- Fluids alone can decrease Ca levels by approximately 1.6–2.4 mg/dL[2].

G. **Increased osteoclastic bone resorption is a major mechanism for severe cases of hypercalcemia. Intravenous bisphosphonates are a first-line medication for hypercalcemia. What are the mechanisms and limitations of intravenous bisphosphonates?**

Add to Fig. 12.2.

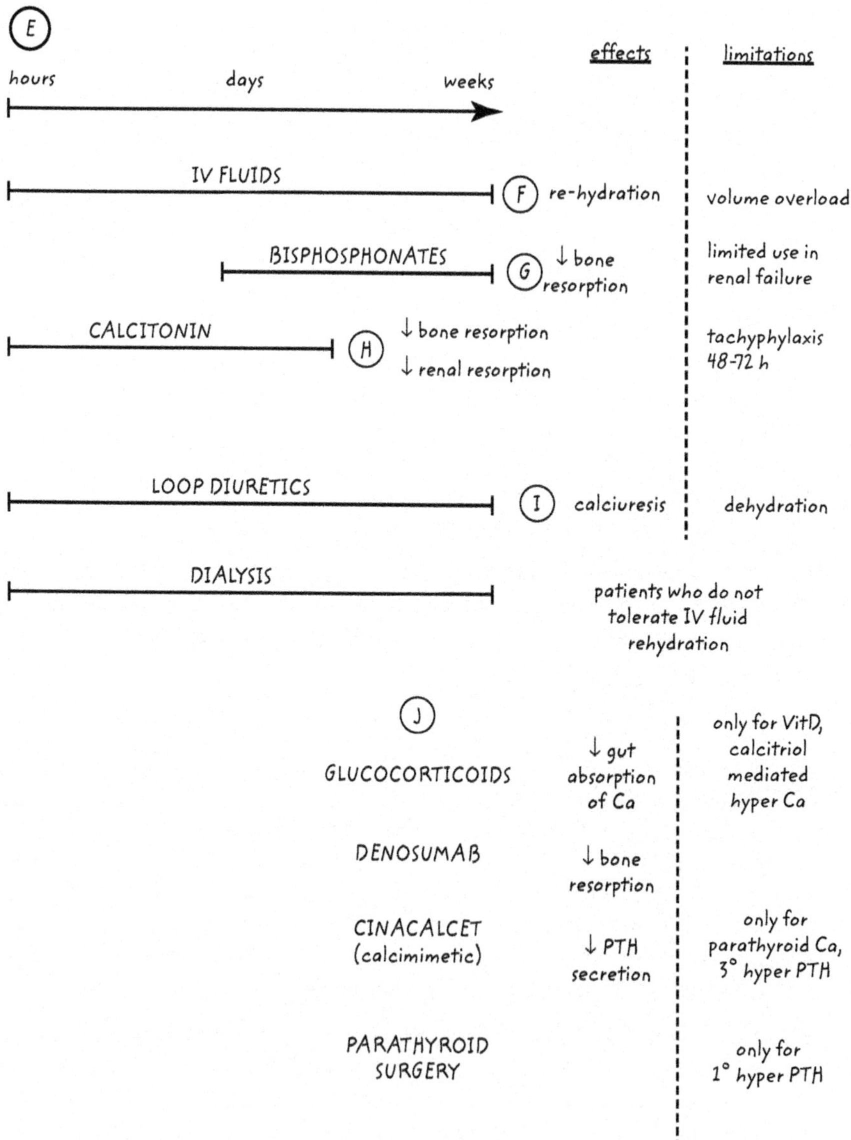

Fig. 12.2 Management of symptomatic hypercalcemia, E–J

Teaching points

- Mechanism: decrease osteoclastic bone resorption.
- Limitations: severe renal insufficiency, relatively contraindicated with CrCl <30 mL/hour.
- Onset of action is 2–4 days, with peak effect at 4–7 days. Duration of action is 1–3 weeks.
- Bisphosphonates are only Food and Drug Administration (FDA)-approved for hypercalcemia of malignancy, but their use can be extrapolated to other causes of hypercalcemia.

H. **Subcutaneous or intramuscular calcitonin can be used as a temporizing measure when Ca levels need to be lowered quickly. What are the mechanisms and limitations of calcitonin?**

Add to Fig. 12.2.

Teaching points

- Mechanism: decreases osteoclastic bone resorption and increases renal excretion of Ca.
- Limitations: tachyphylaxis develops after 48–72 h of use.
- Modestly decreases Ca levels by approximately 1 mg/dL.
- Onset of action is in hours with peak effect at 12–24 h.

I. **The most common therapies for inpatient hypercalcemia management are IV fluids, bisphosphonates, and calcitonin. Loop diuretics can be used if patients become volume overloaded. What are the mechanisms and limitations of loop diuretics?**

Add to Fig. 12.2.

Teaching points

- Mechanism: increase renal excretion of Ca.
- Limitations: worsen dehydration and exacerbate hypercalcemia in volume-depleted patients.
- Thiazide diuretics are always contraindicated in hypercalcemia because they increase renal reabsorption of Ca and increase serum Ca level.
- Patients with heart failure or severe renal insufficiency may require dialysis if they cannot receive intravenous fluids or bisphosphonate therapy.

J. **What are some additional therapies available for hypercalcemia? Our patient has hypercalcemia of malignancy. Hypercalcemia of malignancy can be caused by local bony destruction from metastases, production of parathyroid hormone (PTH)-related protein, and low 1, 25-OH vitamin D. Any additional treatment options?**

Complete Fig. 12.2 *with the list of additional treatment modalities and their effects and limitations.*

Teaching points

- Glucocorticoids and avoiding dietary calcium are effective for controlling the forms of hypercalcemia mediated by vitamin D (hypervitaminosis D, granulomatous diseases, and lymphomas).
- Denosumab, a receptor activator of nuclear factor kappa B ligand (RANK-L) agonist, has been studied in bisphosphonate-refractory hypercalcemia of malignancy. Unlike bisphosphonates, denosumab is not contraindicated in renal failure.
- Calcimimetics such as cinacalcet mimic the effect of Ca and result in decreased PTH secretion. They can be used in hypercalcemia associated with parathyroid cancers, tertiary hyperthyroidism, or in pregnancy.
- Patients with primary hypercalcemia occasionally develop symptomatic moderate or severe hypercalcemia and are treated with urgent parathyroidectomy. Otherwise, an outpatient decision to pursue surgery for parathyroidectomy depends on symptoms, age, and severity of hypercalcemia.

Return to objectives and emphasize the key points

1. Identify patients who require urgent or emergent inpatient treatment of hypercalcemia.
    - Severe hypercalcemia
    - Moderate hypercalcemia with severe symptoms
2. Recognize symptoms of hypercalcemia.
    - Genitourinary (GU)/"stones": kidney stones, acute kidney injury (AKI), nephrocalcinosis
    - "Bones": bone pain
    - Neuropsychiatric/"moans": altered mental status, fatigue, weakness, coma
    - Gastrointestinal (GI)/"groans": nausea/vomiting, constipation, pancreatitis
3. Identify the main treatments for inpatient management hypercalcemia and limitations of their use.
    - IV hydration at a rate of 200–300 cc/hour.
    - If unable, tolerate aggressive fluid repletion and consider dialysis.
    - Loop diuretics should be used only when volume is replete or overloaded.
    - IV bisphosphonates are a cornerstone of therapy but have a long onset of action (2–4 days).
    - Calcitonin can be used as a temporizing measure to lower Ca but its effects only last 48–72 h.

Resources

1. Minisola S, et al. The diagnosis and management of hypercalcaemia. BMJ. 2015;350:h2723.
2. Ahmah S, Kuraganti G, Steenkamp D. Hypercalcemic crisis: a clinical review. Am J Med. 2015;128(3):239–45.

3. Carroll R, Martin G. Endocrine and metabolic emergencies: hypercalcaemia. Ther Adv Endocrinol Metab. 2010;1(5):225–34.
4. Stewart AF. Hypercalcemia associated with cancer. N Engl J Med. 2004;352(4):373–9.
5. Legrand SB, et al. Narrative review: furosemide for Hypercalcemia: an unproven yet common practice. Ann Intern Med. 2008;149(4):259–63.

Chapter 13
Management of Type 2 Diabetes

Anna L. Golob and Sara L. Jackson

Learning Objectives
1. Identify individualized HbA1c targets.
2. Develop a framework for choosing patient-centered glucose-lowering therapy, including therapeutic lifestyle changes and pharmacologic agents.
3. Understand the mechanism, site of action, and efficacy for newer pharmacologic agents.

Teaching Script
Clinical Vignette: A 44-year-old woman with history of hypertension and obesity presents to primary care for routine follow-up. She endorses a general decrease in energy but denies polydipsia or polyuria. Family history is notable for an older brother with type 2 diabetes mellitus (T2DM). Her screening tests for diabetes yield the following results: fasting blood glucose 175 mg/dL and hemoglobin A1c (HbA1c) of 8.0, confirming a new diagnosis of diabetes. She has normal renal function.

A. **What HbA1c level should be targeted?**

Draw Fig. 13.1, *Part A. For our patient, as is the case for many adults, the target HbA1c is <7.0.*

Teaching points
- HbA1c targets must be patient-centered and individualized.
- HbA1c <7% is generally recommended for healthier patients.

A. L. Golob (✉)
VA Puget Sound Health Care System, Department of Medicine, Division of General Internal Medicine, University of Washington, Seattle, WA, USA
e-mail: zilanna@uw.edu

S. L. Jackson
Harborview Medical Center, Department of Medicine, Division of General Internal Medicine, University of Washington, Seattle, WA, USA

S. Mookherjee et al. (eds.), *Chalk Talks in Internal Medicine*,
https://doi.org/10.1007/978-3-030-34814-4_13

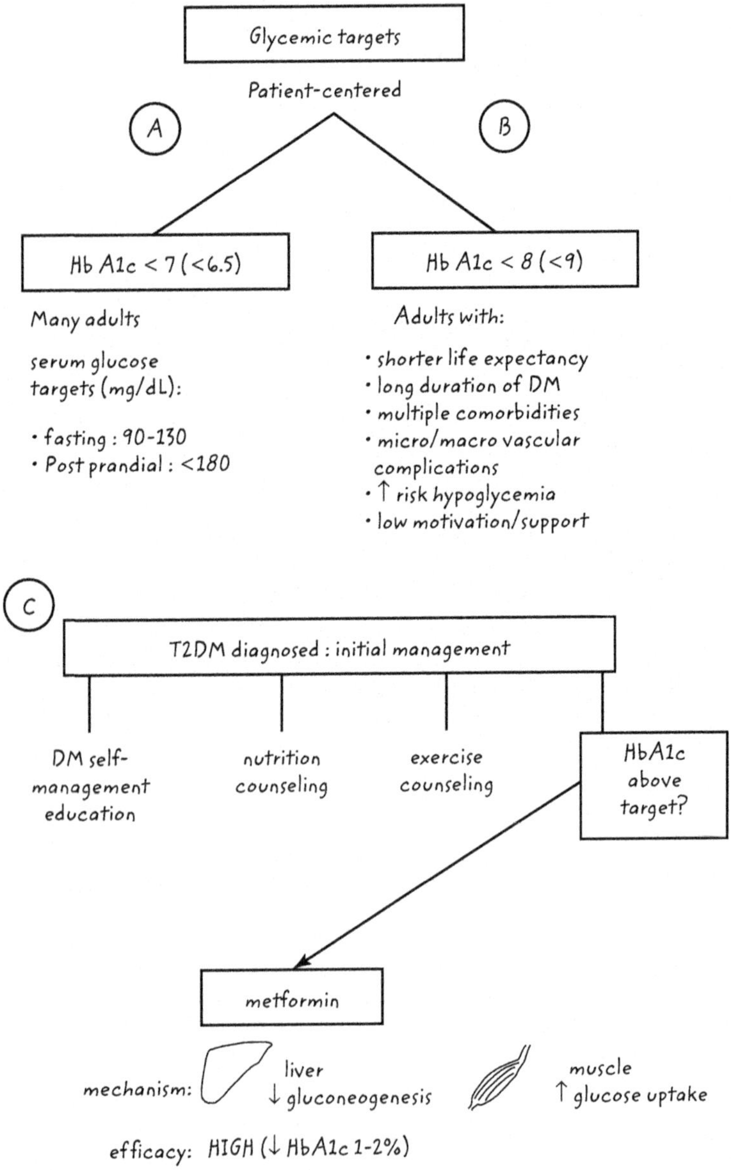

Fig. 13.1 Management of type 2 diabetes, A–C

- Based on population studies, HbA1c of 7.0% correlates to an average serum blood glucose of 150 mg/dL.
- To estimate average serum glucose, add or subtract 30 points from 150 for each additional A1c percentage point.

B. **How would this target differ if she were 82 and had stage 3 chronic kidney disease and heart failure with reduced ejection fraction?**

Draw Fig. 13.1, *Part B. For an 82-year-old woman with T2DM, stage 3 chronic kidney disease (CKD), and heart failure with reduced ejection fraction (HFrEF), the HbA1c goal is <8–9. Feel free to use or substitute your own real-life examples.*

Teaching points

- Less tight control (HbA1c 8–9%) for highly comorbid patients with longer duration of diabetes, shorter-life expectancy, diabetes-related micro- and macrovascular complications, greater risk of hypoglycemia, and lower motivation and support.
- The landmark ACCORD study (NEJM 2008) included ~10 thousand patients with >10-year duration of T2DM randomized to tight (HbA1c 6.0%) versus standard (A1c 7.0–7.9%) glycemic control. It was stopped early because of an increased risk of death from any cause with tight control.
- The ADVANCE and VADT trials showed no improvement in cardiovascular outcomes with tight glycemic control in patients with long-standing T2DM.

C. **What treatment do you recommend for her newly diagnosed diabetes?**

Draw Fig. 13.1, *Part C: Initial Management.*

Teaching points

- All patients should receive diabetes self-management education at the time of diagnosis.
- Overweight or obese patients should be counseled on weight loss, targeting >5% of their body weight: when possible, refer to a dietician or a diabetes nutrition class.
- American Diabetes Association (ADA) guidelines recommend moderate to brisk exercise for at least 30 min five or more days per week.
- If the provider and the patient determine that a medication is indicated to achieve glycemic targets, per ADA guidelines, metformin should be initial therapy unless contraindicated.
- It is OK to start metformin in patients with eGFR >45 and OK to continue it in current users with eGFR >30 if kidney function is stable and metformin is renally dosed.
- Consider sustained release metformin to mitigate gastrointestinal side effects; also consider low/slow up-titration.
- Screen for vitamin B_{12} deficiency in chronic metformin users due to impaired gastric B_{12} absorption.
- In patients with initial HbA1c >10%, consider insulin in addition to metformin as first-line therapy.

D. **Our patient receives diabetes self-management education, meets with a dietician, starts an exercise program, and starts metformin titrated to 1000 mg twice daily. Her HbA1c decreases to 6.7% and is stable for 2 years. However, over time she gains weight and when she is 46, her repeat HbA1c is 8.1% (above target) on full-dose metformin. What are the major classes of medications that can be added to metformin and how much can they be expected to lower her HbA1c?**

Write out the first two columns of Fig. 13.2, *outlining the major classes of DM medications, examples, and expected decrease in HbA1c.*

Teaching points

- Repeat HbA1c every 3–6 months and add additional lifestyle changes and/or pharmacologic agents to metformin if not at target.
- Currently available pharmacologic classes include sulfonylureas, thiazolidinediones (TZD), dipeptidyl peptidase 4 (DPP4) inhibitors, glucagon-like peptide 1 (GLP 1) receptor agonists, sodium-glucose cotransporter 2 (SGLT2) inhibitors, and insulin.

E. **What is the mechanism of action of each of these classes of medications?**

Draw the third column in Fig. 13.2.

F. **With so many options, how should we choose what is the best choice for this patient? She particularly does not want a medication that is likely to cause more weight gain.**

Asterisk the agents that are most associated with weight gain (see Table 13.1). Review other considerations that may influence the choice of an agent.

Teaching points

- Many patients do not want medications that cause weight gain. Options include DPP4-inhibitor (weight neutral), GLP1-RA (weight loss), or an SGLT2-inhibitor (weight loss).
- Other relative advantages and disadvantages for individual patients include expected HbA1c lowering, cost, side effects, risk of hypoglycemia, effect on weight, and cardiovascular effects.
- The information in Table 13.1 is included for the teacher's reference.
- Note that insurers may require a trial and failure of less expensive options before covering newer, more expensive medications.

Return to objectives and emphasize key points

1. Identify individualized HbA1c targets.
    - Glycemic targets must be individualized; with higher HbA1c goals for patients with multiple comorbidities, longer duration DM, shorter life expectancy, end-organ complications of diabetes, and greater risk of hypoglycemia.

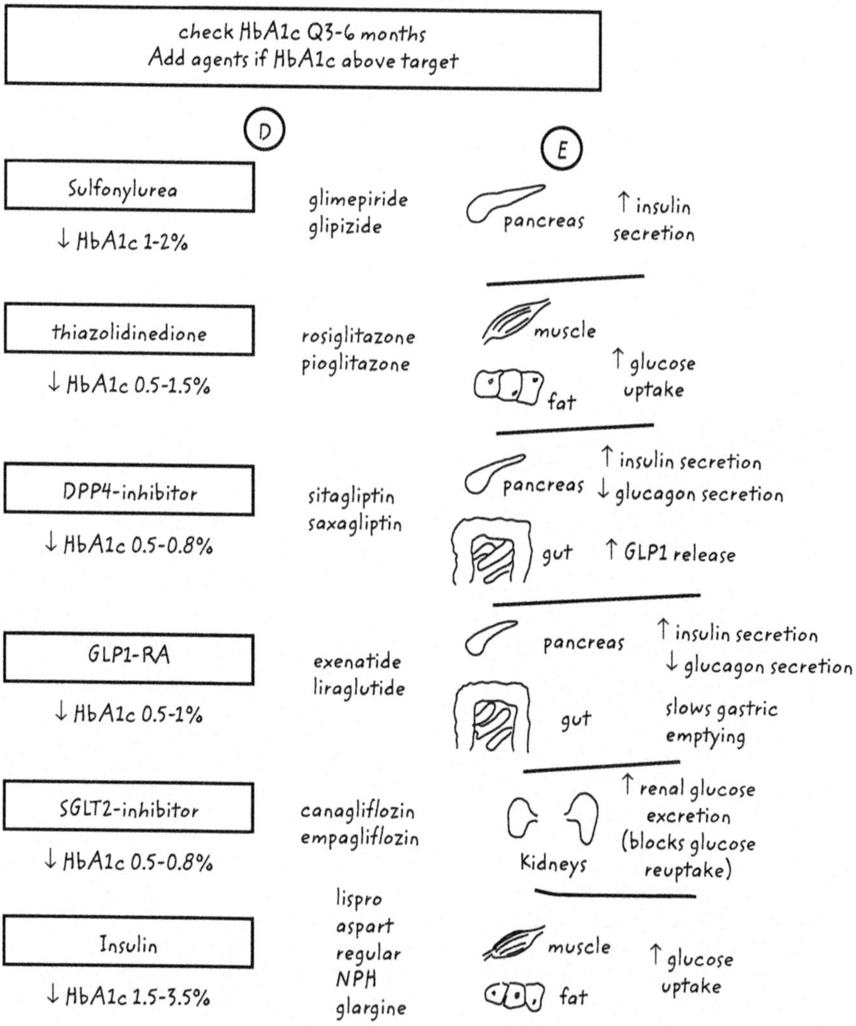

Fig. 13.2 Management of type 2 diabetes, D and E

Table 13.1 Pharmacologic agents for T2DM

	Metformin	Sulfonylurea	TZD	DPP4-I	GLP1-RA	SGLT2-I	Insulin
↓A1c %	1.0–2.0	1.0–2.0	0.5–1.5	0.5–0.8	0.5–1.0	0.5–0.8	1.5–3.5
Hypoglycemia risk	Low	Mod-high	Low	Low	Low	Low	High
Weight	Neutral/loss	Gain	Gain	Neutral	Loss	Loss	Gain
Cost	Low	Low	Low	High	High	High	Variable
Side effects	Gastrointestinal (GI)	Hypos	Edema, heart failure (HF), fracture	Rare	GI	genitourinary (GU) infection, dehydration, fracture	Hypoglycemia
CVD effect	Likely benefit	Neutral	Adverse	Neutral	Liraglutide benefit	Empagliflozin benefit	Neutral

2. Develop a framework for choosing patient-centered glucose-lowering therapy, including lifestyle changes and pharmacologic agents.
    - Must be individualized to the patient.
    - Include self-management education and specific nutrition and exercise counseling.
    - Metformin should be initial therapy unless contraindicated.
    - Additional pharmacologic agents should be added when HbA1c remains above target after initial therapy; consider patient-specific advantages and disadvantages to guide selection.

Resources

1. American Diabetes Association Professional Practice Committee. Standards of medical care in diabetes-2019. Diabetes Care. 2019;42(Suppl 1):S1–2.
2. Gerstein HC, et al. Effects of intensive glucose lowering in type 2 diabetes. N Engl J Med. 2008;358(24):2545–59.
3. Abraira C, Colwell J, Nuttall F, et al. Cardiovascular events and correlates in the Veterans Affairs Diabetes Feasibility Trial. Veterans Affairs Cooperative Study on Glycemic Control and Complications in Type II Diabetes. Arch Intern Med. 1997;157:181.
4. ADVANCE Collaborative Group, Patel A, MacMahon S, et al. Intensive blood glucose control and vascular outcomes in patients with type 2 diabetes. N Engl J Med. 2008;358:2560.
5. Nathan DM, Kuenen J, Borg R, Zheng H, Schoenfeld D, Heine RJ. Translating the A1C assay into estimated average glucose values. Diabetes Care. 2008;31:1473–8.
6. Marso SP, Daniels GH, Brown-Frandsen K, et al. Liraglutide and cardiovascular outcomes in type 2 diabetes. N Engl J Med. 2016;375:311.
7. Zinman B, Wanner C, Lachin JM, et al. Empagliflozin, cardiovascular outcomes, and mortality in type 2 diabetes. N Engl J Med. 2015;373:2117.

Chapter 14
Management of Incidental Thyroid Nodules

Eve Lake and Bradley D. Anawalt

Learning Objectives
1. Describe a systematic approach to the evaluation of incidental thyroid nodules.
2. List at least five possible etiologies of thyroid nodules.
3. List three risk factors for thyroid cancer.
4. List three exam features that suggest possible thyroid malignancy.
5. Demonstrate the thyroid exam.

Clinical Vignette: A 58-year-old man with a history of hypertension and tobacco use presents to your primary care clinic for follow-up of a low-dose chest computed tomography (CT) that was ordered for lung cancer screening. There are no pulmonary nodules, but there is a thyroid nodule noted in the left thyroid lobe measuring 1–2 cm in size. He is feeling physically well with no complaints.

A. **What is the likelihood that this is cancer?**

Draw the thyroid outline and cancer risk estimates.

Teaching points
- Thyroid nodules are found in 1–5% of the population.
- Thyroid cancers occur in 7–15% of nodules, depending on risk factors.
- Most thyroid cancers have an indolent course, and they are usually treatable with excellent long-term survival. For differentiated thyroid cancer, the 10-year survival rate is 95%.

E. Lake (✉)
Harborview Medical Center, Department of Medicine, Division of General Internal Medicine, University of Washington, Seattle, WA, USA
e-mail: evelake@uw.edu

B. D. Anawalt
University of Washington Medical Center, Department of Medicine, Division of General Internal Medicine, University of Washington, Seattle, WA, USA

S. Mookherjee et al. (eds.), *Chalk Talks in Internal Medicine*,
https://doi.org/10.1007/978-3-030-34814-4_14

B. **What are some benign and malignant etiologies in our differential for a thyroid nodule?**

Write down the differential created by the learners. Leave spaces as necessary in the list of malignant etiologies so that they can be ordered by worsening prognosis (Fig. 14.1).

C. **The general approach to the evaluation of an incidental thyroid nodule starts with history and physical exam, followed by labs and appropriate imaging. Let's start with patient history. What are risk factors for thyroid cancer?**

Write down key risk factors as the learners name them.

D. **Our patient tells us that he has no history of head, neck, or chest radiation, and no personal or family history of thyroid cancer. The physical exam is the next important step.**

Draw the important landmarks and list the steps of the thyroid exam as in Fig. 14.2. *If possible, demonstrate the thyroid exam on a volunteer (see Key Resources for links to online demonstrations). Consider demonstrating the size of a palpable nodule using a peanut M&M (about 1 cm).*

Teaching points

- First, look at the patient's neck. Do you see any asymmetry or enlargement?
- Stand behind the patient and find your landmarks.
- Identify the thyroid cartilage (above the thyroid)—it feels like two shields or flat plates stuck together at the top of the trachea. Here you can palpate the thyroid isthmus.
- Move down to the cricoid cartilage. This is just above the first two rings of the trachea.
- Next, firmly palpate each lobe of the thyroid for nodules. The beginner's mistake is to palpate too gently and shallowly—press firmly down to the level of the trachea. Tell the patient that you are going to press firmly into the neck; it may cause mild discomfort but it should not hurt. You can apply firm pressure to one side to make the contralateral lobe easier to palpate.
- Do a lymph node exam of the head and neck. Presence of a palpable Delphian lymph node is highly suggestive of malignancy.
- The Delphian node is centrally located near the thyroid in the prelaryngeal or precricoid nodal tissue. It is associated with increased incidence of metastatic disease spread to central and lateral neck compartments.
- The term "Delphian" was likely derived from the Oracle of Delphi in ancient Greece. The Oracle of Delphi was the most powerful woman of ancient Greece, and her prophecies were thought to be from divine sources. In this case, a Delphian node is a prophesy of malignancy and not so divine.

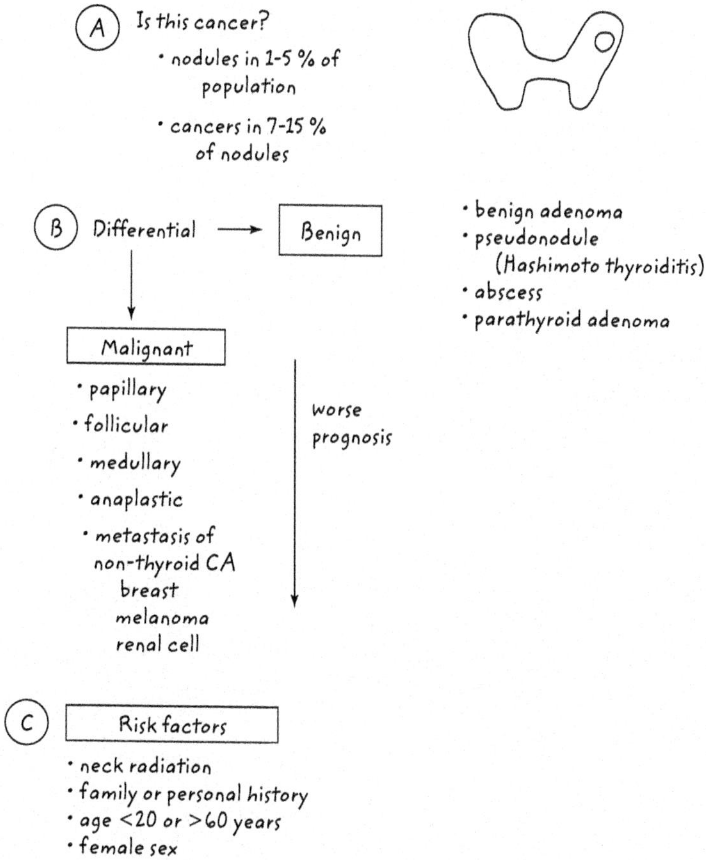

Fig. 14.1 Management of incidental thyroid nodules, A–C

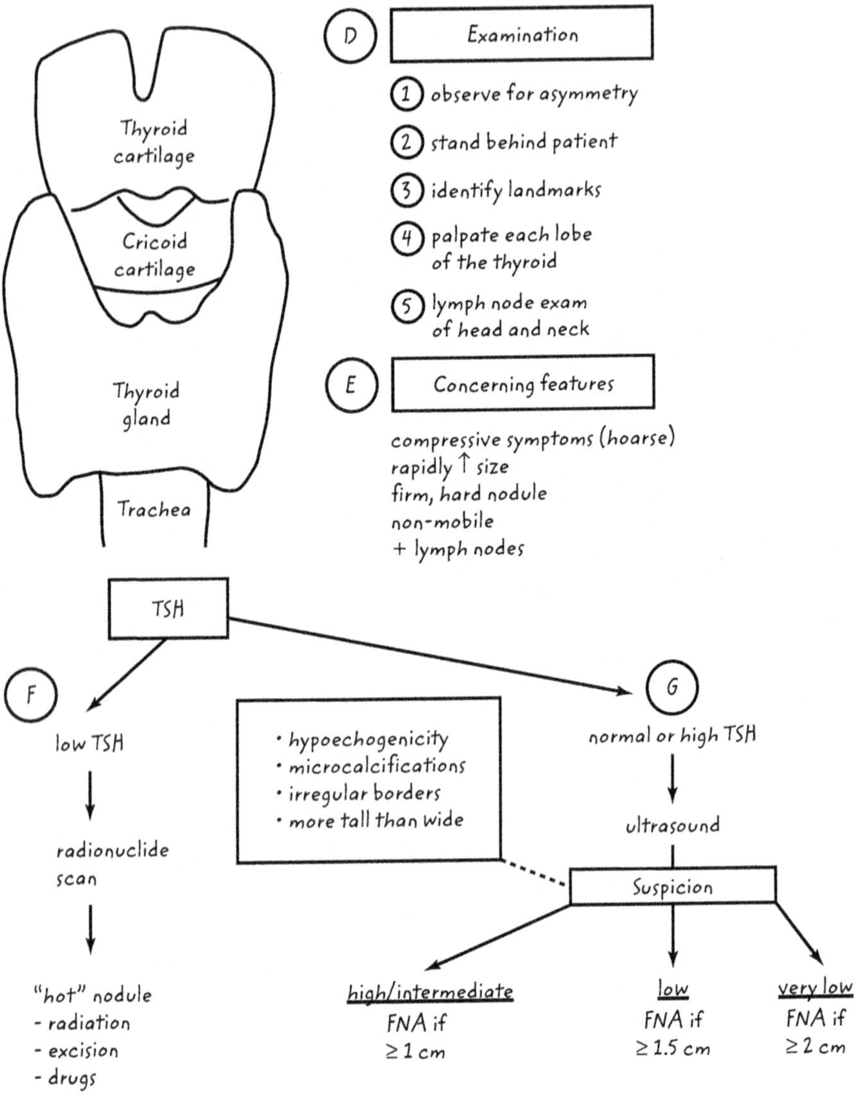

Fig. 14.2 Management of incidental thyroid nodules, D–G

E. **Our patient has a palpable ~1.5 cm nodule in the left thyroid lobe. It is mobile and nontender, and there is no associated lymphadenopathy. What features in the history and on thyroid exam increase the likelihood this is cancer?**

List the concerning features in Fig. 14.2.

F. **The next step is to determine if this is a hyperfunctioning thyroid nodule. A hyperfunctioning thyroid nodule makes thyroid hormone autonomously of serum TSH concentration. If the nodule makes enough thyroid hormone to result in hyperthyroidism, then the serum TSH concentration will be suppressed to below normal. What if this patient's TSH concentration comes back low, and what are the next steps?**

Write the next steps as shown in Fig. 14.2.

Teaching points

- The recommended imaging is a radionuclide scan to identify a hyperfunctioning "hot nodule."
- If a hot nodule is identified with the surrounding thyroid tissue showing no uptake, then treatment with radioiodine or surgical extirpation should be considered.
- Hot nodules do not need a fine-needle aspirate (FNA) because the risk of malignancy is extremely low and because the cytology of a hyperfunctioning thyroid adenoma is difficult to interpret.

G. **What if the patient's TSH concentration is normal or high?**

Write the next steps as shown in Fig. 14.2.

Teaching points

- The recommended imaging is a thyroid ultrasound. This must be a dedicated thyroid ultrasound. If an incidental thyroid nodule is visible on a neck duplex study, the patient still requires a dedicated thyroid ultrasound.
- Two factors are important here: specific features of the nodule on ultrasound that are concerning for malignancy, and size.
- There is practice variation around whether to perform FNA on very low suspicion nodules: simple cysts (without any solid component) or spongiform nodules (look like sponges on ultrasound). Most experts will not FNA these nodules, while others FNA all cysts larger than 2 cm.

H. **Our patient's thyroid ultrasound shows a 1.4 cm nodule with microcalcifications. He should be referred for FNA because of the presence of microcalcifications.**

Circle "high/intermediate risk" in Fig. 14.2.

Return to objectives and emphasize key points

1. Describe a systematic approach to evaluation of incidental thyroid nodules. *Circle or asterisk each of these steps on your diagram: physical exam, checking thyroid function, and determination of appropriate imaging.*
2. List a differential of at least five possible thyroid nodule etiologies.
3. List three risk factors for thyroid cancer and three exam features concerning for malignancy. Risk factors include:
   - Radiation to the head, neck, or upper chest
   - Family or personal history
   - Age <20 years or >60 years
   - Female sex
4. Features on exam that are concerning for malignancy include:
   - Rapid nodule growth
   - Compressive symptoms
   - Firm, hard nodule
   - Nonmobile nodule
   - Lymphadenopathy
5. Demonstrate the thyroid exam

Resources

1. Haugen BR, Alexander EK, Bible KC, Doherty GM, Mandel SJ, Nikiforov YE, et al. 2015 American Thyroid Association management guidelines for adult patients with thyroid nodules and differentiated thyroid cancer: the American Thyroid Association guidelines task force on thyroid nodules and differentiated thyroid cancer. Thyroid [Internet]. 2016;26(1):1–133. https://doi.org/10.1089/thy.2015.0020.
2. Iyer NG, Kumar A, Nixon IJ, Patel SG, Ganly I, Tuttle RM, et al. Incidence and significant of Delphinian node metastasis in papillary thyroid cancer. Ann Surg [Internet]. 2011;253(5):988–91. https://doi.org/10.1097/SLA.0b013e31821219ca. Available from: http://journals.lww.com/annalsofsurgery/Abstract/2011/05000/Incidence_and_Significance_of_Delphian_Node.22.aspx
3. Sciuto R, Romano L, Rea S, Marandino F, Sperduti I, Maini CL. Natural history and clinical outcome of differentiated thyroid carcinoma: a retrospective analysis of 1503 patients treated at a single institution. Ann Oncol [Internet]. 2009;20(10):1728–35. Available from: https://academic.oup.com/annonc/article-lookup/doi/10.1093/annonc/mdp050
4. The thyroid exam: Stanford Medicine 25 [web streaming video]. Palo Alto: Stanford University; 2014 [cited 2017 May 30]. Available from: http://stanfordmedicine25.stanford.edu/videos.html#thyroid-exam

Chapter 15
Management of Osteoporosis

Neha S. Deshpande and Kay M. Johnson

Learning Objectives
1. Determine which patients should receive treatment for osteoporosis.
2. Identify three classes of drugs used for the treatment of osteoporosis.
3. Understand the role of calcium and vitamin D supplementation and lifestyle interventions.
4. Describe recommendations for monitoring and duration of treatment.

Clinical Vignette: A 65-year-old woman undergoes her initial screening dual x-ray absorptiometry (DXA) scan that reports a *T*-score of −2.9. She has never had a low-impact fracture. She smokes one pack of cigarettes per day and drinks two alcoholic drinks per day, with up to four drinks on weekends.

A. **Does this patient have osteoporosis?**

Outline the approach to diagnosing osteoporosis as shown in Fig. 15.1. *Point out that anyone with a fragility fracture should be treated. She has osteoporosis based on her low bone mineral density (BMD).*

N. S. Deshpande (✉)
University of Washington Medical Center, Department of Medicine, Division of General Internal Medicine, University of Washington, Seattle, WA, USA
e-mail: nehasd@uw.edu

K. M. Johnson
VA Puget Sound Health Care System, Department of Medicine, Division of General Internal Medicine, University of Washington, Seattle, WA, USA

S. Mookherjee et al. (eds.), *Chalk Talks in Internal Medicine*,
https://doi.org/10.1007/978-3-030-34814-4_15

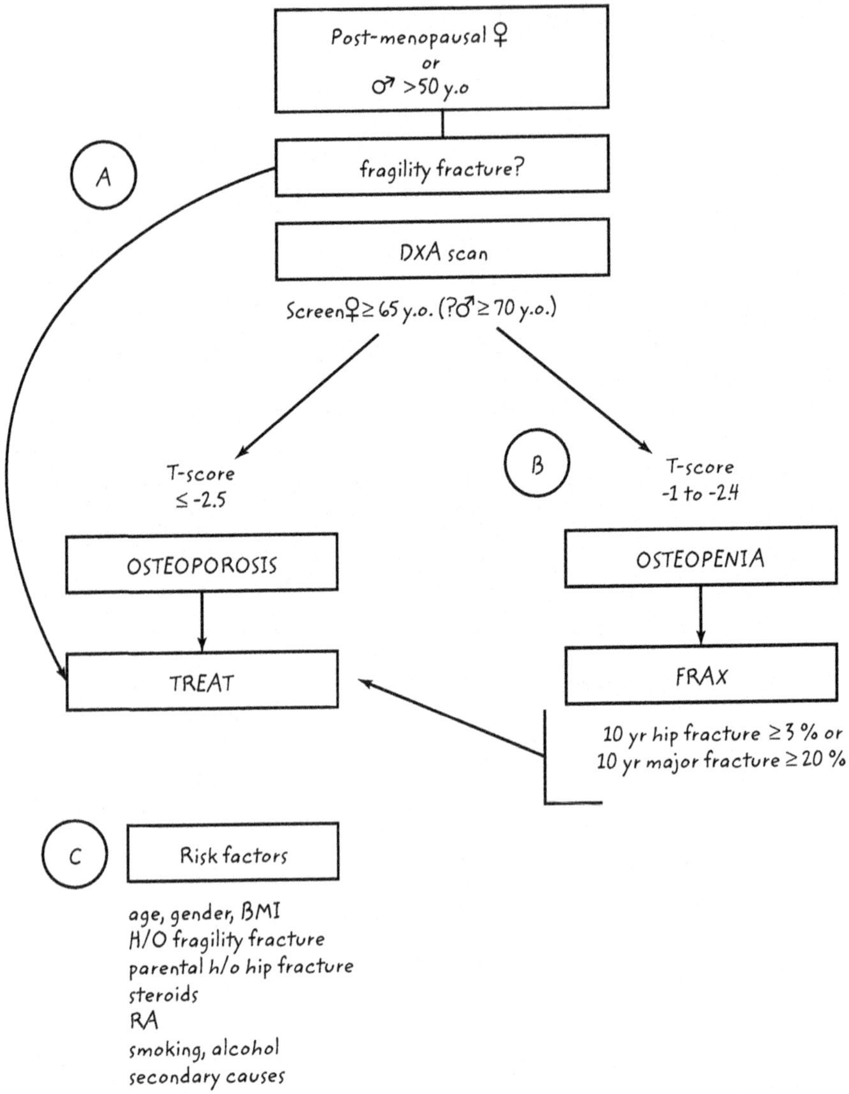

Fig. 15.1 Management of osteoporosis, A–C

Teaching point

- Osteoporosis is diagnosed in postmenopausal women or men aged 50 years or older with a history of a fragility fracture (i.e. low impact fracture of the hip, vertebra, wrist, humerus, or pelvis) **OR** DXA *T*-score ≤ −2.5, indicating bone mineral density (BMD) more than 2.5 standard deviations below the mean BMD of a young adult.

B. **What if her *T*-score was −2.1? How would you decide if she should be treated?**

Outline the diagnosis and evaluation of osteopenia as shown in Fig. 15.1.

Teaching points

- Osteopenia is defined by a *T*-score of −1.0 to −2.4 at the femoral neck or lumbar spine.
- The need to start treatment is determined by estimated probability of a fracture—the Fracture Risk Assessment Tool (FRAX) model is used for this and is accessible online.
- The FRAX model incorporates validated clinical risk factors and BMD for more accurate and individualized fracture risk prediction.
- She should start a medication for fracture prevention if her 10-year probability of a hip fracture is ≥3% or 10-year probability of any major osteoporosis-related fracture is ≥20%.

C. **What clinical risk factors for fracture would you ask our patient about? What are examples of secondary causes of osteoporosis?**

Write down risk factors as they are mentioned in Fig. 15.1. *Emphasize that these are the risk factors included in the FRAX model.*

Teaching point

- Secondary causes of osteoporosis include hypogonadism, premature menopause, inflammatory bowel disease and other causes of malnutrition or malabsorption, type I diabetes mellitus, untreated hyperthyroidism, or postorgan transplant.

D. **What are the classes of pharmacologic treatments for osteoporosis? Which would you recommend to our patient?**

As classes are mentioned, ask about mechanism of action, common side effects, and typical duration of efficacy—write these down as shown in Fig. 15.2.

Teaching points

- Osteonecrosis of the jaw (ONJ) is seen with bisphosphonates and denosumab.
- Teriparatide is a parathyroid hormone analog, and stimulates osteoblastic function.
- Denosumab is a receptor activator of nuclear factor kappa-B ligand (RANKL) inhibitor, and prevents osteoclast activation.
- Nonbisphosphonates have only temporary effects and patients may experience rapid bone loss after treatment discontinuation.

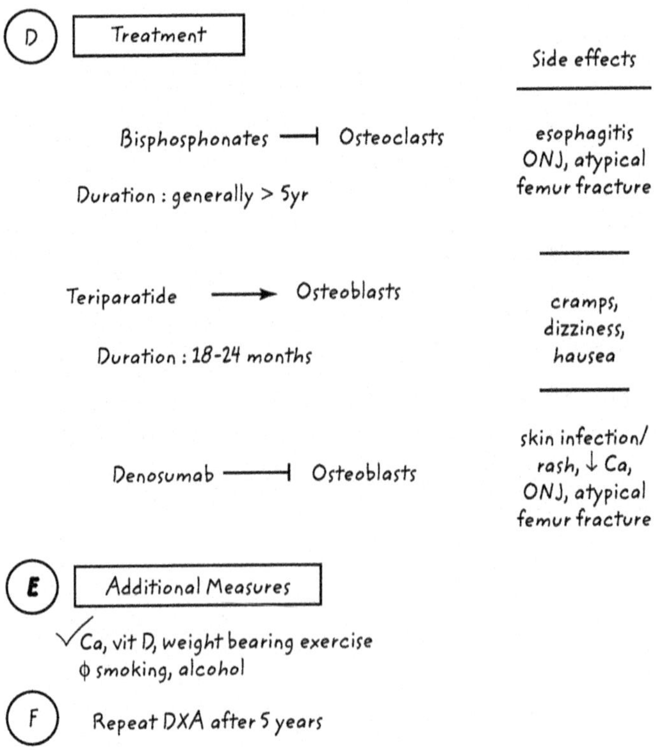

Fig. 15.2 Management of osteoporosis, D–F

- There is limited evidence regarding the benefit of combination therapy, or the optimal sequence of therapy.

For our patient, we would recommend bisphosphonates, which are typically first line and can have beneficial effects that last for years even after the medication is discontinued.

E. **Together, you decide she should start a bisphosphonate. Would you also start her on calcium and vitamin D supplementation? What other lifestyle interventions would you recommend to increase bone density?**

Write down the additional measures as shown in Fig. 15.2.

Teaching points

- Guidelines advise an adequate intake of dietary calcium (1200 mg/day) and vitamin D (800–1000 IU/day). Supplementation is controversial since randomized trial data do not support efficacy for reducing fracture risk.
- Counsel patients to engage in regular weight-bearing activity (e.g., walking, jogging, Tai Chi) and resistive exercises (e.g., yoga, Pilates) to reduce the risk of falls. The evidence regarding fracture risk reduction, however, is limited.
- Counsel patients to quit smoking and moderate their alcohol intake (e.g. less than 3 oz spirits or 12 oz wine per day).
- Avoid the use of medications that can increase falls.

F. **When should you repeat her DXA to monitor her bone density while on treatment?**

Write down "5 years" as shown in Fig. 15.2.

Teaching points

- There is no consensus on optimal monitoring practices.
- The newest American College of Physicians guidelines recommend against repeating a DXA during the initial 5 years of treatment.
- Randomized trial data do not suggest that more frequent DXA scans improve fracture risk prediction or treatment adherence.

Return to objectives and emphasize key points

1. Determine which patients should receive treatment for osteoporosis.
    - State that postmenopausal women, or men older than 50 years, with a history of fragility fracture or *T*-score ≤ -2.5 should be treated for osteoporosis.
2. Identify three classes of drugs used for the treatment of osteoporosis.
    - Draw a star next to bisphosphonates as listed on your board, emphasize that these agents are first line, and that the evidence strongly supports that these agents effectively reduce fracture risk.

3. Understand the role of calcium and vitamin D supplementation and lifestyle interventions.
   - Draw a star next to calcium and vitamin D and exercise as listed on your board and emphasize that these interventions are generally recommended, but there is little evidence to support their efficacy.
4. Describe recommendations for monitoring and duration of treatment.
   - Draw a star next to repeat DXA on your board and emphasize that there is insufficient data regarding the benefit of bisphosphonate treatment beyond 5 years.

Resources

1. Black DM, Rosen CJ. Postmenopausal osteoporosis. N Engl J Med. 2016;374(3):254–62. https://doi.org/10.1056/NEJMcp1513724.
2. Cosman F, de Beur SJ, LeBoff MS, Lewiecki EM, Tanner B, Randall S, et al. Clinician's guide to prevention and treatment of osteoporosis. Osteoporos Int. 2014;25(10):2359–81. https://doi.org/10.1007/s00198-014-2794-2.
3. Ensrud KE, Crandall CJ. Osteoporosis. Ann Intern Med. 2017;167(3):ITC17–32. https://doi.org/10.7326/AITC201708010.
4. Qaseem A, Forciea MA, McLean RM, Denberg TD. Treatment of low bone density or osteoporosis to prevent fractures in men and women: a clinical practice guideline update from the American College of Physicians. Ann Intern Med. 2017;166(11):818–39. https://doi.org/10.7326/M15-1361.
5. Sözen T, Özışık L, Başaran NÇ. An overview and management of osteoporosis. Eur J Rheumatol. 2017;4(1):46–56. https://doi.org/10.5152/eurjrheum.2016.048.
6. FRAX Fracture Risk Assessment Tool https://www.sheffield.ac.uk/FRAX/tool.jsp?locationValue=9.

Chapter 16
Management of Gastrointestinal Bleeding

Daniel Cabrera and Andrew White

Learning Objectives

1. Describe a systematic approach to management of a patient with acute gastrointestinal bleeding.
2. Recognize signs of severe bleeding that may warrant intensive care.
3. List therapeutic and diagnostic management options and which services would perform them.
4. Create patient-specific outpatient management plans after a patient's gastrointestinal bleeding has resolved.

Clinical Vignette: You are evaluating a 58-year-old woman with several days of worsening dark stools. She has a past medical history significant for atrial fibrillation and is currently anticoagulated with warfarin. Three days ago, she noted that her bowel movement was black. Now she describes maroon bowel movements occurring with increasing frequency.

A. **What signs, symptoms, and history can accompany a patient presenting with acute gastrointestinal (GI) bleeding?**

Write out the learner ideas under the categories of "low blood volume symptoms," "evidence of bleeding," and "risk factors," as in Fig. 16.1.

D. Cabrera (✉)
Harborview Medical Center, Department of Medicine, Division of General Internal Medicine, University of Washington, Seattle, WA, USA
e-mail: dancab@u.w.edu

A. White
University of Washington Medical Center, Department of Medicine, Division of General Internal Medicine, University of Washington, Seattle, WA, USA

S. Mookherjee et al. (eds.), *Chalk Talks in Internal Medicine*,
https://doi.org/10.1007/978-3-030-34814-4_16

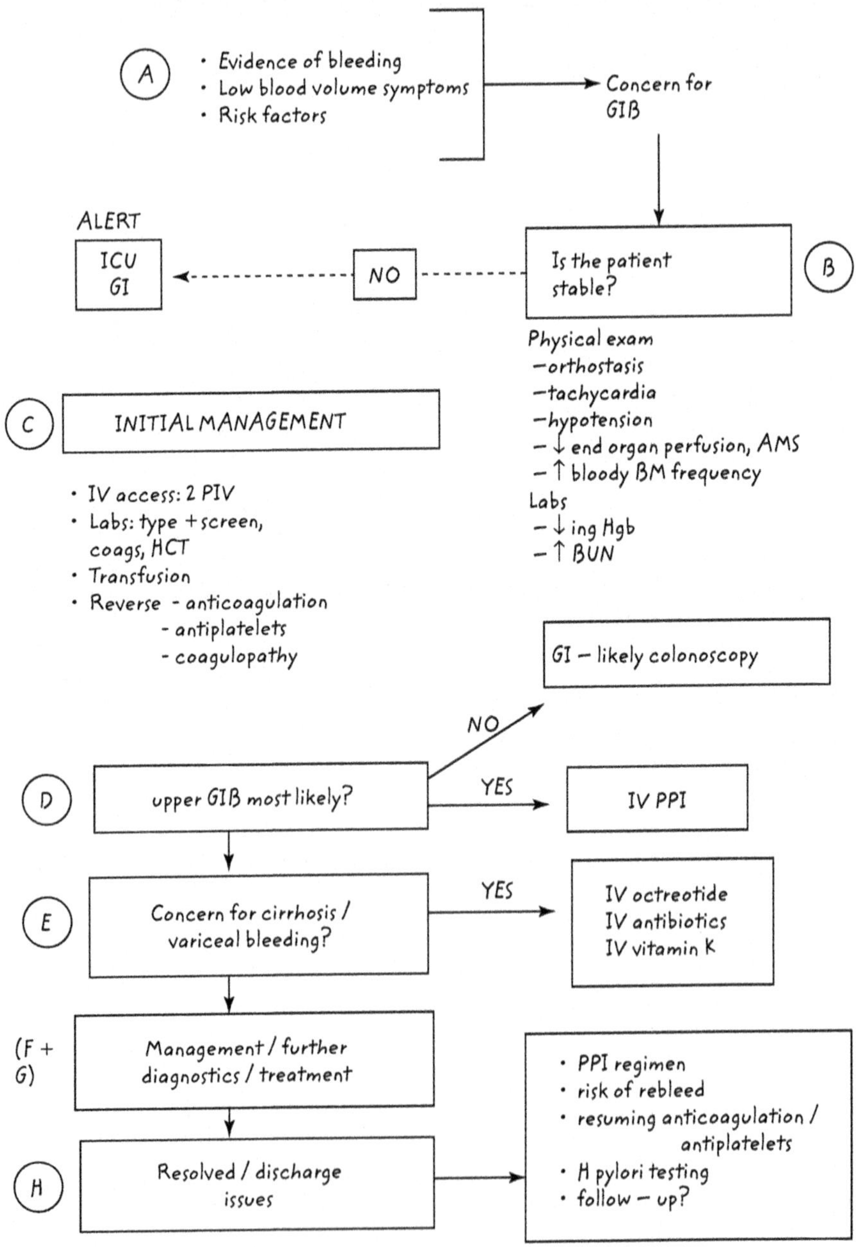

Fig. 16.1 Management of gastrointestinal bleeding, A–H

Teaching points

- Distinguishing between melena and hematochezia can help localize the source of the bleed.
- Low blood volume symptoms: lightheadedness, dizziness, syncope, presyncope, and dyspnea.
- Physical evidence of bleeding: melena, hematochezia, hematemesis, and coffee ground emesis.
- Risk factors: anticoagulation, antiplatelet medications, nonsteroidal anti-inflammatory drugs (NSAIDS), and liver disease.

B. **As you examine the patient, she passes another large maroon stool. It is important to determine that she is clinically stable and does not have ongoing, rapid bleeding. How do you determine if the patient is clinically stable and is not having rapid ongoing bleeding?**

Lead the learners through the physical exam findings and labs under "Is the patient stable?"

Teaching points

- Acute bleeding is not always reflected in the initial hemoglobin (Hgb) check—it is necessary to have serial checks.
- Shock can cause findings of poor perfusion and confusion.
- Hypotension is a late finding of hypovolemia; orthostasis and tachycardia are important preliminary findings of significant volume loss.
- Degrading blood products in the gastrointestinal (GI) tract can cause a rise in blood urea nitrogen (BUN).
- For unstable patients, seek immediate help to support the patient and plan for interventions—contact the intensive care unit (ICU) and gastroenterology service.

C. **Our patient has normal vital signs and is not orthostatic. At the same time as assessing the stability of our patient, it is important to begin the initial management steps. What initial management steps would you take for anyone presenting with a GI bleed?**

Lead the learners through the initial management steps.

Teaching points

- Access: Two large bore IVs. Peripheral IVs (PIV) are more effective than central lines for administering large fluid boluses.
- Labs: Hematocrit (HCT) level, coagulation labs (especially if coagulopathy due to medications or liver disease is suspected), type, and screen.
- Transfusion? Consider transfusing packed red blood cells, especially if there is concern for rapid blood loss. Transfusion thresholds are more restrictive than in years past—a hemoglobin less than 7 is generally considered to be appropriate for most patients. A higher threshold is needed if patients are symptomatic or are suspected of losing blood rapidly.

- Reversal of coagulopathy.
  - Direct oral anticoagulants (DOACs) are increasingly used but are challenging to reverse. In certain conditions and settings, idarucizumab is approved for reversal of dabigatran and andexanet alfa for factor Xa inhibitors (rivaroxaban, apixaban, and edoxaban). Prothrombin complex concentrate (Kcentra) is also used.
  - Patients with known or suspected cirrhosis are a special subgroup at high risk for upper GI bleed and also at risk for coagulopathy due to poor hepatic synthesis of clotting factors. These patients often receive vitamin K for elevated INR, although this typically does not rapidly correct their coagulopathy.
  - Warfarin can be reversed with the infusion of plasma and vitamin K.
  - Platelets can be given if platelet level is low or antiplatelet medications have been given.
- Proton pump inhibitor (PPI) therapy for suspected upper GI bleed.
- Always be ready to contact the gastroenterology service and the ICU!

D. **The initial treatment plan differs on the basis of whether an upper of lower GI bleed is considered most likely. How can you quickly determine whether the GI bleed is from an upper or lower source?**

Explain the need for GI consultation for colonoscopy for suspected lower GI bleed.

Teaching points
- Hematemesis, coffee ground emesis, or melena suggests upper GI source.
- Bright red blood suggests lower GI source.
- Rarely, a slow proximal colonic bleed can mimic maroon-colored melena.
- If the source remains unclear, sometimes nasogastric lavage or aspiration can help localize the bleeding source.
- If a lower GI bleed is most likely, the GI service should be contacted for colonoscopy.
- If an upper GI bleed is suspected, an intravenous (IV) proton pump inhibitor (PPI) should be started and consider GI consultation for upper endoscopy.

E. **How is variceal bleeding managed differently compared to other types of upper GI bleeds?**

Add the additional medical treatments for variceal bleeding.

- IV octreotide reduces portal pressures and lessens variceal bulging.
- IV antibiotics, specifically third-generation cephalosporins or quinolones, confer a mortality benefit for patients with cirrhosis experiencing a GI bleed from *any* cause, not just variceal hemorrhage.

F. **What diagnostic and therapeutic options are there for a GI bleed?**

Prepare Fig. 16.2*: draw an outline of the organs, arteries, varices, ulcer, arteriovenous malformations (AVMs) as shown. Ask the learners to list diagnostic and therapeutic interventions to manage GI bleed.*

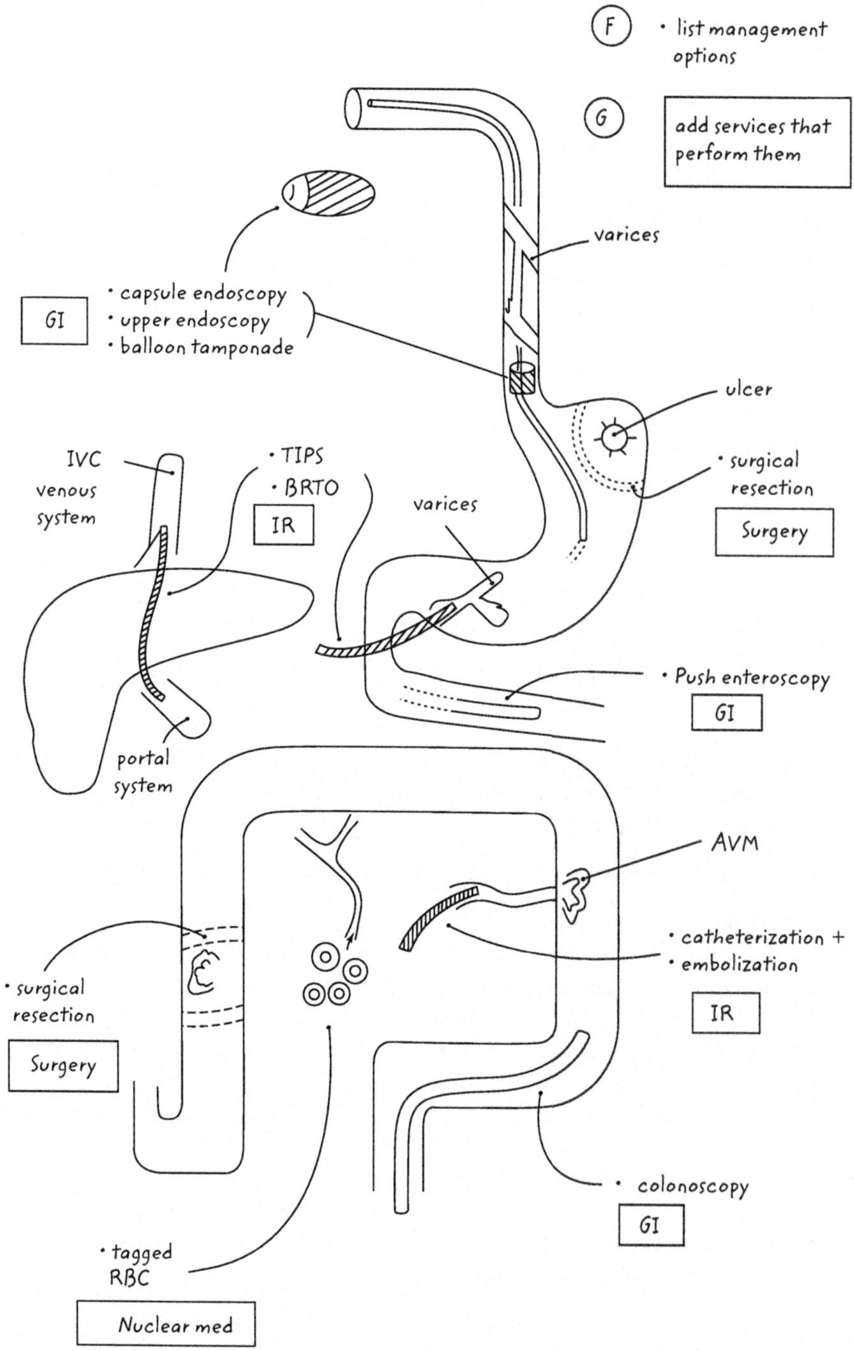

Fig. 16.2 Management of gastrointestinal bleeding, F–G

Teaching points

- Gastroenterology
  - Upper endoscopy (diagnostic and therapeutic)
  - Colonoscopy (diagnostic and therapeutic)
  - Capsule endoscopy (diagnostic)
  - Balloon enteroscopy (diagnostic)
- Interventional radiology (IR)
  - Catheterization (diagnostic) with embolization (therapeutic)
  - Balloon-occluded retrograde transvenous obliteration (BRTO) for gastric variceal hemorrhage
  - Transjugular intrahepatic portosystemic shunt (TIPS) for refractory variceal hemorrhage
- Nuclear medicine
  - Tagged red blood cell scan (diagnostic)
- General surgery
  - Gastric or bowel resection (therapeutic)—VERY RARE!

G. **What services or specialties perform the interventions listed?**

Point to each of the interventions listed and add the name of the appropriate service.

H. **Our patient had an upper GI bleed due to a gastric ulcer, which was treated endoscopically. What issues will you need to address before the patient can be discharged home?**

Return to the algorithm in Fig. 16.1 *and list the key discharge issues.*

Teaching points

- The majority of management strategies are based on evidence from peptic ulcer disease- associated upper GI bleeding.
- Continued outpatient proton pump inhibitors are used primarily when the etiology of GI bleed is peptic ulcer disease. Gastroenterology service often determines dose, frequency, and length of treatment.
- Several scoring systems to assess risk of rebleeding. The modified Glasgow Blatchford Score is more predictive than Rockall.
- For patients on anticoagulation, consider when to resume anticoagulation after hemostasis is achieved. Need for antiplatelet therapy and/or anticoagulation must be balanced against the risk for future GI bleed. May need to create plan with input from other clinical services.
  - In general, aspirin can usually be restarted 1–2 days after hemostasis.
  - Recommendations on clopidogrel (or other antiplatelet medication) are mixed but usually safe to restart 3–5 days after hemostasis.

  - For patients on warfarin or DOACs, the indication for anticoagulation must be weighed against the risk of future GI bleed. This is often a complex decision with individual risk–benefit profiles depending on the situation.

- *Helicobacter pylori* testing is recommended for all patients with new diagnosis of peptic ulcer disease. Typically, this is performed via biopsy of ulcer site during upper endoscopy, and often the results must be followed up after discharge.
- Determine follow-up: likely with the patient's primary care provider (PCP) followed by GI further in the future.

Return to objectives and emphasize key points

1. Describe a systematic approach to management of a patient with acute gastrointestinal bleeding.
   - Emphasize the need to determine clinical stability and potential need for ICU admission.
   - Initial management is the same in all cases: establish large bore IV access, send labs, transfuse if needed, reverse reversible factors such as anticoagulation, antiplatelets, and coagulopathy.
2. Recognize signs of severe bleeding that may warrant intensive care.
   - Circle hypotension, tachycardia, orthostasis in Fig. 16.1.
3. List therapeutic and diagnostic management options and which services would perform them.
   - Circle GI, IR, nuclear medicine, and general surgery in Fig. 16.2.
4. Create patient-specific outpatient management plans after a patient's gastrointestinal bleeding has resolved.

Asterisk PPI, risk of rebleed, resuming medicines, *H. pylori*, and follow-up in Fig. 16.1.

Resources

1. Kim BSM, Li BT, Engel A, Samra JS, Clarke S, Norton ID, et al. Diagnosis of gastrointestinal bleeding: a practical guide for clinicians. World J Gastrointest Pathophysiol. 2014;5(4):467–78.
2. Laine L, Jensen DM. Management of patient with ulcer bleeding. Am J Gastroenterol. 2012;107:345–60.
3. Cheng DW, Lu YW, Teller T, Sekhon HK, Wu BU. A modified Glasgow Blatchford Score improves risk stratification in upper gastrointestinal bleed: a prospective comparison of scoring systems. Aliment Pharmacol Ther. 2012;36(8):782–9.
4. Qureshi W, Mittal C, Patsias I, Garikapati K, Kuchipudi A, Cheema G, et al. Restarting anticoagulation and outcomes after major gastrointestinal bleeding in atrial fibrillation. Am J Cardiol. 2014;113(4):662–8.
5. Sengupta N, Feuerstein JD, Patwardhan VR, Tapper EB, Ketwaroo GA, Thaker AM, et al. The risks of thromboembolism vs. recurrent gastrointestinal bleeding after interruption of systemic anticoagulation in hospitalized inpatients with gastrointestinal bleeding: a prospective study. Am J Gastroenterol. 2015;110:328–35.

Chapter 17
Management of *Clostridium difficile* Infection

Allison Himmel and Jill Watanabe

Learning Objectives

1. Differentiate between nonsevere, severe, and fulminant *Clostridium difficile (C. difficile)* infections.
2. Treat an initial episode of *C. difficile* infection.
3. Recommend treatment for recurrent *C. difficile* infection.
4. Recognize indications for evaluation for surgical management of *C. difficile* infection.

Clinical Vignette: A 59-year-old woman was admitted to the hospital for acute respiratory failure due to community-acquired pneumonia. She was intubated and treated with bronchodilators, steroids, and broad-spectrum antibiotics. She was stable for discharge on hospital day 4 and given oral antibiotics to complete her course at home. She now presents to her primary care provider 1 week after discharge with copious watery stools and abdominal cramping. She has a temperature of 38.1 °C and normal pulse rate and blood pressure. Abdominal exam reveals normal bowel tones and no tenderness or distention. Laboratory results are notable for a white blood cell count of 13,000 mm^3, creatinine of 0.9 mg/dL, and stool polymerase chain reaction (PCR) positive for toxigenic *Clostridium difficile (C. difficile).*

A. **Does this patient have *C. difficile* infection (CDI)?**

Write the definition of CDI as in Fig. 17.1*—she does have CDI.*

A. Himmel (✉) · J. Watanabe
Harborview Medical Center, Department of Medicine, Division of General Internal Medicine, University of Washington, Seattle, WA, USA
e-mail: ahimmel@uw.edu

S. Mookherjee et al. (eds.), *Chalk Talks in Internal Medicine*,
https://doi.org/10.1007/978-3-030-34814-4_17

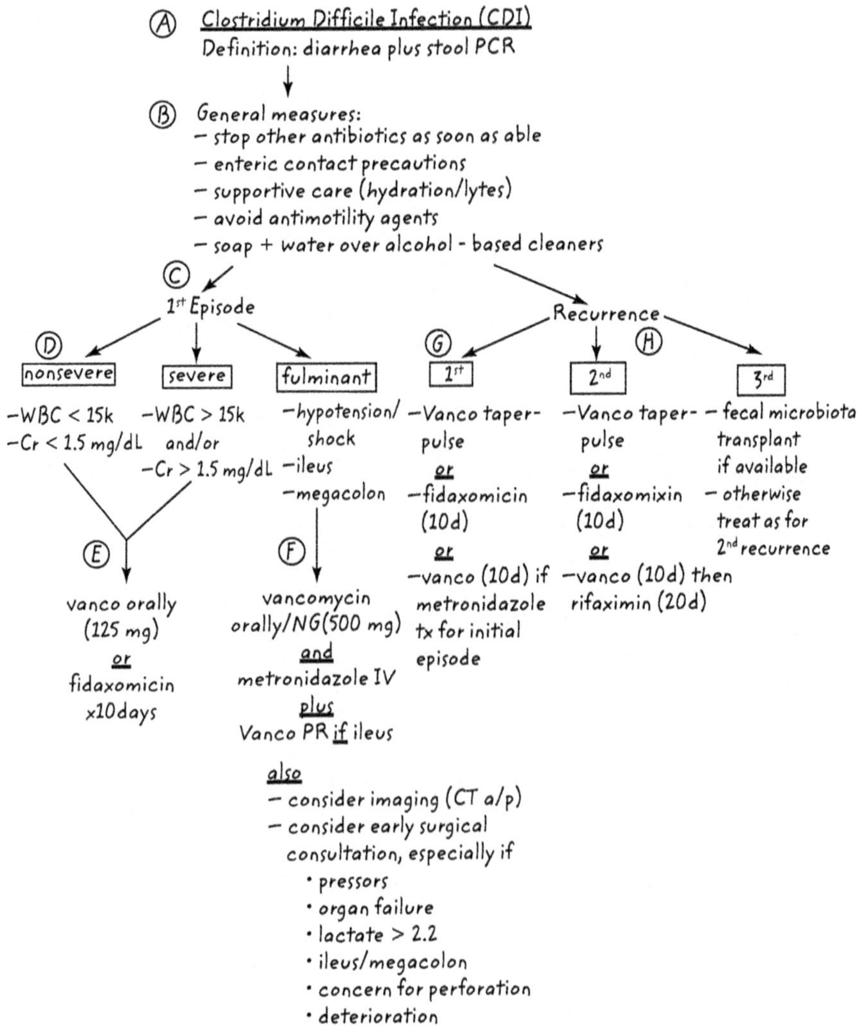

Fig. 17.1 Management of *Clostridium difficile* infection, A–H

Teaching points

- CDI is defined by having both:
    1. Diarrhea (three or more unformed stools in a 24-h period)
    2. Positive stool polymerase chain reaction (PCR) for *C. difficile* strain with toxin genes—highly sensitive but limited positive predictive value due to colonization
- Colonization occurs in up to 25% of hospitalized patients (compared to <2% of adults without recent health care exposure); do NOT treat asymptomatic patients.
- If PCR is negative, consider alternate diagnoses (e.g., norovirus, noninfectious postantibiotic diarrhea, osmotic diarrhea from tube feeds, laxatives, inflammatory bowel disease).

B. **Our patient's symptoms and stool test are consistent with CDI. Before we consider specific treatment, what general management strategies should be used for all patients?**

Write general measures as shown in Fig. 17.1.

C. **What are the two key questions that determine the best treatment of *C. difficile* infection for individual patients?**

Write "1st episode" and "recurrence" as shown in Fig. 17.1.

Teaching points

- A recurrence is considered to be within 8 weeks of completion of anticlostridial therapy.
- Severity of infection is the second main determinant of treatment

D. **This is our patient's first episode of CDI. The next task is to determine the severity of her infection. The most recent specialty society guidelines specify three levels of severity: nonsevere, severe, and fulminant. What criteria would generally indicate a more severe infection?**

Write down nonsevere, severe, and fulminant as shown in Fig. 17.1 *and add the criteria as they are mentioned.*

Teaching points

- It is challenging to precisely differentiate nonsevere CDI from severe CDI. Various guidelines use different criteria to assess severity. The ones listed in the figure are from the most recently published guidelines, the 2017 Update by the Infectious Diseases Society of America (IDSA) and Society for Healthcare Epidemiology of America (SHEA). The most recent guidelines from the American College of Gastroenterology were published in 2013.
- Several international guidelines also mention imaging and colonoscopy findings as criteria for severe infection (i.e., pericolonic fat stranding, pseudomembranes).

- Older age, serious comorbid illness, and immune compromise are other predictors of unfavorable outcome.

E. **How would you classify the severity of our patient's infection? What treatment is recommended?**

Our patient has nonsevere CDI—complete the algorithm as shown in the Fig. 17.1.

- The most appropriate therapy is oral vancomycin (125 mg q6h × 10 days).
- Fidaxomicin is also considered first-line therapy (200 mg twice daily × 10 days). Trials show that fidaxomicin has a similar rate of diarrhea resolution compared to vancomycin as well as a significant decrease in the rate of recurrence at 1 month. The main downside is cost.
- In contrast to previous guidelines, oral metronidazole is now considered second-line therapy, even for nonsevere disease, given decreased efficacy versus vancomycin. However, it may still be used in settings where the first-line agents are not available or contraindicated, at a dose of 500 mg q8h × 10 days.

F. **Patients meeting criteria for fulminant CDI require more aggressive treatment. What are the key additional management steps in fulminant CDI?**

Complete the algorithm as shown in Fig. 17.1.

Teaching points

- Although there is limited data, the IDSA/SHEA guidelines recommend increasing the vancomycin dose to 500 mg q6h in the fulminant setting.
- Intravenous metronidazole 500 mg q8h should also be given to all patients with fulminant infection.
- In patients with ileus or significant abdominal distention, start rectal vancomycin 500 mg q6h.
- Consider computed tomographic (CT) scan of the abdomen and pelvis.
- Strongly consider early surgical consultation in all patients with fulminant disease and some patients with severe disease; criteria are listed in the figure.
- Traditional surgical approach is subtotal colectomy, which can improve mortality if performed early.
- Diverting loop ileostomy with colonic lavage is a newer technique that spares the colon and has shown improved historical survival versus colectomy in preliminary studies, but needs further study.

G. **Our patient's diarrhea resolves shortly after starting vancomycin. She returns 1 month later with recurrent watery stools and abdominal cramping. Stool is again positive for *C. difficile* PCR. She again has no indicators of severe disease. Since this is a recurrence within 8 weeks of completion of therapy, this is considered a first recurrence of CDI. How should she be treated?**

Complete the first recurrence treatment algorithm as shown in Fig. 17.1.

Teaching points

- Ten percent to 30% of patients will have a recurrence after the first episode and 40–65% of those with one recurrence will have subsequent recurrence.
- Repeat stool tests should NOT be done in asymptomatic patients (up to 50% have positive tests up to 6 weeks after treatment completion).
- Risk factors for recurrent CDI include age >65 years, continued use of antibiotics, severe comorbidities, more than 1 prior CDI episode, use of PPIs (controversial), severe initial infection, and Nap1/B1/027 subtype (a hypervirulent strain associated with more treatment failures).
- Several vancomycin taper/pulse regimens exist. The IDSA/SHEA recommends 125 mg orally Q6h × 10–14 days, 125 mg twice daily × 1 week, 125 mg daily × 1 week, and then 125 mg q2–3 days for 2–8 weeks.
- A standard 10-day course of vancomycin is recommended for recurrence only if metronidazole was used for the initial treatment.

H. **Our patient again does well with retreatment, but unfortunately develops a second recurrence 6 weeks later. What are her options for retreatment? What if she has a third recurrence despite treatment?**

Complete the second and third recurrence treatment algorithm as shown in Fig. 17.1.

- For the second recurrence, vancomycin taper/pulse is generally preferred.
- Other options with more limited data for multiply recurrent CDI include 10 days of fidaxomicin or 10 days of vancomycin followed by 20 days of rifaximin.
- The monoclonal antibody bezlotoxumab neutralizes *C. difficile* toxin B. It decreases the rate of recurrent infection when given in combination with antibiotic therapy and is approved by the U.S. Food and Drug Administration (FDA) for secondary prevention in patients at high risk of recurrence. It is expensive and its role remains unclear.
- For a third recurrence of CDI, fecal microbiota transplant (FMT) is the treatment of choice where available.

Return to objectives and emphasize key points

1. Differentiate between nonsevere, severe, and fulminant *C. difficile* infection—*circle the criteria for each category in* Fig. 17.1.
2. Treat an initial episode of *C. difficile* infection—*circle these in* Fig. 17.1.
   - Oral vancomycin or fidaxomicin for nonsevere and severe CDI
   - Oral vancomycin plus intravenous metronidazole for fulminant CDI (plus rectal vancomycin if concern for ileus) and surgical consultation
3. Recommend treatment for recurrent *C. difficile* infection—*circle these in* Fig. 17.1.
   - First recurrence: vancomycin taper/pulse (or fidaxomicin or 10-day vancomycin in certain patients)

- Second recurrence: vancomycin taper/pulse (or fidaxomicin or 10-day vancomycin followed by rifaximin)
- Fecal microbiota transplant for third or more recurrences

4. Recognize indications for evaluation for surgical management.

- Consider surgical consultation in all patients with fulminant CDI.
- Surgery for CDI is most frequently performed in cases with the following: *Asterisk this section in the figure*:

  - Hypotension requiring pressors
  - Organ failure from severe sepsis
  - Serum lactate >2.2 despite treatment
  - Ileus/megacolon
  - Bowel perforation
  - Deterioration despite optimal medical therapy

Resources

1. Curry S. Clostridium difficile. Clin Lab Med. 2017;37:341–69.
2. Feher C, Mensa J. A comparison of current guidelines of five international societies on *Clostridium difficile* infection management. Infect Dis Ther. 2016;5:207–30.
3. Hrebinko K, Zuckerbraun B. *Clostridium difficile:* what the surgeon needs to know. Semin Colon Rectal Surg. 2018;29:28–36.
4. McDonald L, Gerding D, Johnson S, Bakken J, Carroll K, Coffin S, et al. Clinical practice guidelines for *Clostridium difficile* infection in adults and children: 2017 update by the Infectious Diseases Society of America (IDSA) and Society for Healthcare Epidemiology of America (SHEA). Clin Infect Dis. 2018;66:e1–e48.
5. Nelson R, Suda K, Evans C. Antibiotic treatment for *Clostridium difficile*-associated diarrhea in adults. Cochrane Database Syst Rev 2017;(3): CD004610. https://doi.org/10.1002/14651858.CD004610.pub5.
6. Stevens V, Nelson R, Schwab-Daugherty E, Khader K, Jones M, Brown K, et al. Comparative effectiveness of vancomycin and metronidazole for the prevention of recurrence and death in patients with *Clostridium difficile* infection. JAMA Intern Med. 2017;177:546–53.
7. Surawicz C, Brandt L, Binion J, Ananthakrishnan A, Curry S, Gilligan P, et al. Guidelines for diagnosis, treatment, and prevention of *Clostridium difficile* infections. Am J Gastroenterol. 2013;108:478–98.
8. Vindigni S, Surawicz C. Fecal microbiota transplantation. Gastroenterol Clin North Am. 2017;46:171–85.

Chapter 18
Evaluation of Dysphagia

Sabeena Setia and Heidi Powell

Learning Objectives
1. Describe a systematic approach to the evaluation of dysphagia.
2. Distinguish the difference between oropharyngeal and esophageal dysphagia.
3. Understand which tests to order to evaluate a structural abnormality and a motility disorder.
4. Recognize "red flag" signs and symptoms that would warrant urgent endoscopic evaluation or suggest esophageal cancer.

Clinical Vignette: A 53-year-old man reports "trouble swallowing" intermittently over the past year. He has no associated pain or weight loss. Lisinopril is his only medication.

A. **Does this patient have dysphagia?**

Write the definition of "dysphagia" as shown in Fig. 18.1.

Teaching points
- Dysphagia is difficulty with swallowing. Objectively, there is an abnormal delay in transit of liquid or solid bolus during the oropharyngeal or esophageal stages of swallowing.
- If symptoms are not clearly associated with swallowing, then other causes such as xerostomia or globus sensation should be considered.
- Prevalence is about 16% in the elderly but >60% for those who live in long-term care facilities.

S. Setia (✉)
Landmark Health, Seattle, WA, USA

H. Powell
University of Washington Medical Center, Department of Medicine, Division of General Internal Medicine, University of Washington, Seattle, WA, USA

S. Mookherjee et al. (eds.), *Chalk Talks in Internal Medicine*,
https://doi.org/10.1007/978-3-030-34814-4_18

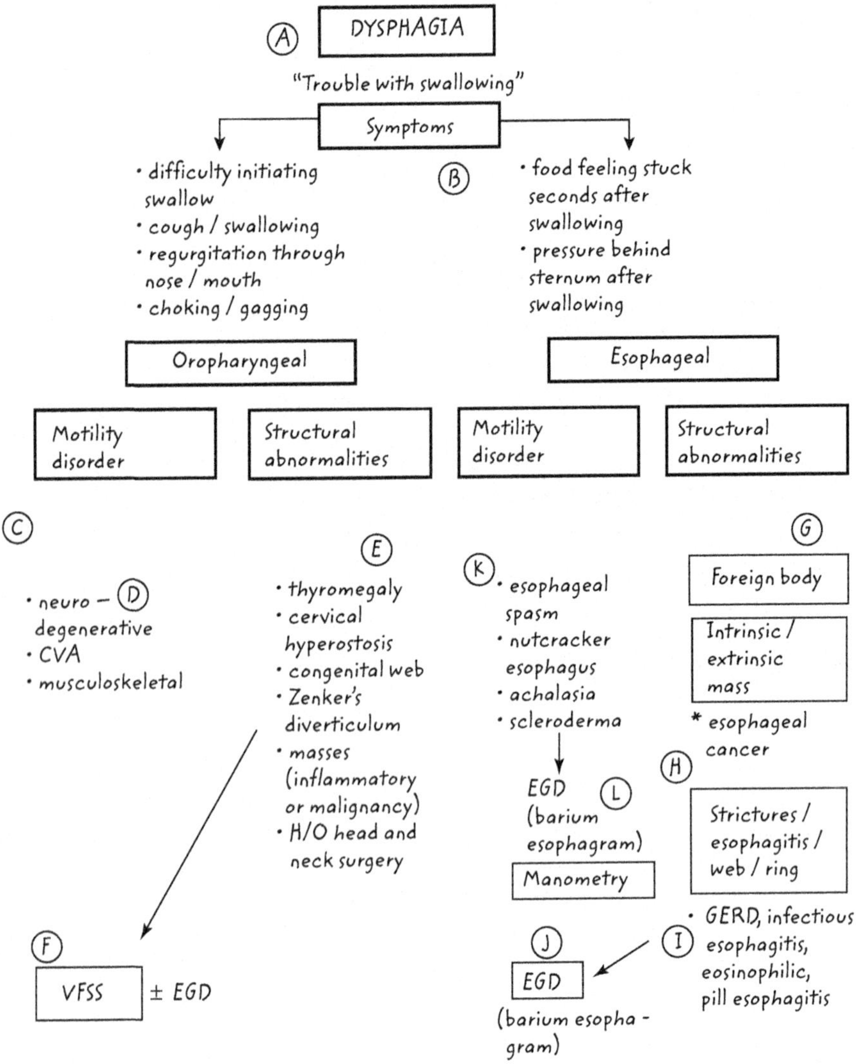

Fig. 18.1 Evaluation of dysphagia, A–L

B. **Dysphagia can be caused by oropharyngeal or esophageal disorders. It is important to distinguish between these two types of disorders early in the evaluation as different diagnostic tests are required to determine their causes. On further questioning, our patient reports that he swallows food without any problems but then feels that it gets stuck lower down in his chest. What symptoms help to differentiate oropharyngeal versus esophageal dysphagia?**

Write down symptoms for oropharyngeal and esophageal dysphagia in two columns as they are listed by the learners.

C. **Both oropharyngeal and esophageal dysphagia can be caused by a motility disorder or a structural abnormality. What key question helps differentiate between the two?**

Write down "motility disorders" and "structural abnormalities" below "oropharyngeal" and "esophageal" and draw visual cues for liquids and solids below "motility disorder" and structural abnormalities."

Teaching points

- Ask the patient if the symptoms occur with both liquids and solids.
- Motility disorders cause difficulty in swallowing both liquids and solids.
- Structural abnormalities usually cause problems with swallowing solids only. When structural abnormalities become more advanced, swallowing liquids is affected as well.

D. **Oropharyngeal dysphagia is more often caused by a motility disorder (associated with a systemic disorder) rather than a structural abnormality. What are the main motility causes of oropharyngeal dysphagia?**

Write down main categories of causes in Fig. 18.1.

Teaching points

- Neurologic conditions (Parkinson's disease, multiple sclerosis, amyotrophic lateral sclerosis (ALS), dementia, polio, supranuclear palsy)
- Stroke (cerebral infarct, intracranial hemorrhage)
- Brain stem tumors
- Musculoskeletal diseases (polymyositis, dermatomyositis, muscular dystrophy, and myasthenia gravis)

E. **What are structural abnormalities that can cause oropharyngeal dysphagia?**

Write down the common causes in Fig. 18.1.

F. **Which is the best diagnostic test to identify the cause of oropharyngeal dysphagia?**

- A video fluoroscopic swallowing study (VFSS) is the test of choice.
- VFSS helps to identify normal and abnormal anatomy and physiology of the swallow in patients with oropharyngeal disorders. It can evaluate the integrity of airway protection before, during, and after swallowing.

- With the aid of a speech pathologist, the effectiveness of postures, maneuvers, bolus modifications, and sensory enhancements in improving swallowing safety and efficiency can be evaluated. They can recommend therapeutic techniques for oral and pharyngeal disorders.
- Esophagogastroduodenoscopy (EGD) is sometimes necessary, especially if a mass is suspected.

G. **For our patient, liquids and food "go down" fine but then food gets stuck lower in his chest. He most likely has esophageal dysphagia suggestive of a structural abnormality. What are causes of structural esophageal dysphagia?**

Write down the three main categories on Fig. 18.1, *leaving room to add additional text under "masses" and "strictures."*

- Structural abnormalities can be caused by three major processes: (1) foreign objects, (2) masses causing frank obstruction (extrinsic or intrinsic), or (3) strictures or inflammatory processes that alter the mucosal surface and block passage of solids.

H. **Our patient has had intermittent symptoms. If our patient had rapidly progressive symptoms, what should we be the most concerned about?**

Write down esophageal cancer under "intrinsic or extrinsic mass."

- Esophageal cancer: It is the leading cause of mechanical obstruction for those aged >50 years.
- Red flag signs and symptoms include weight loss, anemia, anorexia, hematemesis, and rapidly progressive symptoms.
- Risks include a smoking history and family history.
- Urgent EGD is indicated.

I. **Our patient denies weight loss or chest pain. If he had retrosternal chest pain with swallowing, what would you be concerned about?**

Write down causes of strictures and esophagitis as shown in Fig. 18.1.

Teaching points

- Medications can cause direct injury to the esophageal mucosa—a thorough history of medication use (both prescribed and over-the-counter [OTC]) is important in the evaluation of dysphagia.
- Common pills include nonsteroidal anti-inflammatory drugs (NSAIDS), bisphosphonates, trimethoprim-sulfamethoxazole, ferrous sulfate, potassium chloride tablets, doxycycline, and tetracycline.

J. **What is the best diagnostic test for evaluating structural esophageal abnormalities?**

Write down EGD—put barium esophagram in parentheses as a noninvasive option in selected circumstances.

Teaching points

- An EGD is the best test to evaluate an obstructive esophageal problem. The mucosa can be directly visualized and evaluated for webs/rings/masses. Biopsies and dilation can be performed if indicated.
- A barium esophagram is another option to help determine the cause of the obstruction but interventional procedures cannot be performed at the same time.

K. **Our patient has problems with swallowing solids and his symptoms are consistent with esophageal dysphagia, but if he had problems swallowing both liquids and solids, we would be concerned about a motility disorder. What are common causes of esophageal motility disorders?**

Write down the common causes under "motility disorders."

- Primary esophageal motility disorders include diffuse esophageal spasm, nutcracker esophagus, achalasia.
- Secondary motility disorders include systemic sclerosis.

L. **EGD or an esophagram (barium swallow) should be initially ordered for evaluating esophageal motility disorders. EGDs not only are important for the evaluation for dangerous structural processes but also may reveal findings that can help diagnose motility disorders. During the endoscopy, biopsies can be collected, which may aid in diagnosis. Esophagrams may offer a visual representation of a patient's esophageal motility that can aid in diagnosis. What test should be done after anatomic abnormalities are ruled out by EGD?**

Write "EGD, barium esophagram, manometry" under motility disorders.

- Evaluates how well the esophageal muscles sequentially contract and function, and how well the upper and lower esophageal sphincters function.
- Manometry is useful for diagnosing:
  - Diffuse esophageal spasm: multiple forceful poorly coordinated muscle contractions of the esophagus.
  - Achalasia: Lower esophageal sphincter doesn't relax properly and muscles in the wall of the esophagus are weakened. This can cause regurgitation of food/liquids back up into the throat.
  - Systemic sclerosis: Muscles in the lower esophagus stop contracting, leading to severe gastroesophageal reflux.

In summary, our patient describes a sensation of food getting stuck in his chest, his symptoms are intermittent and he doesn't have any "red flags" for esophageal cancer. He underwent an EGD and was found to have a Schatzki's ring—this is a common type of esophageal ring—which was dilated resulting in resolution of his symptoms.

Return to objectives and emphasize key points

1. Describe symptoms that distinguish oropharyngeal dysphagia from esophageal dysphagia:
   - Feeling of choking/gagging when trying to swallow
   - Inability to control saliva in mouth
   - Coughing with swallowing
   - Regurgitation through nose/mouth
   - Difficulty initiating a swallow
   - Conversely, the symptom of "food getting stuck" in the chest suggests esophageal dysphagia.

2 & 3. Recognize the difference between a motility disorder and a structural abnormality and which tests to order:
   - Difficulty with swallowing both liquids and solids suggests a motility disorder and is best evaluated with a VFSS for oropharyngeal disorders. For esophageal motility disorders, manometry often is performed once an EGD or barium study has ruled out a structural problem.
   - Difficulty with swallowing food and not liquids suggests a structural abnormality and is best evaluated with an EGD.

4. Recognize signs and symptoms of esophageal cancer:
   - Rapidly progressive symptoms
   - Anemia, weight loss, hematemesis, and anorexia

Resources

1. Spieker MR. Evaluating dysphagia. Am Fam Physician. 2000;61(12):3639–48.
2. Cook IJ. Diagnostic evaluation of dysphagia. Nat Clin Pract Gastroenterol Hepatol. 2008;5(7):393–403.
3. Jalil AAA, Katzka DA, Castell DO. Approach to the patient with dysphagia. Am J Med. 2015;128:1138.e17–22.
4. Jansson-Knodell CL, Codipilly C, Legget CL. Making dysphagia easier to swallow: a review for the practicing clinician. Mayo Clin Proc. 2017;92(6):965–72.

Chapter 19
Approach to Abnormal Liver Blood Tests

Sylvia Mollerstrom and Lauren A. Beste

Learning Objectives

1. Implement a systematic approach to the interpretation of abnormal liver blood tests.
2. Describe the workup of liver test abnormalities, including indications for liver biopsy.
3. Describe worrisome liver blood test results that require urgent evaluation.

Clinical Vignette: An asymptomatic 50-year-old woman presents to clinic for a new patient evaluation. She brings in laboratory results obtained a few months ago from another provider, including liver blood tests notable for elevated aspartate aminotransferase (AST) of 45 international units (IU)/L (reference range 9–38 U/L) and an alanine aminotransferase (ALT) of 60 international units/L (reference range 7–33 U/L). Alkaline phosphatase (alk phos) is within the normal range at 100 international units/L (reference range 34–121 U/L). Total bilirubin and gamma-glutamyltransferase (GGT) are normal.

A. **To understand the significance of her abnormal liver blood test results, it is useful to review the important functional units of the liver: the liver lobule and portal triad. What are the components of each?**

Draw the schematic of the liver lobule and the portal triad, labeling the components as they are named.

S. Mollerstrom (✉)
Harborview Medical Center, Department of Medicine, Division of General Internal Medicine, University of Washington, Seattle, WA, USA
e-mail: sylvie@uw.edu

L. A. Beste
VA Puget Sound Health Care System, Department of Medicine, Division of General Internal Medicine, University of Washington, Seattle, WA, USA

S. Mookherjee et al. (eds.), *Chalk Talks in Internal Medicine*,
https://doi.org/10.1007/978-3-030-34814-4_19

Teaching points

- Venous blood from the gut flows to the liver from the portal vein.
- Oxygenated blood flows to the liver through the hepatic artery.
- These two sources of blood mix in the sinusoid and drain to the central vein, which drains to the IVC.
- Conjugated bilirubin travels from the hepatocytes toward the portal triad and exits the liver via the bile ducts.

B. **What is the source of the "liver function test (LFT)" results given above (AST, ALT, alkaline phosphatase, bilirubin, GGT)?**

List the lab values to the right and draw arrows to indicate their source. Key teaching points are tabulated below for reference (the table does not need to be reproduced on the white board). Add albumin and INR to the list of labs if they are not mentioned by the learners.

Teaching points

<table>
<tr><th>Lab</th><th colspan="2">Notes</th><th>Significance</th></tr>
<tr><td>AST</td><td rowspan="2">Also called "transaminases," "aminotransferases," or "liver enzymes"
Intracellular enzymes that convert amino acids into high-energy molecules</td><td>90% from liver
Also found in skeletal muscle, heart, brain, gastric mucosa, kidney, pancreas, spleen, lung, red blood cells</td><td rowspan="2">Released from injured hepatocytes</td></tr>
<tr><td>ALT</td><td>Almost 100% from liver
Very small amounts come from kidney and muscle</td></tr>
<tr><td>Alk Phos</td><td colspan="2">Found in liver, bone, gut, and placenta
In the liver, it is produced by the canalicular membrane (hepatocytes next to bile canaliculi).
Alk phos production is induced by high levels of bile acids.</td><td>Bile duct obstruction or hepatocyte injury</td></tr>
<tr><td>GGT</td><td colspan="2">Active in biliary epithelial cells.
More specific to the liver than alk phos.
Supports a hepatic source of the elevated alk phos (as opposed to bone or other source).</td><td>Bile duct dysfunction</td></tr>
<tr><td>Bilirubin</td><td colspan="2">Produced by the breakdown of hemoglobin.
Conjugated in the hepatocyte.
After conjugation, bilirubin is called "direct bilirubin".</td><td>Bile duct obstruction or hepatocyte injury</td></tr>
<tr><td>Albumin, INR</td><td colspan="2">Albumin and clotting factors are proteins synthesized in the liver.
Albumin production is inhibited by physiologic stress and advanced liver disease.
Most of the body's clotting factors (II, V, VII, IX, X, XI, and XII) are made by the liver.
A rise in INR reflects deficient production of at least one of the extrinsic cofactors (or vitamin K deficiency).</td><td>Decreased hepatic synthetic ability</td></tr>
</table>

C. **While we often refer to "liver function tests," not all of these labs actually reflect liver function. Which of these labs actually reflect liver function?**

Put a box around albumin and INR.

D. **It is useful to think of liver blood test abnormalities as being "cholestatic" (primarily a bile duct problem) or "hepatocellular" (primarily a hepatocyte problem). Our patient has a mild elevation in AST and ALT—how would you categorize her liver test abnormalities? What is your differential diagnosis?**

Complete the "hepatocellular" side of abnormal liver tests.

Teaching points

- There are many causes of drug-induced liver injury; Livertox.nih.gov is a useful resource for both hepatocellular and cholestatic causes.
- Common drugs include trimethoprim-sulfamethoxazole, isoniazid, methotrexate, valproic acid, herbal supplements (e.g., body-building products, green tea extract)
- Iron overload = hemochromatosis, copper overload = Wilson disease
- A few etiologies can cause severe elevations in transaminases with ALT and AST >1000. Examples include:
  - Hypotension/shock
  - Toxic ingestion (e.g., acetaminophen overdose, amanita phalloides ["death cap"] mushroom poisoning)
  - Acute infection
  - Acute Budd–Chiari syndrome
  - Flares of autoimmune hepatitis
  - HELLP (Hemolysis, Elevated Liver enzymes, Low Platelet count) syndrome

E. **An elevated bilirubin and alkaline phosphatase would be more characteristic of cholestatic injury. What are some of the main causes of cholestatic liver injury?**

Complete the "cholestatic" side of abnormal liver tests.

Teaching points

- There are many causes of drug-induced liver injury. A few classic culprits include amoxicillin-clavulanate, trimethoprim-sulfamethoxazole, and amiodarone.
- PBC = primary biliary cholangitis, PSC = primary sclerosing cholangitis.
- Cholelithiasis may cause isolated elevated alkaline phosphatase unless also associated with bile duct obstruction.

F. **Our patient is asymptomatic, does not take any medications or supplements, and does not drink alcohol. Her liver tests are repeated and the results are unchanged from previous. What labs or diagnostic studies should we send to work up her mild aminotransferase elevation?**

Add check marks next to the items on the differential diagnosis that you're are going to test the patient for.

- Viral hepatitis (hepatitis C antibody, hepatitis B surface antigen, hepatitis B core antibody, hepatitis B surface antibody), hemochromatosis (iron, ferritin, transferrin saturation).
- If these are normal: ultrasound to look for fatty infiltration, masses, or obstruction.
- In a patient with suggestive risk factors or symptoms, consider selective workup for rarer causes such as autoimmune hepatitis (antinuclear antibody, antismooth muscle antibody, serum immunoglobulin levels), Wilson disease (ceruloplasmin level), alpha-1 antitrypsin deficiency (alapha-1-antitrypsin level), thyroid dysfunction (thyroid-stimulating hormone), or celiac disease (tissue transglutaminase).

G. **If our patient had an isolated elevated alkaline phosphatase on labs, what labs or studies should we send?**

Write out the algorithm shown in Fig. 19.1.

Teaching points

- First, check GGT to confirm hepatic source of alkaline phosphatase.
- If GGT is elevated, evaluate for hepatic sources with an ultrasound. If biliary obstruction or mass is seen:
  - Obtain additional imaging with computed tomography (CT) or magnetic resonance imaging (MRI).
  - Consider endoscopic retrograde cholangiopancreatogram (ERCP) or magnetic resonance cholangiopancreatography (MRCP) if signs of biliary tract disease.
  - For masses without obvious source, check alpha-fetoprotein (AFP), CA 19-9, carcinoembryonic antigen (CEA), and consider biopsy of the mass.
- If no evidence of biliary obstruction:
  - Exclude primary biliary cholangitis (check antimitochondrial antibody).
  - Exclude hepatocellular carcinoma (check liver protocol CT or MRI, and AFP).
  - Consider liver biopsy if suspicion for infiltrative disease persists.
  - Consider need for MRCP if clinical suspicion for ductal abnormality persists.

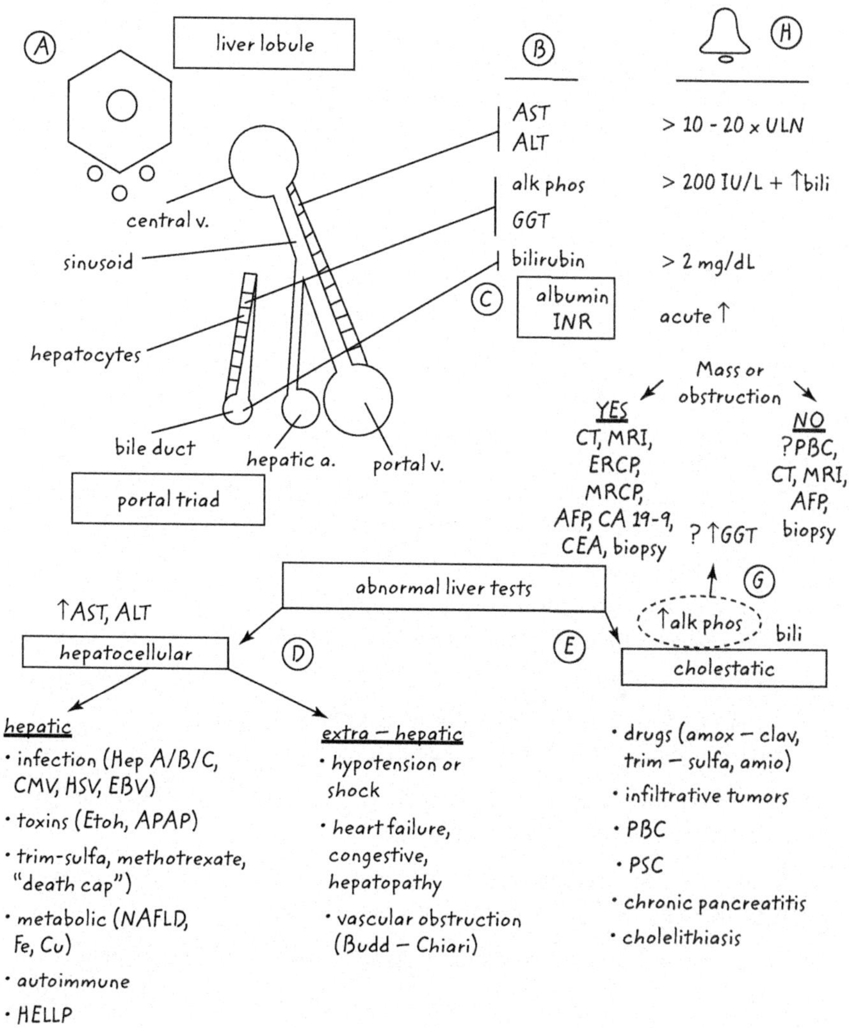

Fig. 19.1 Approach to abnormal liver blood tests, A–H

H. **Keeping in mind that acute changes in labs or symptoms are generally more worrisome than chronic laboratory abnormalities, what lab abnormalities should prompt an urgent evaluation?**

Fill out the alarming lab levels as shown in Fig. 19.1.

Teaching points

- Patients with severe liver test abnormalities often require hospitalization, especially if there are also clinical signs of decompensation (e.g., new encephalopathy, new ascites, gastrointestinal bleeding).
- Examples of situations where you would likely monitor closely with serial labs:
  - AST, ALT >10–20 times the upper limit of normal but no other liver test abnormalities, and no concerning symptoms
  - Total bilirubin >2 mg/dL in the setting of new medications, and no concerning symptoms
- Examples of situations where you would almost always hospitalize the patient:
  - Alk phos >200 IU/L with newly elevated total bilirubin, +/– fever or chills (i.e., acute cholangitis)
  - AST, ALT >10–20 times the upper limited of normal, plus newly elevated INR or total bilirubin
  - INR >1.5, newly elevated total bilirubin, new encephalopathy (i.e., acute liver failure). Patients like this ideally should be transferred to a facility capable of performing liver transplantation.

Return to objectives and emphasize key points

1. Identify which LFT abnormalities reflect liver injury rather than true dysfunction
   - Liver injury—AST, ALT, bilirubin, alk phos
   - Liver dysfunction—albumin and clotting factors
2. Distinguish between hepatocellular and cholestatic patterns of injury and highlight some of the common causes of each
   - Hepatocellular—Hepatitis A/B/C, alcohol, fatty infiltration, iron overload
   - Cholestatic—cholelithiasis, infiltrative tumors, PBC
3. Highlight worrisome liver blood test results that require urgent evaluation
   - Liver test abnormalities in the setting of new symptoms of hepatic decompensation
   - AST, ALT >10–20 times the upper limit of normal
   - Acute increase in total bilirubin >2 mg/dL, especially in the setting of new medications or additional symptoms
   - Alk phos >200 IU/L with elevated total bilirubin, +/– fever or chills (i.e., acute cholangitis)
   - INR >1.5, acutely elevated total bilirubin, new encephalopathy (i.e., acute liver failure)

Resources

1. American Gastroenterological Association. American Gastroenterological Association medical position statement: evaluation of liver chemistry tests. Gastroenterology. 2002;123(4):1364–6.
2. Kwo PY, Cohen SM, Lim JK. ACG clinical guideline: evaluation of abnormal liver chemistries. Am J Gastroenterol. 2017;112(1):18–35.
3. Livertox.nih.gov.

Chapter 20
Workup of Diarrhea

Maralyssa Bann and Deborah Greenberg

Learning Objectives

1. Identify most common causes of acute and chronic diarrhea in North America.
2. Recognize when additional workup is warranted in patients with acute or chronic diarrhea.
3. Systematically evaluate a patient presenting with diarrhea.
4. Distinguish between functional, inflammatory, osmotic, secretory, and malabsorption diarrhea.

Clinical Vignette: A 50-year-old woman presents to your clinic reporting four loose, watery stools per day for the past 6 weeks. This is a change from her baseline of a regular, formed brown stool every 2 days. She has not seen any blood in the toilet bowel, and she denies fevers or abdominal pain. She has lost around five pounds unintentionally. She does not think the diarrhea is associated with eating or fasting.

A. **Does this patient have diarrhea?**

Write the definition of diarrhea on the whiteboard.

Teaching points

- Patients may use the word "diarrhea" to describe many different types of stool changes—diarrhea is defined as:
  - Increased stool water content (>200 g in a 24-h period)

M. Bann (✉)
Harborview Medical Center, Department of Medicine, Division of General Internal Medicine, University of Washington, Seattle, WA, USA
e-mail: mbann@uw.edu

D. Greenberg
University of Washington Medical Center, Department of Medicine, Division of General Internal Medicine, University of Washington, Seattle, WA, USA

S. Mookherjee et al. (eds.), *Chalk Talks in Internal Medicine*,
https://doi.org/10.1007/978-3-030-34814-4_20

– Abnormal looseness and/or frequency of bowel movements (>3 above baseline in a 24-hour period)

B. **It is useful to think of diagnosing the cause of diarrhea in terms of the five major mechanisms by which diarrhea can occur.**

Leaving space under the definition of diarrhea, draw cylinders representing the mechanisms of diarrhea. Put the first letter of each (F, I, O, S, M) by each cylinder to serve as prompt as well as to maintain the order to facilitate the rest of the teaching script. Draw the notations on each cylinder as you fill out the names.

Teaching points

- It is important to acknowledge that more than one mechanism can occur at a time!
- Functional: Transit time impacts the ability of the intestinal wall to absorb water.
- Inflammatory: Mucosal injury results in leakage of proteins, mucus, and fluid into the lumen.
- Osmotic: Excess solute draws more water into the lumen.
- Secretory: Inappropriate ion transport into the lumen.
- Malabsorption: Impaired absorption of nutrients, especially fat (steatorrhea).

C. **The time course of diarrheal illness is an important diagnostic component. How do you define acute and chronic diarrhea? Does our patient have acute or chronic diarrhea?**

Move back to the definition of diarrhea and continue the algorithm with "time course," as shown in Fig. 20.1.

Teaching points

- Presence of symptoms longer than 2 weeks but less than 4 weeks should be evaluated in the context of severity of illness and underlying risk factors.
- Our patient's symptoms have lasted longer than 4 weeks, consistent with chronic diarrhea.

D. **Our patient has chronic diarrhea; but how would you evaluate her if she had acute diarrhea? What are some signs, symptoms, or risk factors that would warrant workup of acute diarrhea?**

Complete the algorithm on the "acute" side, as shown in Fig. 20.1.

Teaching points

- Acute diarrhea is often caused by viral infection, is generally self-limited and mild in severity, and often does not require further medical evaluation.
- Warning signs include:
  - Fever, systemic toxicity, or bloody stool
  - Recent hospitalization or antibiotic use
  - Patient comorbidities such as inflammatory bowel disease, pregnancy, severe chronic illness, advanced age, or immune compromise including HIV
  - Exposure via travel history or recent outbreak

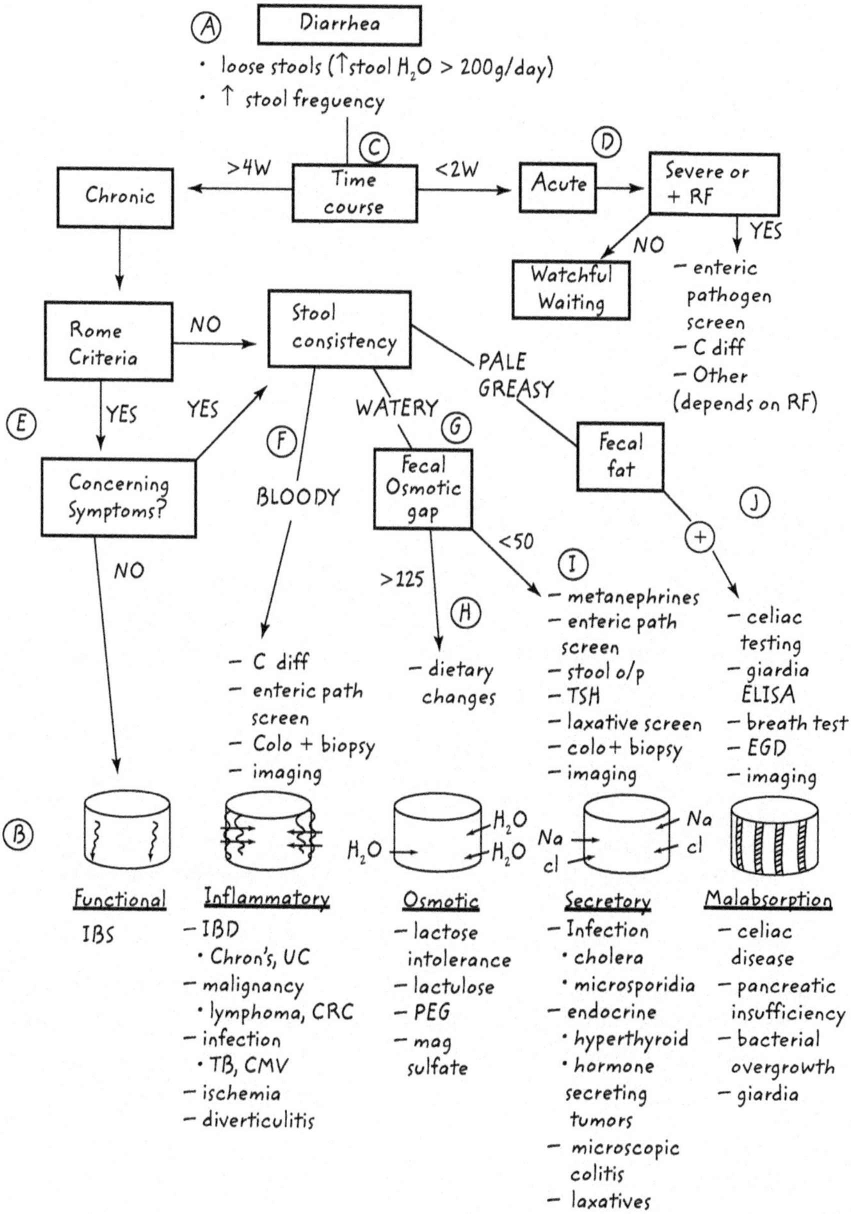

Fig. 20.1 Workup of diarrhea, A–J

E. **What is the most common cause of chronic watery diarrhea in North America?**

Complete the algorithm from "chronic" to "functional," adding IBS below "functional."

Teaching points

- Diagnosis of irritable bowel syndrome (IBS) is made by symptoms using the Rome criteria: recurrent abdominal pain that is associated with change in stool frequency and change in stool form, and improves with defecation (must involve two of three).
- Signs or symptoms NOT consistent with IBS should prompt evaluation for a different etiology of chronic diarrhea.
  - Anorexia
  - Unintentional weight loss
  - Malnutrition
  - Severe symptoms that awaken the patient from sleep
- No defined organic cause.
- Prevalence of IBS is 10–15% in North America.
- Should be considered in the differential diagnosis for all patients with watery chronic diarrhea.

F. **Our patient has lost weight, and therefore requires further workup. Consistency of stool is an important consideration: bloody, watery, or pale/greasy. What differential diagnosis would you have and what workup would you do if the stools were bloody?**

Complete the algorithm for "bloody," including the workup and differential diagnosis under "inflammatory".

Teaching points

- Chronic diarrhea associated with bloody stools should raise concerns for inflammatory cause, especially if associated with crampy abdominal pain, tenesmus, weight loss, or fever.
- Other important considerations are malignancy, ischemic colitis, and infection.

G. **Our patient describes a chronic watery diarrhea with unintentional weight loss. What laboratory value calculation can distinguish between osmotic and secretory causes of diarrhea?**

Continue the algorithm to the branch point for the fecal osmotic gap.

Teaching points

- Calculation of the fecal osmotic gap: stool osmolality = (2∗(Stool Na + Stool K)).
- High osmotic gap (>125) indicates osmotic cause.
- Low osmotic gap (<50) indicates secretory cause.

H. **What are some causes of osmotic diarrhea—what is the most important strategy to determine if the patient has osmotic diarrhea?**

Complete the algorithm for "osmotic," listing etiologies.

Teaching points

- Osmotic diarrhea will typically improve when fasting.
- Osmotic laxatives: lactulose, polyethylene glycol, or magnesium sulfate.
- Inability to digest sugars: lactose intolerance.

I. **Our patient has watery diarrhea that does not improve with fasting, which could be consistent with secretory diarrhea. What workup and differential should be considered?**

Complete the algorithm for "secretory," listing the workup and etiologies.

J. **If our patient had described pale, greasy, and foul-smelling stools, instead of watery diarrhea, what would have been your next steps?**

Complete the algorithm for "pale/greasy," listing the workup and etiologies.

Teaching points

- In summary, our patient has chronic watery diarrhea and weight loss, the diarrhea does not improve with fasting, and her symptoms are consistent with secretory diarrhea.
- Further workup reveals hyperthyroidism. With treatment her symptoms improve.

Return to objectives and emphasize key points

1. Identify the most common causes of acute and chronic diarrhea in North America.
   Circle on your algorithm
   - Viruses are the most common cause of acute diarrhea.
   - IBS is the most common cause of chronic diarrhea.
2. Recognize when additional workup is warranted in patients with acute or chronic diarrhea.
   Reinforce arrows along the algorithm:
   - If acute, more severe symptoms (fever, blood, vital signs) and associated risk factors should prompt additional testing.
   - If chronic, the absence of Rome criteria and/or the presence of concerning symptoms (blood, anorexia, weight loss) warrants further evaluation.
3. Systematically evaluate a patient presenting with diarrhea.
   Reinforce arrows along the algorithm:
   - Categorize as acute vs. chronic diarrhea.
   - Discuss IBS with patients who fit the Rome criteria and have no concerning symptoms.
   - Further distinguish between fatty, watery, and bloody diarrhea to direct further specific testing.

4. Distinguish between functional, inflammatory, osmotic, secretory, and malabsorption diarrhea.
    - Chronic diarrhea meeting the Rome criteria in the absence of concerning symptoms is likely functional and requires no further workup.
    - If bloody diarrhea is present, consider inflammatory causes.
    - If fatty diarrhea is present, consider malabsorptive causes.
    - If watery diarrhea is present, categorize further as osmotic or secretory based on the fecal osmotic gap and/or response to dietary changes.

Resources

1. Shane AL, Mody RK, Crump JA, Tarr PI, Steiner TS, Kotloff K, et al. Infectious Diseases Society of America clinical practice guidelines for the diagnosis and management of infectious diarrhea. Clin Infect Dis. 2017;65(12):e45–80.
2. Riddle MS, DuPont HL, Connor BA. ACG clinical guideline: diagnosis, treatment, and prevention of acute diarrheal infections in adults. Am J Gastroenterol. 2016;111:602–22.
3. Engsbro AL, Begtrup LM, Kjeldsen J, Larsen PV, deMuckadell OS, Jarbol DE, et al. Patients suspected of irritable bowel syndrome – cross-sectional study exploring the sensitivity of Rome III criteria in primary care. Am J Gastroenterol. 2013;108(6):972–80.
4. Eherer AJ, Fordtran JS. Fecal osmotic gap and pH in experimental diarrhea of various causes. Gastroenterology. 1992;103(2):545–51.
5. Juckett G, Trivedi R. Evaluation of chronic diarrhea. Am Fam Physician. 2011;84(10):1119–26.
6. Schiller LR, Pardi DS, Sellin JH. Chronic diarrhea: diagnosis and management. Clin Gastroenterol Hepatol. 2017;15(2):182–93.

Chapter 21
Approach to the Care of the Solid Organ Transplant Recipient

Joana Lima Ferreira and Christopher Wong

Learning Objectives

1. Take a focused history of a solid organ transplant (SOT) recipient, using a lung transplant recipient as an example.
2. Use the timeline for infectious complications after transplant as a tool to develop the differential diagnosis.
3. Recognize common noninfectious complications after transplant.

Clinical Vignette: A 54-year-old woman who is 9 months post bilateral lung transplant for idiopathic pulmonary fibrosis presents with a three-day history of progressive dyspnea, productive cough, and fever.

A. **Organ transplant history has a major impact on the evaluation of an acute medical problem. What information should we gather pertaining to the patient's transplant?**

List the major components of the transplant history as shown in Fig. 21.1.

Teaching points

- Why: The reason for the transplant can affect current management in several ways. For example, some conditions can recur in the transplanted organ—for example, hepatitis C virus in a liver transplant recipient or sarcoidosis in a lung transplant recipient.
- When: The amount of time elapsed since transplant affects the likelihood of certain complications, including the type of infection and malignancy.
- Viral serologies: Epstein-Barr Virus (EBV) and Cytomegalovirus (CMV) antibody status, often listed as "D" for Donor and "R" for recipient. For example,

J. Lima Ferreira (✉) · C. Wong
University of Washington Medical Center, Department of Medicine, Division of General Internal Medicine, University of Washington, Seattle, WA, USA

S. Mookherjee et al. (eds.), *Chalk Talks in Internal Medicine*,
https://doi.org/10.1007/978-3-030-34814-4_21

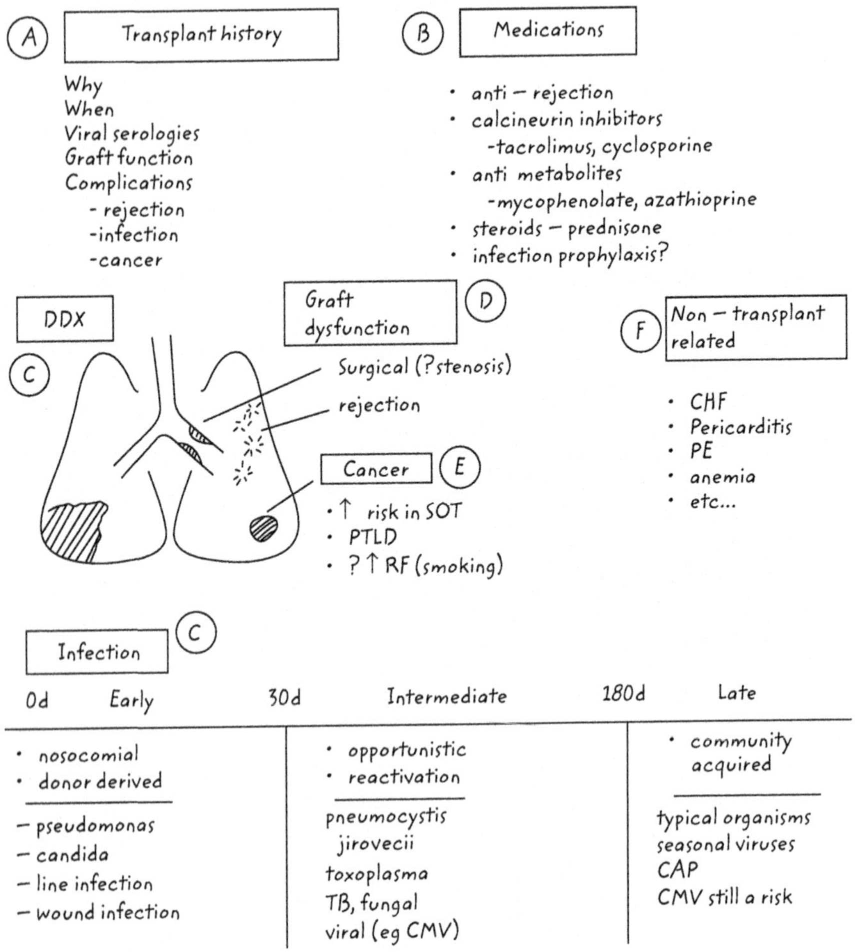

Fig. 21.1 Approach to the care of the solid organ transplant recipient: A–F

"EBV D+/R-" means that the donor was positive for EBV but the recipient (the patient) was negative. The risk for complications related to these viruses is higher if the donor is positive and the recipient is negative.

- Graft function: SOT recipients will have periodic tests to assess graft function. This may include laboratory studies (e.g., creatinine for a renal transplant recipient), functional testing (e.g., pulmonary function testing for lung transplant recipients, echocardiogram for heart transplant recipients), and surveillance biopsies.
- Complications: A history of post-transplant complications can help form the differential diagnosis of a patient's current presentation. For example, a history of graft rejection treated with additional immunosuppression can increase the risk of opportunistic infections.

B. **What types of medications would you expect this patient to be taking?**

Antirejection medications and possibly infection prophylaxis medications. Write down the major categories of medications and examples, as shown in Fig. 21.1.

- Antirejection medications can themselves cause side effects that may confound a presentation of new symptoms. Knowing target drug levels (typically drawn as trough levels) can be helpful in managing the medication's dose, as well as in assessing for the possibility of rejection.
- Calcineurin inhibitors such as tacrolimus or cyclosporine are the mainstay of most antirejection medication regimens.
- Antimetabolites such as mycophenolate and azathioprine may also be used concurrently, or instead of, calcineurin inhibitors.
- Prednisone is commonly used; many patients who have been stable for a long time without rejection may be maintained on very low doses, or, in some cases, none at all.
- Infection prophylaxis: Most SOT recipients receive prophylaxis against viral and fungal infections for the first several months (e.g., 0–6 months post-transplant), and potentially longer depending on their level of immunosuppression and whether they have a history of infections.

C. **Our patient presents with progressive dyspnea, cough, and fever. Let's walk through this patient's differential diagnosis. The first concern in this patient will likely be the possibility that she has an infection (pulmonary or otherwise) causing her symptoms. What types of infections would you be most likely to see depending on how long it has been since her transplant?**

Draw the lungs in the figure under "Differential", draw an infiltrate indicating "pneumonia" and then draw the "Infection" table: include the categories of timing and the broad categories of types of infection under each period of time. Ask learners to list the types of infections and that they would expect to see under each column and add them as mentioned.

Teaching points

- Infectious complications can occur at any time after that transplant, but the timing for specific infections developing after SOT follows some common patterns.
- An episode of rejection that was treated with an increase in immunosuppression can be considered to "reset" the timeline with regard to risk of infections.
- Early infections (0–30 days after transplant):
  - Nosocomial bacteria and yeast are the most common pathogens.
  - Superficial and deep surgical-site infections, donor-derived infections, or patient's pre-existing conditions (e.g., cystic fibrosis patients colonized by *Pseudomonas*).
- Intermediate period (31–180 days after transplant):
  - The high level of immunosuppression allows reactivation of latent pathogens transmitted from donor organs and the ones within the recipient.
  - Most patients receive prophylaxis against *Pneumocystis jirovecii* and CMV.
  - Opportunistic infections during this period include viral (CMV, EBV, VZV), fungal (*Pneumocystis jirovecii*, *Cryptococcus*, *Coccidioides*, *Histoplasma*, *Blastomyces*, and others), parasitic (*Toxoplasma gondii*), and mycobacterial (e.g., TB reactivation), as well as continued risk for bacterial infections.
- Late infections (beyond 180 days after transplant):
  - Type of infection varies depending on prior exposures, need for increased immunosuppression and development of other complications such as malignancy and rejection.
  - Community-acquired viral and bacterial infections are considerations, as well as CMV (late manifestation after discontinuation of prophylactic therapy).
  - Other infections may be organ-specific. For example, in this case of a lung transplant recipient, if there has been chronic rejection, there is an increased risk of *Aspergillus* infection.

D. **In addition to infectious processes, there are several other possible processes that could lead to our patient's presentation. What are the possible causes of graft dysfunction, and how might they present?**

Using the drawing of the lungs, indicate "surgical" and "rejection" as causes of graft dysfunction.

Teaching points

- Surgical:
  - Immediate postoperative complications can cause significant morbidity in the first days to months after transplant.
  - Airway stenosis at the site of anastomosis is the most common airway complication related to lung transplant.
  - Airway complications should be suspected when patients present with recurrent pneumonia or persistent airflow obstruction after lung transplant.

- Rejection:
  - Acute cellular rejection (ACR) occurs when recipient lymphocytes react against donor antigens. It is commonly seen in the first year after transplant and can present with dyspnea, hypoxemia, cough, and fever.
  - It may be difficult to distinguish acute rejection from infection on clinical grounds alone.
  - ACR is the most significant risk factor for the development of chronic lung allograft rejection, which is caused by progressive obliterative bronchiolitis.
  - Chronic rejection is typically more subacute and chronic, characterized by a gradual decline in FEV1 and dyspnea on exertion.

E. **Another potential cause of our patient's symptoms could be a malignancy. What are the most common malignancies related to solid-organ transplant?**

Using the drawing of the lungs, indicate "cancer" as a possible cause of the symptoms.

Teaching points

- Increased cancer risk in SOT recipients may result from immunosuppression as well as other risk factors, such as prior/current smoking history.
- The most common post-transplant de novo malignancies are associated with chronic infections by known oncogenic viruses, including human papillomavirus (HPV) causing nonmelanoma skin cancers, Epstein-Barr virus (EBV) causing post-transplant lymphoproliferative disorder (PTLD), and hepatitis B and C virus causing hepatocellular carcinoma.
- Post-transplant lymphoproliferative disorder (PTLD) is a heterogeneous group of lymphoproliferative disorders, ranging from reactive polyclonal hyperplasias to aggressive non-Hodgkin lymphomas.

F. **It is important to consider nontransplant related causes of her symptoms. What other conditions may be causing this patient's symptoms?**

Write out some nontransplant-related causes of dyspnea.

Return to objectives and emphasize key points

1. Take a focused history of a SOT recipient.
   - Circle "why, when, viral serologies, graft function, and complications."
2. Use the timeline for infectious complications after transplant as a tool to develop the differential diagnosis.
   - Circle "community acquired" in the late period—emphasize that stable transplant patients are susceptible to the same infectious issues as the rest of the community.
3. Recognize common noninfectious complications after transplant
   - asterisk: "graft dysfunction" and "cancer"

Resources

1. Wong CJ, Krug MF. Pearls for the internist taking care of the patient with a solid organ transplant. SGIM Forum. 2016;39(7):1–3.
2. Fishman JA, Issa NC. Infection in organ transplantation: risk factors and evolving patterns of infection. Infect Dis Clin North Am. 2010;24(2):273–83. https://doi.org/10.1016/j.idc.2010.01.005.
3. Pagalilauan GL, Limaye AP. Infections in transplant patients. Med Clin North Am. 2013;97(4):581–600. https://doi.org/10.1016/j.mcna.2013.03.002.
4. Green M. Introduction: infections in solid organ transplantation. Am J Transplant. 2013;13(Suppl 4):3–8. https://doi.org/10.1111/ajt.12093.
5. Tejwani V, Panchabhal TS, Kotloff RM, Metha AC. Complications of lung transplantation, a roentgenographic perspective. Chest. 2016;149(6):1535–45. https://doi.org/10.1016/j.chest.2015.12.019.
6. Ahmad S, Shlobin OA, Nathan SD. Pulmonary complications of lung transplantation. Chest. 2011;139(2):402–11. https://doi.org/10.1378/chest.10-1048.
7. Dantal J, Campone M. Daunting but worthy goal: reducing the de novo cancer incidence after transplantation. Transplantation. 2016;100(12):2569–83. https://doi.org/10.1097/TP.0000000000001428.
8. Jagadeesh D, Woda BA, Draper J, Evens A. Post-transplant lymphoproliferative disorders: risk, classification and therapeutic recommendations. Curr Treat Options Oncol. 2012;13(1):122–36. https://doi.org/10.1007/s11864-011-0177-x.

Chapter 22
Screening for Lung Cancer

Ronald Huang and Barak Gaster

Learning Objectives

1. Identify which patients benefit most from low-dose CT (LDCT) for lung cancer screening.
2. Discuss the risks and benefits of LDCT for lung cancer screening.
3. List the components of shared decision-making for lung cancer screening.

Clinical Vignette: A 66-year-old woman is seen in clinic for an annual wellness visit. She has no symptoms. She has no medical history. She does not take medications. She smokes one pack of cigarettes per day. She has smoked for 40 years. It occurs to you that maybe you should screen her for lung cancer.

A. **What is the most important topic to discuss with her, even before talking about screening?**

Write "SCREEN?" vertically on the white board and fill out "smoking cessation."

Teaching points

- Smoking cessation is the best-studied and most-effective way to prevent dying from lung cancer.
- Make sure to keep this the highest priority with patients whether they are currently smoking or have already quit.
- Lung cancer screening is not a replacement for smoking cessation.

R. Huang (✉) · B. Gaster
University of Washington Medical Center, Department of Medicine, Division of General Internal Medicine, University of Washington, Seattle, WA, USA
e-mail: RLHuang@evergreenhealthcare.org

S. Mookherjee et al. (eds.), *Chalk Talks in Internal Medicine*,
https://doi.org/10.1007/978-3-030-34814-4_22

B. **What are the risks of screening that should be discussed with her?**

Write down the risks, as shown in Fig. 22.1.

Teaching points

- False positives are common with screening. Almost 25% of all screening tests will find a nodule, but over 95% of those nodules will turn out not to be cancer. Most nodules can be classified as benign after follow-up CT scans, but 6% of positive screening tests will require an invasive procedure.
- Overdiagnosis: Diagnosing lung cancer that would never have affected the patient if it were not for screening. Many older patients eligible for screening might die of other causes before their lung cancer would have caused any problems.
- Radiation from a LDCT is less than from a regular chest CT, but this exposure is still important to mention. LDCT is a specialized non-contrast study obtained during a single breath hold. The radiation exposure from LDCT is 1.5 mSv. In comparison, the radiation from a regular chest CT is 8 mSv, while the average adult in the US is exposed to about 2.4 mSv per year from background radiation.

C. **What is the efficacy of screening? How much will screening with an LDCT lower her risk of dying from lung cancer?**

Write down the efficacy information, as shown in Fig. 22.1.

Teaching points

- In terms of efficacy, lung cancer is an ideal disease for screening. It has a high prevalence; the population at risk is identifiable; it usually presents in later stages when mortality is high; and patients with early-stage disease fare better.
- LDCT was proven effective in the National Lung Screening Trial (NLST, reference below), which was published in 2011.
- The NLST randomized over 53,000 patients to annual LDCT for 3 years or annual chest x-ray (CXR) for 3 years and followed patients for a median duration of 6.5 years.
- The NLST found over the period of the study that 13 out of 1000 people died of lung cancer when they were screened with LDCT compared to 16 out of 1000 screened with CXR. The relative reduction in mortality from lung cancer was 20%. The number needed to screen with LDCT to prevent one lung cancer death was 320.

D. **Is this patient eligible for lung cancer screening?**

Write down the eligibility information, as shown in Fig. 22.1.

Teaching points

- Under US Centers for Medicare & Medicaid guidelines, adults aged 55–77 who have more than a 30-pack-year smoking history and are currently smoking or have quit within the past 15 years are eligible for screening.

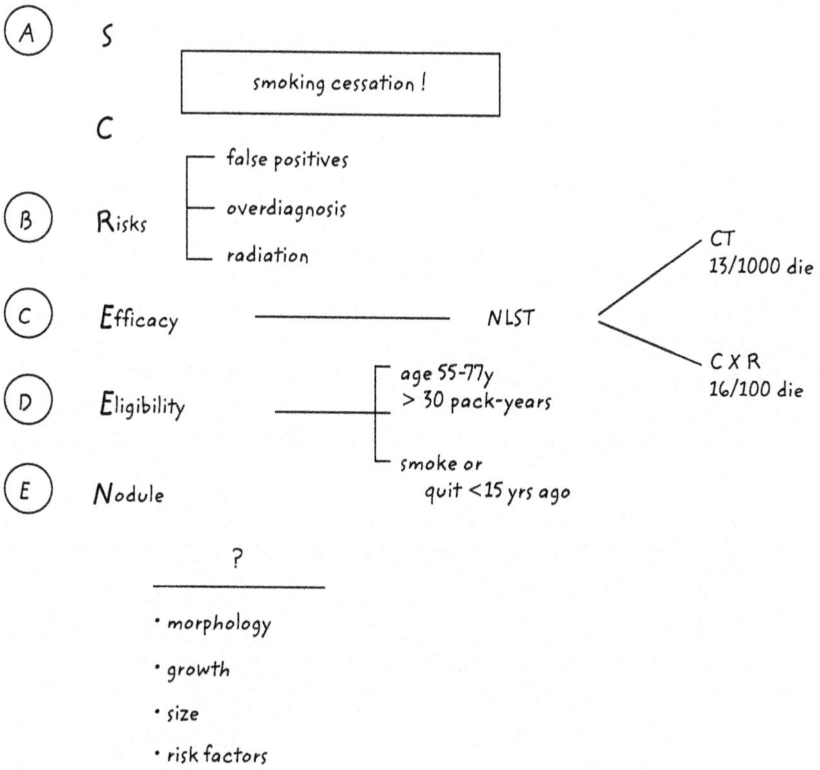

Fig. 22.1 Screening for lung cancer, A–E

- Private insurers will cover screening up to age 80 based on the US Preventive Services Task Force recommendations.
- Patients should be asymptomatic. If a patient has symptoms of lung cancer, then an LDCT is not appropriate.
- Before embarking on screening, patients should be counseled that screening is meant to be performed annually until the patient no longer meets the eligibility criteria.

E. **The patient has an LDCT and is found to have a 3 mm nodule in her left lower lobe. What are the most important factors determining the follow-up plan?**

List the important nodule and patient characteristics, as shown in Fig. 22.1.

Teaching points

- Morphology: Nonsolid nodules or nodules with fat or calcifications are more likely to be benign (consult with radiologist).
- Growth: It is concerning if the nodule has increased in size or is new compared with a prior scan.
- Absolute size: Solid nodules <6 mm are more likely to be benign.
- Patient factors: Other comorbidities, age, current smoking.
- For this patient, offer reassurance that most nodules are benign but emphasize the need for additional follow-up given the risk of cancer.
- The use of standardized follow-up protocols for nodules helps to avoid unnecessary biopsies and missed diagnoses (see references). Many health systems have specialty or multidisciplinary clinics that follow lung nodules found by screening.

Return to objectives and emphasize key points

1. Identify which patients benefit the most from low-dose CT for lung cancer screening.
   - Aged 55–77
   - More than 30 pack-year smoking history
   - Current smoker or quit smoking within the past 15 years
2. Discuss the risks and benefits of LDCT for lung cancer screening.
   - The risks of LDCT are false positives, overdiagnosis, and radiation exposure.
   - The benefit of LDCT is that 3 people out of every 1000 screened will avoid dying of lung cancer.
3. List the components of shared decision-making for lung cancer screening.
   - Counsel about smoking cessation.
   - Discuss the risks and benefits of LDCT.
   - Determine eligibility.

- Counsel that screening is meant to be performed annually and assess willingness to proceed with follow-up testing if needed.
- Many decision aids are available to help with shared decision-making (see references).

Resources

1. National Lung Screening Trial Research Team, Aberle DR, Adams AM, Berg CD, Black WC, Clapp JD, Fagerstrom RM, Gareen IF, Gatsonis C, Marcus PM, Sicks JD. Reduced lung-cancer mortality with low-dose computed tomographic screening. N Engl J Med. 2011;365(5):395–409.
2. Bach PB, Mirkin JN, Oliver TK, Azzoli CG, Berry DA, Brawley OW, Byers T, Colditz GA, Gould MK, Jett JR, Sabichi AL, Smith-Bindman R, Wood DE, Qaseem A, Detterbeck FC. Benefits and harms of CT screening for lung cancer: a systematic review. JAMA. 2012;307(22):2418–29.
3. National Lung Screening Trial Research Team, Church TR, Black WC, Aberle DR, Berg CD, Clingan KL, Duan F, Fagerstrom RM, Gareen IF, Gierada DS, Jones GC, Mahon I, Marcus PM, Sicks JD, Jain A, Baum S. Results of initial low-dose computed tomographic screening for lung cancer. N Engl J Med. 2013;368(21):1980–91.
4. Moyer VA, U.S. Preventive Services Task Force. Screening for lung cancer: U.S. Preventive Services Task Force recommendation statement. Ann Intern Med. 2014;160(5):330–8.
5. Gould MK. Clinical practice. Lung-cancer screening with low-dose computed tomography. N Engl J Med. 2014;371(19):1813–20.
6. Centers for Medicare & Medicaid Services. Decision Memo for Screening for Lung Cancer with Low Dose Computed Tomography (LDCT) (CAG-00439N). 2015. https://www.cms.gov/medicare-coverage-database/details/nca-decision-memo.aspx?NCAId=274.
7. Shieh Y, Bohnenkamp M. Low-dose computed tomography for lung cancer screening: clinical and coding considerations. Chest. 2017;152(1):204–9.
8. Lung Cancer CT Screening: Should I Get Screened? http://www.shouldiscreen.com/lung-cancer-risk-calculator/.
9. Decision Aid For Lung Cancer Screening with Computerized Tomography (CT) https://www.thoracic.org/professionals/clinical-resources/disease-related-resources/decision-aid-for-lung-cancer-screening-with-ct.php.
10. Is Lung Cancer Screening Right for Me? A Decision Aid for People Considering Lung Cancer Screening With Low-Dose Computed Tomography. https://effectivehealthcare.ahrq.gov/decision-aids/lung-cancer-screening/patient.html.
11. Lung CT Screening Reporting & Data System. https://www.acr.org/Clinical-Resources/Reporting-and-Data-Systems/Lung-Rads.
12. NCCN Clinical Practice Guidelines in Oncology: Lung Cancer Screening Versuib 2.2018. https://www.nccn.org/professionals/physician_gls/pdf/lung_screening.pdf.

Chapter 23
Approach to Hemolytic Anemia

Brandon Fainstad and Leslie Enzian

Learning Objectives
1. Develop a systematic approach to evaluating anemia based on the reticulocyte index and basic hemolysis labs.
2. Identify the cause of hemolytic anemia based on a peripheral blood smear and one unique clinical feature.

Clinical Vignette: A 28-year-old woman with *systemic lupus erythematosus* (*SLE*) presents with fatigue and shortness of breath. She denies any signs of bleeding. Medications: Hydroxychloroquine, mycophenolate, dapsone (recently initiated). Labs: Hemoglobin 5 g/dl, Hematocrit 15% (previously 32%), platelets normal, reticulocyte index 4.2%.

A. **What is a reticulocyte index (RI) and why is the RI such an important tool for differentiating the causes of anemia?**

Write the formula for reticulocyte count on the white board.

Teaching points
- When you order a reticulocyte count, you are provided with a total reticulocyte count and percentage.
- However, these values are only useful when the degree of anemia is taken into account.

B. Fainstad (✉)
Veterans Affairs, Rocky Mountain Regional Medical Center, Aurora, CO, USA
e-mail: brandon.fainstad@va.gov

L. Enzian
Harborview Medical Center, Department of Medicine, Division of General Internal Medicine, University of Washington, Seattle, WA, USA
e-mail: enzian@uw.edu

S. Mookherjee et al. (eds.), *Chalk Talks in Internal Medicine*,
https://doi.org/10.1007/978-3-030-34814-4_23

- The RI equation determines whether or not the degree of reticulocytosis is appropriate.

B. **The reticulocyte index helps differentiate between underproduction anemia and anemia from destruction or loss of red blood cells. What does an RI less than 2% suggest?**

Add "<2%" and "underproduction" to the white board.

Teaching points

- As a patient becomes increasingly anemic, a normally functioning bone marrow will increase the rate of red blood cell maturation by producing more reticulocytes. Thus, the reticulocyte count and percentage will increase relative to the degree of anemia (RI > 3%) in order to compensate appropriately.
- A dysfunctional bone marrow will not generate an adequate reticulocytsis (RI < 2%) to correct the anemia.
- If a patient is anemic with a low RI, then underproduction is at least contributing to their anemia.
- The differential for underproduction is broad and will not be covered here—major causes include micronutrient deficiency, chornic inflammaiton, malignancy, and bone marrow suppression from a variety of causes.

C. **What would the reticulocyte index be in the setting of acute blood loss or red blood cell destruction?**

Complete the algorithm for ">3%."

Teaching points

- Assuming the bone marrow is functioning appropriately, the RI should be >3% within 24 hours after the development of anemia.
- The history and exam may still help you identify the source of blood loss or further investigation may be warranted if laboratory testing excludes hemolysis as the cause of anemia.
- Note that the RI may be <3% if the blood loss started within less than 24 hours, as there may not have been enough time for the marrow to generate sufficient reticulocytosis. However, an acute blood loss anemia of that extent would typically be clinically apparent without additional laboratory testing.

D. **Our patient has an elevated reticulocyte index but no signs or symptoms of acute blood loss. What additional laboratory tests help confirm that an anemia is due to hemolysis?**

Add labs pointing to hemolytic anemia, as shown in Fig. 23.1.

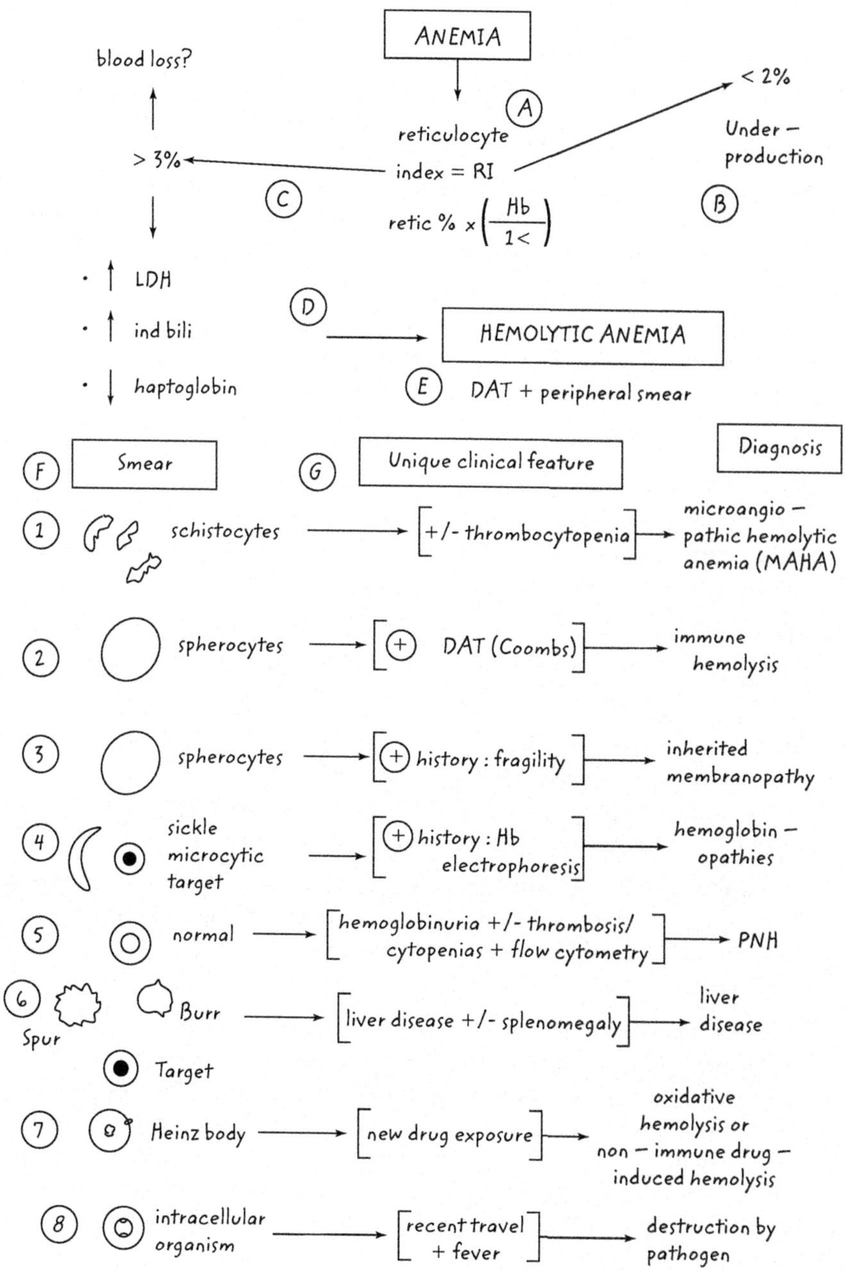

Fig. 23.1 Approach to Hemolytic Anemia, A–G

Teaching points

- Elevated lactate dehydrogenase (LDH): Released from the hemolyzed RBC. Elevation is not specific to hemolytic anemia as LDH is found in many types of cells in the body (e.g., WBC, myocytes).
- Elevated indirect bilirubin: Hemoglobin released from hemolyzed RBCs is broken down into bilirubin but, again, elevated bilirubin is not specific for hemolysis.
- Low haptoglobin: Haptoglobin is an acute phase reactant generated in the liver. Levels could either be inappropriately normal due to inflammation despite ongoing hemolysis, or low in the setting of liver dysfunction in the absence of hemolysis.

E. **Our patient is found to have elevated LDH and indirect bilirubin, and a low haptoglobin level. We continue to suspect hemolytic anemia. What additional tests should we order?**

Write down "DAT" and "peripheral smear," as shown in Fig. 23.1.

- Direct Antiglobulin Test (DAT), also known as a Coombs test, is typically positive in patients with an autoimmune process leading to their anemia.
- A peripheral blood smear is critical in assessing the characteristic changes in RBC morphology that help make the appropriate diagnosis.

F. **The peripheral smear is extremely useful in figuring out the cause of hemolytic anemia. What are some RBC abnormalities you can see in patients with hemolytic anemia?**

Draw the common abnormalities as listed by learners (1–8 in the figure). Group spur cells (acanthocytes), burr cells (echinocytes), and target cells together. Also draw two spherocytes (for immune hemolysis and inherited membranopathy), as shown in Fig. 23.1. *Consider drawing these before starting your talk.*

G. **It is useful to think of the common causes of hemolytic anemia in terms of their characteristic peripheral smear findings and at least one "unique clinical feature." What is the most likely diagnosis in each case with the associated clinical feature?**

Write down the key clinical features next to each peripheral smear. Ask learners to provide the most likely diagnosis in each case. The table below provides helpful notes. Focus primarily on microangiopathic hemolytic anemia (MAHA) and immune mediated. These are the two most common, acute, and urgent groups of diseases. If time is limited, it is reasonable to address these two entities exclusively while mentioning that the complete differential is quite broad including many rarer, less acute, and less severe diseases. See Teaching Points below for further details, although this table does not need to be written on the white board.

Teaching Points

Smear + Clinical Feature → likely diagnosis	Further differential/notes
Schistocytes +/− thrombocytopenia → Microangiopathic Hemolytic Anemia (MAHA)	• Thrombotic thrombocytopenic purpura (TTP) most commonly due to an inherited deficiency of ADAMTS13 (enzyme responsible for cleaving vWF). The classic pentad of MAHA, thrombocytopenia, altered mental status fever, and acute kidney injury (AKI) is not necessary for the diagnosis, only MAHA and a confirmed ADAMTS13 activity level <10%. • Hemolytic Uremic Syndrome—most commonly presenting in children due to Shiga toxin producing E. coli (STEC) infections. More rarely due to complement dysregulation related to other infection or medications. Diagnosed by the classic triad of MAHA, thrombocytopenia, AKI with either evidence of STEC infection or compliment dysregulation • Disseminated intravascular coagulation (DIC)—coagulopathy, thrombocytopenia, and low fibrinogen • Malignant hypertension • Prosthetic valve • Pre-eclampsia
Spherocytes + positive Direct Antiglobulin Test (DAT) → Immune-mediated Hemolysis	• Most commonly idiopathic, but consider the following potential underlying causes: • Medications—antibiotics, NSAIDs, chemotherapy and quinine • Infectious—e.g., HIV, EBV • Autoimmune disease—e.g., lupus, rheumatoid arthritis, scleroderma, dermatomyositis • Lymphoprolipherative disease • Immunodeficiency—e.g., combined variable immune deficiency • Transfusions/transplant
Spherocytes, negative DAT and personal or family history of anemia → Inherited membranopathy	• Hereditary spherocytosis(elevated mean corpuscular hemoglobin concentration + positive fragility test)
Sickle cells or microcytosis and target cells + personal or family history of anemia → Hemoglobinopathy	• Sickle Cell • Thalassemia: Alpha thalassemia more common in people of Southeast Asian descent, and • Beta thalassemia in people of African and Mediterranean descent.
Normal smear + hemaglobinuria +/− unexplained thrombosis or cytopenias → Paroxysmal Nocturnal Hemoglobinuria (PNH)	• PNH is a rare clonal disorder that presents with hemolysis, thrombosis, and bone marrow failure. Confirmed with flow cytometry.

Smear + Clinical Feature → likely diagnosis	Further differential/notes
Spur, burr or target cells + liver disease +/− splenomegaly → Hemolysis of liver disease	• This is a commonly misdiagnosed as DIC (for example, low fibrinogen, low platelets, and elevated INR). However, these abnormalities are due to liver synthetic dysfunction rather than consumption. • Alterations in the cholesterol to lipid content of the RBC membrane make the RBCs less deformable and more fragile. • Hypersplenism leads to increased RBC sequestration and can also result in increased RBC clearance within the enlarged spleen.
+/− Heinz bodies + new drug exposure → Non-immune drug induced hemolysis	• Oxidative hemolysis, more common in the setting of G6PD deficiency—e.g., • Dapsone, nitrofurantoin, and primaquine • Other mechanisms—e.g., heavy metals, interferon, and insect or snake bites
+/− Intracellular organism + recent travel and fever → Destruction by pathogen	• Malaria • Babesiosis • Clostridial sepsis

Returning to Our Case

Based on concerns for active hemolysis, a peripheral blood smear was performed, revealing numerous spherocytes and her DAT returned positive the next day. She was diagnosed with acute immune-mediated hemolytic anemia related to her SLE.

Return to Objectives and Emphasize Key Points

1. Develop a systematic approach to evaluating anemia based on the reticulocyte index and basic hemolysis labs.

   - When the cause for anemia is not clear, use the RI as the initial step in evaluating the etiology—The Reticulocyte Index (RI) determines if the reticulocytosis is appropriate for the degree of anemia, thus differentiating underproduction anemia from blood loss or hemolytic anemia.
   - Hemolysis labs—RI of >3%, an elevated LDH and indirect bilirubin, and a low haptoglobin will establish hemolysis as the cause of anemia.
   - Smear and DAT—Always obtain a peripheral blood smear and DAT to help identify the etiology of hemolysis.

2. Identify the cause of hemolytic anemia based on a peripheral blood smear and one unique clinical feature.

   - The most common causes for clinically significant acute hemolytic anemia are MAHA and immune-mediated hemolysis.
   - MAHA is diagnosed by schistocytes on the peripheral smear and is often associated with thrombocytopenia.
   - Immune hemolysis will often have spherocytes on peripheral smear and is confirmed with a positive DAT.

Resources

1. Hutchinson RE, Davey FR. Hematopoiesis. In: Henry JB, editor. Clinical diagnosis and management by laboratory methods. 19th ed. Philadelphia: WB Saunders; 1996.
2. Dhaliwal G, Cornett P, Tierney L Jr. Hemolytic anemia. Am Fam Physician. 2004;69(11):2599–607.
3. Sabatine MS. "Anemia" 5.1. In: Pocket medicine: the Massachusetts General Hospital handbook of internal medicine. Philadelphia: Wolters Kluwer; 2017.
4. George JN, Nester CM. Syndromes of thrombotic microangiopathy. N Engl J Med. 2014;371(7):654–66.
5. Owen JS, et al. Erythrocyte echinocytosis in liver disease. Role of abnormal plasma high density lipoproteins. J Clin Invest. 1985;76(6):2275–85.
6. Cooper RA, et al. Role of the spleen in membrane conditioning and hemolysis of spur cells in liver disease. N Engl J Med. 1974;290(23):1279–84.

Chapter 24
Management of Monoclonal Gammopathy of Uncertain Significance

Mahri Haider and Mehraneh Khalighi

Learning Objectives

1. Identify the appropriate studies to evaluate patients with monoclonal gammopathy of uncertain significance (MGUS).
2. Describe the diagnostic criteria for MGUS.
3. Recognize the laboratory abnormalities indicative of organ or tissue damage recalled by the acronym CRAB (hyperCalcemia, Renal insufficiency, Anemia, Bone lesions), which are concerning for progression to a malignant stage.

Clinical Vignette: A 65-year-old woman with peripheral neuropathy had an serum protein electrophoresis (SPEP) and immunofixation sent as part of her work-up. Her results indicate an IgG kappa monoclonal component.

A. **Our patient had an SPEP ordered as part of neuropathy work-up. What are some of the clinical scenarios that might trigger a lab evaluation for monoclonal protein?**

Write down symptoms/scenarios as suggested by learners as shown in Fig. 24.1.

Teaching points

- Neuropathy, usually thoracic or lumbosacral radiculopathy, caused by compression of the nerve by a paravertebral plasmacytoma (bone or soft tissue tumor of plasma cells). Less likely to present as spinal cord compression or peripheral neuropathy (the mechanism of the latter may be paraneoplastic, especially in IgM cases).

M. Haider (✉)
Harborview Medical Center, Department of Medicine, Division of General Internal Medicine, University of Washington, Seattle, WA, USA
e-mail: mhaider@uw.edu

M. Khalighi
VA Puget Sound Health Care System, Department of Medicine, Division of General Internal Medicine, University of Washington, Seattle, WA, USA
e-mail: Mehraneh.Khalighi@va.gov

S. Mookherjee et al. (eds.), *Chalk Talks in Internal Medicine*,
https://doi.org/10.1007/978-3-030-34814-4_24

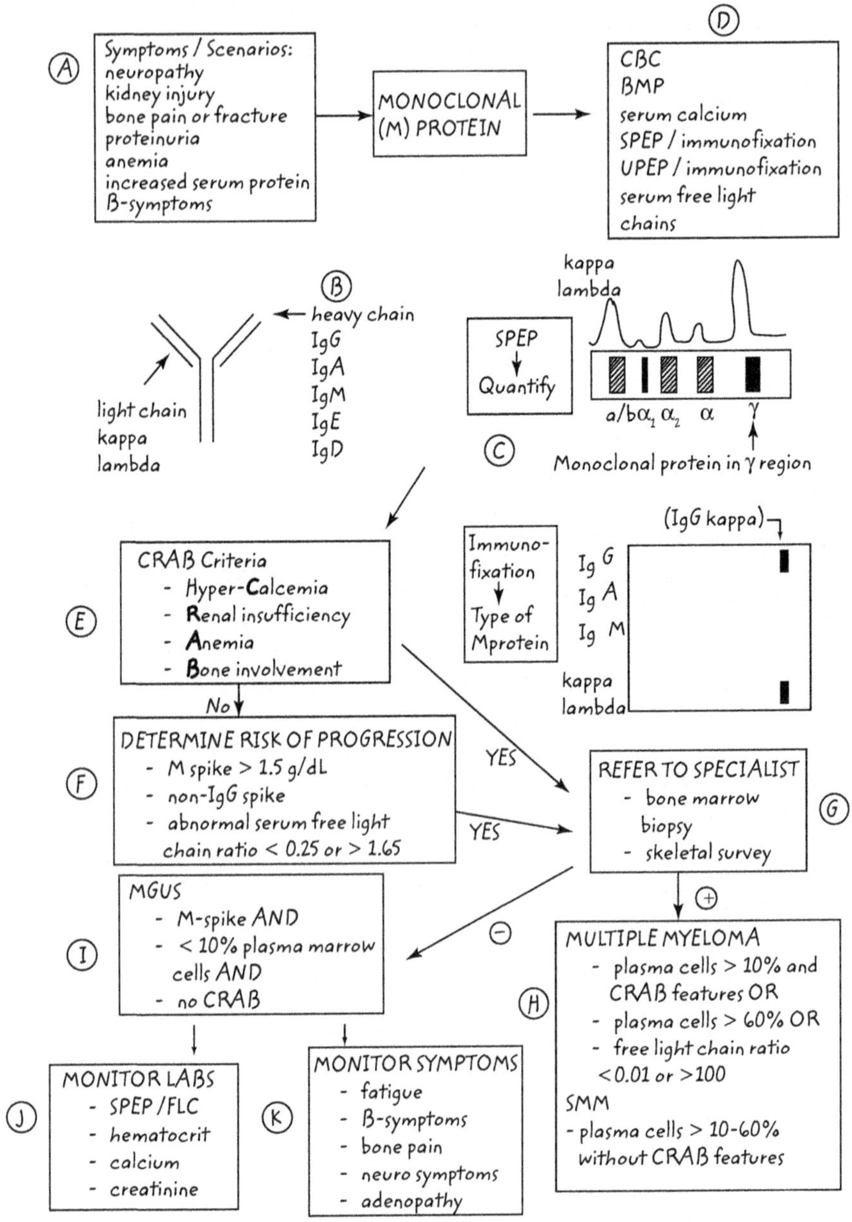

Fig. 24.1 Management of monoclonal gammopathy of uncertain significance: A–K

- Renal disease resulting from light chain nephropathy or hypercalcemia.
- Bone disease presenting with bony pain due to osteolysis or from bone fracture (axial > distal).
- Proteinuria is a common feature with AL amyloid deposition.
- Normocytic, normochromic anemia, due to bone marrow replacement by plasma cells, chronic inflammation.
- Protein gap or "gamma gap" is the difference between the total serum protein and serum albumin.
- B-symptoms of fever, night sweats, and weight loss.

B. **The patient asks you what it means to have an IgG kappa monoclonal component. How can you explain "IgG kappa monoclonal protein" to your patient?**

Draw an immunoglobulin and label light and heavy chains as shown in Fig. 24.1.

Teaching points

- Plasma cells are a type of white blood cells that make immunoglobulin, also called antibodies.
- Each immunoglobulin is made up of two heavy chains (IgG, IgA, IgM, IgE, or IgD) and two light chains (kappa or lambda).
- The immunoglobulin made by a clonal plasma cell is called a monoclonal protein (aka M-protein).

C. **What tests were used to detect and quantify her monoclonal protein?**

Draw the SPEP and immunofixation schematics as shown in Fig. 24.1.

Teaching points

- SPEP: Detects possible monoclonal protein components and quantifies them.
- Serum immunofixation: Identifies the immunoglobulin heavy and light chain sub-type associated with the M-spike.
- Urine protein electrophoresis (UPEP)/urine immunofixation: 24-hour urine collection is preferred to spot urine. Detects and quantifies urinary free kappa or lambda light chains (Bence Jones protein) that might be missed by SPEP, especially in light-chain-only disease.
- Serum free light chains: Detects and measures free kappa and free lambda light chains in the serum and is more sensitive than urine immunofixation. The ratio (kappa/lambda), rather than individual levels, is the key (normal is generally 0.26–1.65). The free light chain ratio has both diagnostic and prognostic significance.
- 20% of multiple myeloma cases are light chain only (negative SPEP/immunofixation).

D. **All patients with a monoclonal gammopathy require further evaluation to determine the cause. Monoclonal proteins are associated with a clonal process that is either potentially or frankly malignant. Monoclonal gammopa-**

thy of undetermined significance (MGUS) is an asymptomatic premalignant disorder. It needs to be distinguished from plasma cell malignancies, the most common of which is multiple myeloma (MM). Other, less common potential malignancies that could present this way are AL amyloidosis, Waldenstrom's macroglobulinemia, and non-Hodgkin lymphoma. What labs should be sent next to help distinguish pre-malignant from malignant conditions?

Write out appropriate labs as listed by learners.

Teaching points

- Complete blood count (CBC): Detects anemia that suggests bone marrow infiltration and possible malignancy, especially when hemoglobin is <10 g/dL or a 2-point drop from the baseline.
- Basic metabolic panel (BMP): Elevated creatinine suggests renal insufficiency and end organ damage, possibly related to light chain deposition or hypercalcemia.
- Serum calcium: The presence of high calcium suggests possibility of osteolytic bone disease and associated malignancy.

E. **Our patient's serum immunofixation shows an IgG level of 1.9 g/dL. Her UPEP shows no M-spike and urine immunofixation shows oligoclonal banding restricted to kappa free light chains. Her serum free light chains show a kappa/lambda ratio of 1.45. Other pertinent labs include a hemoglobin of 13 g/dL, creatinine of 1.1 mg/dL, and serum calcium of 10.1 mg/dL. She heard about the CRAB criteria and is wondering if she meets any of them.**

Write out the CRAB criteria as shown in Fig. 24.1.

Teaching points

- CRAB criteria are specific lab or imaging abnormalities that indicate organ or tissue damage and are concerning for malignancy.
- CRAB = hyper**C**alcemia, **R**enal insufficiency, **A**nemia, **B**one lesions.
  - Hypercalcemia (calcium >11.5 mg/dL).
  - Renal insufficiency (creatinine >2 mg/dL).
  - Anemia (hemoglobin <10 g/dL).
  - Bone involvement (requires imaging to assess for osteolytic lesions).
- Patients with monoclonal gammopathy and any CRAB criteria should be referred for a bone marrow biopsy.
- Our patient does not meet any of the laboratory CRAB criteria.

F. **On average, patients with MGUS have a 1% per year risk of progression to MM. However, certain patients are considered at high risk of progression. What can you tell our patient about her risk of progression?**

Ask learners for risk factors for progression and write them on the white board as shown in Fig. 24.1.

Teaching points

- Risk factors that indicate a higher risk of progression to multiple myeloma include:
  - Level of M-spike, serum monoclonal protein level >1.5 g/dL.
  - Non-IgG MGUS (i.e., IgA, IgM, IgD MGUS).
  - Abnormal serum free light chain ratio (i.e., the ratio of kappa/lambda free light chains <0.25 or >1.65).
- At 20 years, the risk of progression for no risk factors, 1 risk factor, 2 risk factors, and 3 risk factors is 5%, 20%, 40%, and 60%, respectively.
- Our patient has 1 risk factor (level of M-spike is >1.5 g/dL), and, therefore, she has 20% risk of progression to multiple myeloma in the next 20 years.

G. **Patients with a monoclonal protein should be referred for a bone marrow biopsy and skeletal imaging if they have CRAB features or any of the above criteria that increase the risk of progression to malignancy. What is the appropriate skeletal imaging study to evaluate for lytic bone involvement in patients with monoclonal gammopathy?**

Continue the algorithm as shown in Fig. 24.1.

Teaching points

- In high-risk patients, skeletal x-ray, also known as a skeletal survey, is the first-line imaging study for detecting lytic bone lesions (note – these lesions are not detected on bone scan).
- The more sensitive skeletal MRI should be considered if there is clinical concern for bone disease despite negative skeletal x-ray.

H. **She is referred for bone marrow biopsy and skeletal survey based on the elevation in her M-spike >1.5 g/dL. Her bone marrow biopsy showed <10% plasma cells; her skeletal survey was normal. But let us say her biopsy had had an elevated percentage of plasma cells, 30%—what are the diagnostic criteria for smoldering myeloma (SMM) and MM?**

Continue the algorithm as shown in Fig. 24.1.

Teaching points

- Smoldering MM is a premalignant condition with an elevated risk of progression to MM. Patients with SMM are not immediately treated with chemotherapy, but due to their high risk of progression they are monitored much more closely.
- SMM: Bone marrow plasma cells 10–60% and/or M-spike, serum monoclonal protein >3 g/dL without CRAB features.
- MM: Bone marrow plasma cells >10% AND CRAB features OR bone marrow plasma cells >60% OR free light chain ratio <0.01 or >100.

I. **What are the diagnostic criteria for MGUS?**

List the criteria as shown in Fig. 24.1.

J. **Which labs should be used for following patients with MGUS and how frequently?**

List the labs as shown in Fig. 24.1.

- Labs: SPEP, free light chains, hematocrit, calcium, creatinine
- Frequency: Intermediate or high risk (2–3 high-risk criteria) → 6 months, then follow labs yearly; Low risk (0–1 high risk criteria) → 6 months, then follow SPEP every 1–2 years

K. **What clinical symptoms or physical exam findings would you monitor for in-patients with MGUS?**

List appropriate symptoms as listed by learners.

Teaching points
- Fatigue/generalized weakness
- Constitutional symptoms, also known as B-symptoms, (weight loss, fever, night sweats)
- Bone pain
- Neurologic symptoms (neuropathy, headache, dizziness, loss of vision/hearing)
- Lymphadenopathy, hepatosplenomegaly, restrictive cardiomyopathy, macroglossia

Return to objectives and emphasize key points
1. Identify the appropriate studies to evaluate and follow patients with MGUS
   - SPEP: Detects possible monoclonal protein components
   - Serum immunofixation: Determines immunoglobulin heavy and light chain associated with the M-spike
   - UPEP/urine immunofixation: Detects urine free kappa or lambda light chains (Jones Bence protein) that could potentially be nephrotoxic
   - Serum free light chains: Measures free kappa and free lambda in the serum. The ratio is the key. Helps in determining prognosis
   - CBC: Anemia
   - BMP: Creatinine
   - Serum calcium
   - Skeletal survey (can be deferred in asymptomatically low-risk patients)
2. Describe the diagnostic criteria for monoclonal gammopathy of uncertain significance (MGUS).
   - M-spike, serum monoclonal protein <3 g/dL (serum) AND
   - <10% clonal plasma cells in the bone marrow AND
   - no evidence of CRAB (hypercalcemia, renal insufficiency, anemia, or bone lesions)

3. Recognize the clinical features and laboratory manifestations concerning for progression to malignant stage (CRAB).
    - HyperCalcemia (calcium >11.5 mg/dL)
    - Renal insufficiency (creatinine >2 mg/dL)
    - Anemia (hemoglobin <10 g/dL)
    - Bone involvement (one or more osteolytic lesions detected on skeletal radiography)

Resources

1. Bird J, Behrens J, Westin J, et al. UK myeloma forum (UKMF) and Nordic myeloma study group (NMSG): guidelines for the investigation of newly detected M-proteins and the management of monoclonal gammopathy of undetermined significance (MGUS). Br J Haematol. 2009;147:22.
2. Kyle RA, Durie BG, Rajkumar SV, et al. Monoclonal gammopathy of undetermined significance (MGUS) and smoldering (asymptomatic) multiple myeloma: IMWG consensus perspectives risk factors for progression and guidelines for monitoring and management. Leukemia. 2010;24:1121.
3. Maciocia N, Wechalekar A, Yong K. Monoclonal gammopathy of uncertain significance (MGUS) and smoldering myeloma (SMM): a practical guide to management. Hematol Oncol. 2017;35(4):432–9. https://doi.org/10.1002/hon.2345.
4. Rajan AM, Rajkumar SV. Diagnostic evaluation of monoclonal gammopathy of undetermined significance. Eur J Haematol. 2013;91:561.
5. Rajkumar SV, Kyle RA, Therneau TM, Melton LJ 3rd, Bradwell AR, Clark RJ, Larson DR, Plevak MF, Dispenzieri A, Katzmann JA. Serum free light chain ratio is an independent risk factor for progression in monoclonal gammopathy of undetermined significance. Blood. 2005;106(3):812.

Chapter 25
Approach to Unintentional Weight Loss

Alexander Pratt and Caroline Rhoads

Learning Objectives

1. Identify when weight loss is clinically concerning.
2. Describe the necessary elements of a tailored review of systems (the 3Ms) and physical exam intended to elucidate the most common causes of unintentional weight loss.
3. Order necessary screening tests when no cause for the weight loss is apparent on review of systems or exam.
4. Formulate a management plan of careful monitoring if there is an absence of positive history, exam, or laboratory/imaging workup.
5. Explain to patients that after a negative preliminary workup, unintentional weight loss can be safely monitored over a period of 3–6 months.

Clinical Vignette: A 59-year-old male presents to your clinic for an annual wellness exam. On review of his vital signs you notice he has lost 9 kg since his last visit 4 months ago, dropping from 74 kg to 65 kg. You see the patient and find he was not aware of his weight loss and has no insights as to its cause.

A. **When is unintentional weight loss clinically significant?**

Write the definition on the white board.

Teaching points

- A loss of >5% body weight over a period of 6–12 months is significant.
- Unintentional weight loss is common, with 15–20% of adults experiencing it in their lifetime. Age-related physiologic changes typically result in no more than a loss of 0.1–0.2 kg/year after the age of 65 years.

A. Pratt (✉) · C. Rhoads
Harborview Medical Center, Department of Medicine, Division of General Internal Medicine, University of Washington, Seattle, WA, USA
e-mail: aepratt@uw.edu

S. Mookherjee et al. (eds.), *Chalk Talks in Internal Medicine*,
https://doi.org/10.1007/978-3-030-34814-4_25

- In several studies evaluating large cohorts of representative samples of adults in the United States and Israel, clinically significant weight loss resulted in an 18–24% increase in mortality over a follow-up period.

B. **What's the first step in evaluating unintentional weight loss?**

Start writing the algorithm as shown in Fig. 25.1.

Teaching points
- Most patients with unintentional weight loss do not have undiagnosed cancer.
- In the undifferentiated patient with unintentional weight loss, a good place to start is assessing for occult psychiatric disease or for the presence of a difficult psychosocial situation.
- Psychiatric illness, specifically depression, anorexia, or substance abuse disorders, is a very common cause of unintentional weight loss, accounting for 15-25% of cases.
- A focused assessment of the patient's psychiatric health should cover the following elements:
  - Does the patient pass screening for depression?
  - History of eating disorders?
  - Alcoholism or other substance abuse disorders?
  - Paranoia related to dementia or latent psychosis?
- In the absence of psychiatric illness, a quick assessment of the patient's psychosocial situation is also necessary, as several psychosocial problems can lead to weight loss:
  - Has the patient lost housing or their job recently?
  - Is the patient being abused?
  - Is the patient grieving?

C. **If there is no identifiable psychiatric illness or psychosocial issue, what are the elements of a high-yield focused history that is likely to yield an explanation?**

Continue the algorithm with the focused history; write the 3M's on the white board as shown in Fig. 25.1.

Teaching points
- The focused history can be organized into the 3Ms: Meds, Metabolism, and Major Organ Systems.
- A focused history in these areas is most likely to suggest an organic cause of the patient's weight loss.

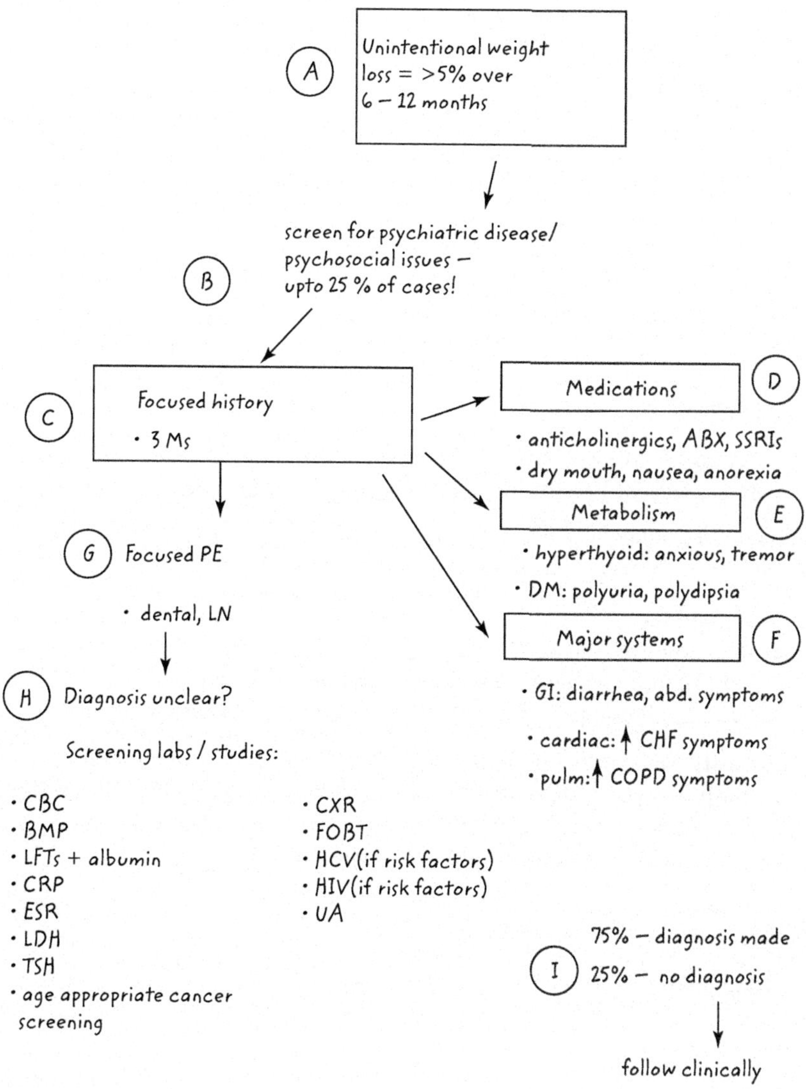

Fig. 25.1 Approach to unintentional weight loss, A–I

D. **The first of the "3Ms" is medications. Review of the patient's current medications and any side effects they may be causing. What are some common medications and medication side-effects that could result in unintentional weight loss?**

Ask learners for examples of medications that could be associated with weight loss and add them as appropriate.

Teaching points

- Anorexia—amantadine, antibiotics, antipsychotics, anticonvulsants, benzodiazepines, digoxin, metformin, opiates, selective serotonin reuptake inhibitors (SSRIs)
- Dry mouth—clonidine, loop diuretics, anticholinergics, antihistamines
- Dysphagia—doxycycline, iron, non-steroidal anti-inflammatory drugs (NSAIDs), potassium, bisphosphonates
- Nausea and vomiting—amantadine, antibiotics, digoxin, dopamine agonists, SSRIs, statins, metformin, bisphosphonates
- Dysgeusia—allopurinol, angiotensin converting enzymes (ACE) inhibitors, antibiotics, anticholinergics, antihistamines, calcium channel blockers (CCBs), spironolactone

E. **The second "M" is for metabolism. What are some common endocrine disorders that could result in weight loss, and what are their symptoms?**

Ask learners for examples of metabolic issues that could be associated with weight loss and add them as appropriate.

Teaching points

- Hyperthyroidism—anxiety, emotional lability, weakness, tremor, palpitations, heat intolerance, increased perspiration, increased appetite
- Diabetes Mellitus—polyuria, polydipsia, polyphagia, blurred vision

F. **The last "M" stands for major organ systems. Perform a focused review of the major organ systems to rule out new or worsening chronic conditions. Which organ systems are most likely to be contributing to worsening weight loss, and what symptoms would you assess for?**

Ask learners for examples of symptoms that could be associated with weight loss and add them under organ systems as appropriate.

Teaching points

- Gastrointestinal—abdominal pain, early satiety, dysphagia/odynophagia, diarrhea, steatorrhea
- Cardiac—worsened dyspnea on exertion, refractory angina, orthopnea, paroxysmal nocturnal dyspnea, and edema. Cardiac cachexia is an underappreciated cause of unintentional weight loss (e.g., New York Heart Association Class 4 heart failure)
- Pulmonary—worsening dyspnea, chronic cough, wheezing, hemoptysis, increasing O2 needs. Similar to cardiac issues, severe pulmonary disease will lead to weight loss (e.g., FEV1 <1 L in COPD)

G. **In addition to the usual physical exam, there are areas of focus that are more likely to suggest a cause of unintentional weight loss. What are some key exam maneuvers that are likely to yield a diagnosis?**

Teaching points

- Gastrointestinal: abdominal tenderness or mass
- Dental examination: loose teeth
- Lymphatics: cervical, clavicular, axillary, and inguinal lymph node examinations

H. **If your focused history and exam have not yielded any clues as to the cause of unintentional weight loss, it is reasonable to proceed to a screening laboratory workup. What labs and studies would you consider?**

Write down labs and studies as suggested by learners.

Teaching points

- In large cohorts of individuals with clinically significant unexplained weight loss and no historical/exam findings to suggest a cause, a negative laboratory workup was an effective way to "rule out" patients that did not require further invasive workup.
- Only in cases of a positive result should you consider a more extensive and focused (and expensive) workup that would include advanced imaging (CT, MRI, PET) or procedures (endoscopy/colonoscopy).
- It is also appropriate to assure that the patient is up to date on age-appropriate cancer screening.

I. **What's the likelihood that this combination of history, exam, and labs is going to yield a clue as to the cause of my patient's weight loss?**

Write down "75%" as shown in Fig. 25.1.

Teaching points

- Current research suggests that a focused history and exam, as well as the screening labs shown above, will identify a finding suggestive of an underlying organic cause in ~75% of the patients assessed.
- What about the patients that might have cancer? In the study referenced above, ALL patients that would later be found to have an occult malignancy had a positive finding either on history, exam or after bloodwork.

J. **What about the remaining ~25% of patients whose workup is completely negative? Is further testing indicated?**

Write "follow clinically" as shown in Fig. 25.1.

Teaching points

- Compared to patients with abnormal history/exam/laboratory findings, patients with a normal workup have a favorable prognosis.
- Studies have investigated the group of patients with a negative history/exam/laboratory workup by performing computed tomography, endo/colonoscopy, MRI, and radionuclide imaging. None of these patients were found to have an occult malignancy.

- It is appropriate and reasonable to carefully observe patients and follow-up on an interval of 3–6 months rather than initiate costly and invasive further workup.

Return to objectives and emphasize key points

1. Identify when weight loss is clinically important.
   - Highlight that only weight loss >5% over a period of 6–12 months is clinically relevant.
   - Remind learners that after the age of 65, a progressive loss of 0.1–0.2 kg/year is normal.
2. Describe the necessary elements of a tailored review of systems (the 3Ms) and physical exam intended to elucidate the most common causes of unintentional weight loss.
   - Highlight the necessity of screening for psychiatric illness and psychosocial challenges in the workup of unintentional weight loss.
   - Highlight the 3Ms as part of a focused history that should be conducted in any patient with unintentional weight loss.
   - Review the pertinent organ systems that should be examined closely (dental, gastrointestinal, lymphatic) in cases of unintentional weight loss.
3. Order necessary screening tests when no cause of the weight loss is apparent on history or exam.
   - Highlight the list of screening testing that should be considered when your review of systems is negative.
4. Recognize that in the absence of positive history, exam, or laboratory/imaging workup, unintentional weight loss can be safely observed over a period of 3–6 months.
   - Highlight that about 25% of all patients with unintentional weight loss will have no identifiable cause and that this generally portends a favorable prognosis.
   - Reinforce that these patients can be carefully observed for a period of 3–6 months before follow-up.

Resources

1. McMinn J, et al. Investigation and management of unintentional weight loss in older adults. BMJ. 2011;342:d1732.
2. Vanderschueren S, et al. The diagnostic spectrum of unintentional weight loss. Eur J Intern Med. 2005;16:160–4.
3. Gaddey H, et al. Unintentional weight loss in older adults. Am Fam Physician. 2014;89(9):718–22.

Chapter 26
Approach to Sepsis

Daniel Santovasi and Paul Cornia

Learning Objectives
1. Define sepsis
2. Stratify patients with sepsis according to the degree/level of risk
3. Describe the initial treatment strategies for sepsis

Clinical Vignette: A 61-year-old woman presents to your local emergency department with two days of cough, fever, and chills. At triage, her "sepsis screen" is positive.

A. **In broad terms, what is sepsis?**

Ask learners how they would define sepsis and then write down the accepted two-component definition.

Teaching points
- Historical context: The word sepsis dates back to the poems of Homer. It is derived from the word "sepo" meaning "I rot", speaking to the life-threatening nature of this condition.
- Per the Surviving Sepsis Campaign 2016, sepsis is defined as "Life-threatening organ dysfunction caused by dysregulated host response to infection."
- The consensus definition has changed over time, most recently moving on from a definition based on the systemic inflammatory response syndrome (SIRS). This does not require specific mention, but it is prudent to point out the definition is evolving.

B. **"Severe inflammatory response" sure sounds bad, again in broad strokes. Let's talk about what this means.**

Highlight the main components of the pathophysiology of sepsis as shown in Fig. 26.1.

D. Santovasi (✉) · P. Cornia
VA Puget Sound Health Care System, Department of Medicine, Division of General Internal Medicine, University of Washington, Seattle, WA, USA
e-mail: dsantov@uw.edu

S. Mookherjee et al. (eds.), *Chalk Talks in Internal Medicine*,
https://doi.org/10.1007/978-3-030-34814-4_26

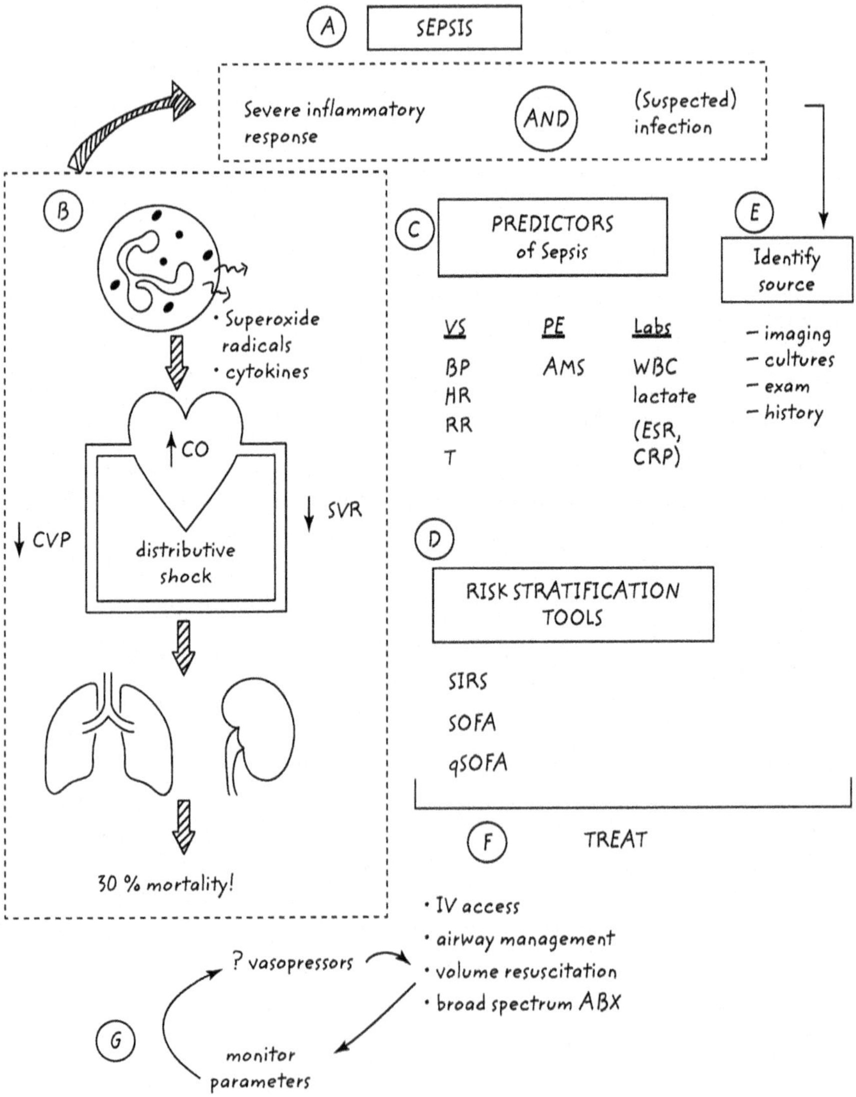

Fig. 26.1 Approach to sepsis: A–G

Teaching points

- The process begins with the neutrophil (the drawing shows toxic granulation), which releases superoxide radicals and causes the release of cytokines, which in the case of persistent and widespread inflammation….
- … results in distributive shock: low systemic vascular resistance (SVR), high cardiac output (CO), low central venous pressure (CVP)
- … and drives organ failure: the most commonly affected organs are the kidney (acute kidney injury) and lung (acute respiratory distress syndrome)
- The mortality rate of septic shock is high (> 30% in most studies) and increases with the number of organs involved, but is not related to the site of infection or to the causative organism

C. **Our patient had a positive "sepsis screen." What does this mean? No single test is sufficiently sensitive and specific to risk stratify patients with sepsis according to mortality risk. What markers do you think may be useful in identifying patients with sepsis?**

Start with the broad categories of vital signs, physical exam, and labs, and write down specific key indicators as the learners volunteer them.

Teaching points

- Key vital signs include blood pressure (BP), heart rate (HR), respiratory rate (RR), and temperature (T).
- Physical exam: Altered mental status (AMS) is a poor prognostic sign.
- Labs: Commonly followed labs include WBC, lactate, and acute-phase reactants, though changes in these labs are not specific for sepsis.

D. **Time is central in the recognition and management of sepsis. As such, a number of risk stratification tools are used to help rapidly identify sepsis using a combination of the vital signs, physical exam, and lab findings we just discussed. What tools have you seen used?**

List tools as they are suggested. Three key tools are SIRS, SOFA, and qSOFA.

Teaching Points

SIRS— VS + leukocytosis *Need 2 or more:*	**qSOFA**—VS and AMS *Need 2 or more:*	**SOFA**—complex, requires arterial blood gas results, performs better in ICU than qSOFA *Need increase in 2 or more:*
RR HR Temp Leukocytosis or bands	RR>22 Altered mentation Systolic BP<100	Respiratory: arterial pO2/ FiO2 ratio ("P/F ratio") Neuro: Glasgow coma scale (GCS) Cardiac: mean arterial pressure (MAP) Renal: creatinine Hepatic: bilirubin Heme: platelets

E. **Our patient's triage vital signs are blood pressure 90/60 mmHg, heart rate 110 beats per minute, respiratory rate 24 breaths per minute, and temperature 38.0 degrees Celsius.**

Overall, a combination of an assessment tool and clinical judgment are required for risk stratification. Are we worried about sepsis in our patient? Yes! But we also need to identify infection or suspicion of infection to diagnose this patient with sepsis—not all hypotension is caused by infection. How might you "search" for infection in this patient?

List the possible means by which an infectious source could be identified in this patient.

F. **On further history, the patient reports dyspnea in addition to cough. Portable chest X-ray is notable for an opacified right middle lobe. Blood cultures are obtained. She now definitely has sepsis. Let's treat her! What are the cornerstones of early sepsis management?**

Write down the key elements of early sepsis management.

Teaching points
- Treatment must begin with appropriate intravenous access and airway management.
- This is immediately followed by volume resuscitation and broad-spectrum antibiotic therapy.
- This treatment paradigm is based on the 2001 Early Goal Directed Therapy of sepsis and septic shock trial.

G. **Our patient receives two liters of crystalloid fluid, plus intravenous vancomycin and piperacillin/tazobactam. Her tachycardia improves to 100 bpm but her blood pressure is now 85/50 mmHg. What should be done next?**

Write down the next steps as shown in Fig. 26.1.

Teaching points
- Patients need to be monitored closely for their response to therapy; at a minimum, this will typically include monitoring of vital signs, mental status, and labs including lactate and markers of organ function (creatinine, liver function tests, among others).
- In this patient with persistent hypotension, the clinician needs to determine if the patient needs vasopressors and to what level of care the patient should be admitted (i.e., acute care vs. intensive care unit) to ensure adequate ongoing monitoring.

Our patient was started on norepinephrine and was admitted to the medical intensive care unit for continued monitoring and treatment.

Return to objectives and emphasize key points
1. Define sepsis. Return to the figure and emphasize that it is life-threatening sequelae of dysregulated inflammation in response to infection. Draw X's over the lungs and kidney to emphasize that these organ systems are commonly effected.

2. Identify components of the rapid risk stratification for sepsis.
   - Vital sign abnormalities, physical exam findings, lab tests
3. Identify the key early treatments of sepsis:
   - Rapid antibiotic administration
   - Fluid resuscitation with crystalloid and assessment of hemodynamic response

Resources

1. Seymour C, Liu V, Iwashyna T, Brunkhorst F, Rea T, Scherag A, et al. Assessment of clinical criteria for sepsis. JAMA. 2016;315(8):762.
2. Raith E, Udy A, Bailey M, McGloughlin S, MacIsaac C, Bellomo R, et al. Prognostic accuracy of the SOFA score, SIRS criteria, and qSOFA score for in-hospital mortality among adults with suspected infection admitted to the intensive care unit. JAMA. 2017;317(3):290.
3. Funk D, Parrillo J, Kumar A. Sepsis and septic shock: a history. Crit Care Clin. 2009;25(1):83–101.
4. Wanahita A, Goldsmith E, Musher D. Conditions associated with leukocytosis in a tertiary care hospital, with particular attention to the role of infection caused by Clostridium difficile. Clin Infect Dis. 2002;34(12):1585–92.
5. Rivers E, Nguyen B, Havstad S, Ressler J, Muzzin A, Knoblich B, et al. Early goal-directed therapy in the treatment of severe sepsis and septic shock. N Engl J Med. 2001;345(19):1368–77.
6. Marino PL. The ICU book. Philadelphia: Lippincott Williams & Wilkins; 2014.
7. Rhodes A, Evans L, Alhazzani W, Levy M, Antonelli M, Ferrer R, et al. Surviving sepsis campaign: international guidelines for management of sepsis and septic shock: 2016. Intensive Care Med. 2017;43(3):304–77.
8. Zahar J-R, et al. Outcomes in severe sepsis and patients with septic shock: pathogen species and infection sites are not associated with mortality. Crit Care Med. 2011;39:1886–95.

Chapter 27
Approach to Fever in the Hospitalized Patient

Meghaan Hawes and Alexandra Moretti Morrison

Learning Objectives

1. Develop a differential diagnosis for infectious and non-infectious causes of fever in a hospitalized patient.
2. Describe the diagnostic approach to determining the cause of fever in the hospital.
3. Explain the initial management of fever in a hospitalized patient.

Clinical Vignette: A 75-year-old man with a history of hypertension and gout is admitted to the hospital after a motor vehicle accident. He has no known allergies and takes only aspirin and lisinopril. He is diagnosed with a right femur fracture and undergoes surgical repair of his fracture. A Foley catheter is placed prior to his surgery due to immobility. Following surgical blood loss, he requires a blood transfusion on post-operative day 1. On post-operative day 3, he develops a temperature of 39.2 °C with a heart rate of 118 and a new oxygen requirement.

A. **How do we define fever? Does our patient have a fever?**

Write down the definition to start the algorithm in Fig. 27.1.

Teaching points

- Fever is defined as body temperature of 38.3 °C (101 °F) or higher.
- In hospitalized patients, a sustained change in baseline temperature, including what would be considered "low grade" fevers (less than 38.3 °C), would be cause for further evaluation.

M. Hawes (✉) · A. M. Morrison
Harborview Medical Center, Department of Medicine, Division of General Internal Medicine, University of Washington, Seattle, WA, USA
e-mail: meghaan@uw.edu

S. Mookherjee et al. (eds.), *Chalk Talks in Internal Medicine*,
https://doi.org/10.1007/978-3-030-34814-4_27

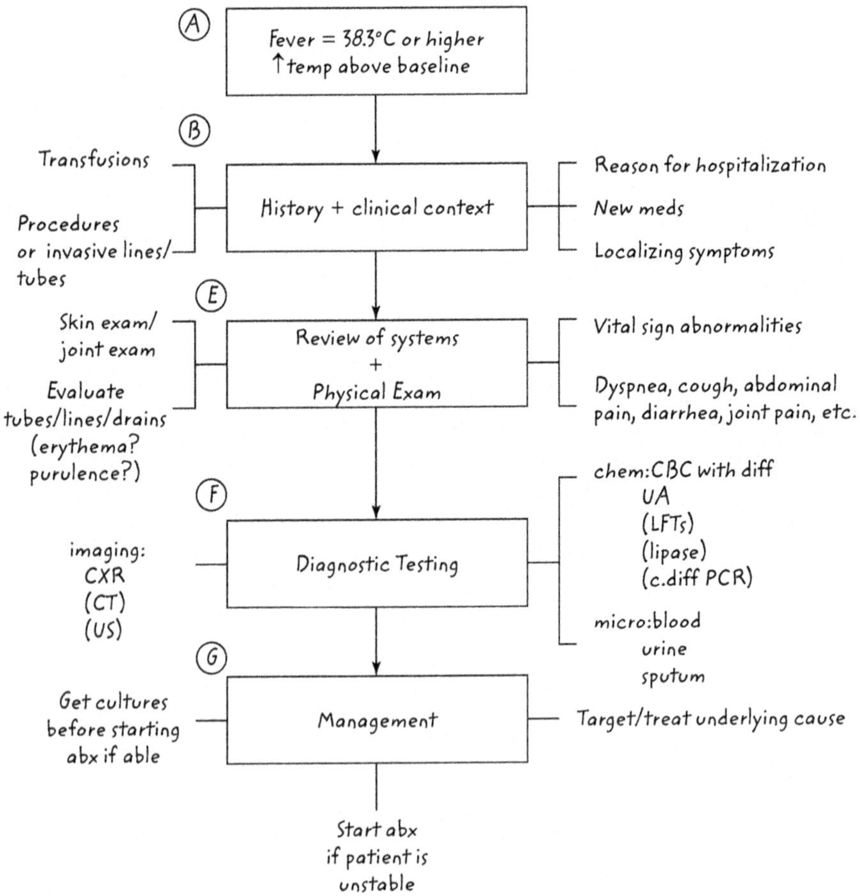

Fig. 27.1 Fever in a hospitalized patient, A, B, E–G

B. **Our patient's temperature of 39.2 °C meets criteria for a fever. When assessing the cause of a fever in a hospitalized patient, consider the patient's clinical context. What additional information would you want to know?**

Write down relevant suggestions from the learners.

Teaching points

- Why is the patient in the hospital?
- Is there hemodynamic or respiratory instability in addition to a fever?
- Does the patient have any new symptoms that might localize a fever source?
- Has the patient had any recent procedures or indwelling lines that might predispose them to infection risk? (e.g., surgery, prior or current CVC or urinary catheter)
- Has the patient started any new medications or received blood products?
- Are there any aspects of the patient's history that might put them at risk for fever? (e.g., substance use, history of rheumatologic condition or malignancy, recent sick contacts, recent trauma)

C. **When developing a differential diagnosis for fever in the hospital, consider both infectious and non-infectious etiologies. What are some potential infectious causes of fever in the hospital? Based on our patient's clinical presentation, which infections could be causing his fever?**

Draw the human body diagram as shown in Fig. 27.2 *to identify areas potentially affected by infections as they are mentioned, adding any that are missed.*

Teaching points

- "Healthcare-associated infections" include hospital-acquired pneumonia, ventilator-associated pneumonia, catheter-associated urinary tract infection (UTI), central line-associated bloodstream infection, and surgical-site infection. This group of infections affects 1 in 25 hospitalized patients on any given day, based on CDC estimates.
- By definition, hospital-acquired pneumonia occurs ≥48 h after admission in non-ventilated patients; ventilator – associated pneumonia develops ≥48 h after tracheal intubation.
- Other infections that can develop or present in the hospital setting:
  - *C. diff* colitis.
  - Urinary tract infection (UTI).
  - Soft tissue infection (abscess, cellulitis).
  - Bloodstream infection not related to a central line.
  - Spontaneous bacterial peritonitis.
  - Endocarditis (less likely, but should be considered in a patient with a history of a bloodstream infection or risk factors such as intravenous drug use).
  - Viral infections (upper respiratory, meningitis) occurring prior to hospital admission may present with fever in the hospital, given potential delays in symptom onset after an incubation period.

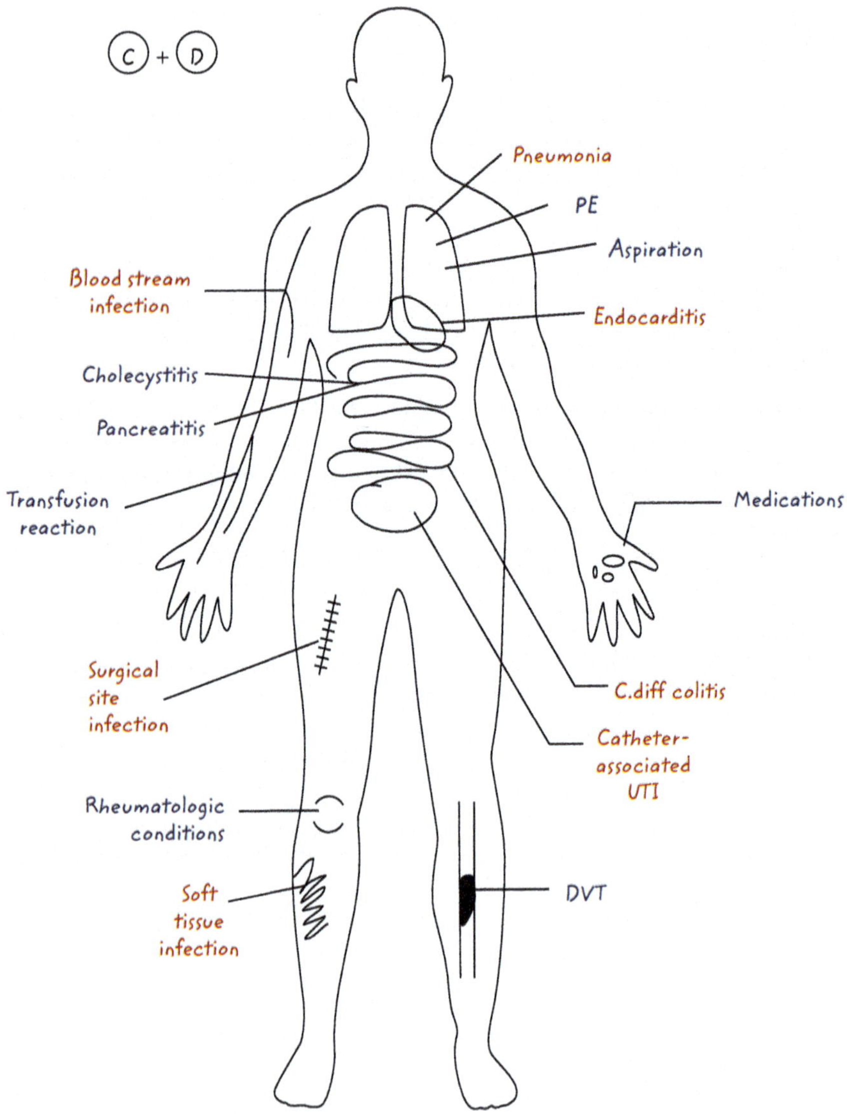

Fig. 27.2 Fever in a hospitalized patient, C, D

- For our patient, intubation during his surgery puts him at risk for developing pneumonia, and urinary catheterization puts him at risk for a catheter-associated UTI. Surgical-site infection should also be considered, given his recent femur fracture repair.

D. **What are some non-infectious causes of fever in the hospital? Are there any non-infectious causes of fever to consider in our patient?**

Use Fig. 27.2 *to identify areas of the body affected by non-infectious causes of fever as they are mentioned, adding any that are missed.*

Teaching points

- Medications/"drug fever"—common culprit medication categories included antibiotics (penicillins, cephalosporins, minocycline, TMP-SMX, vancomycin, nitrofurantoin), anticonvulsants (carbamazepine, phenytoin), immunosuppressants (azathioprine, mycophenolate mofetil, sulfasalazine), and others (allopurinol, metoclopramide).
- More severe complications related to medications that also cause fever include serotonin syndrome, neuroleptic malignant syndrome, and malignant hyperthermia.
- Inflammatory conditions (e.g., pancreatitis, acalculous cholecystitis, alcoholic hepatitis, post-operative inflammation, aspiration).
- Thromboembolic disease (DVT, PE).
- Fat embolism.
- Transfusion reactions.
- Rheumatologic conditions (gout flare, vasculitis).
- Substance use or withdrawal (alcohol withdrawal, methamphetamine intoxication).
- Severity of fever may help distinguish potential etiology. For example, fevers >41 °C (106 °F) are often due to non-infectious causes, like medications.
- Our patient is at risk for venous thromboembolism (VTE), following his traumatic injury and immobility from his fracture. He could also have developed a fat embolism after his trauma and long bone fracture. A transfusion-related fever should be considered, but is less likely, since his fever occurred 2 days after he received blood. Based on his medical history, a gout flare is also possible, although would be low on the differential unless he had associated joint symptoms. His medication list should be reviewed to assess for any new medications that could cause drug fever.

E. **After reviewing the patient's history, clinical context, and potential exposures in the hospital that would put him at risk for a fever, the next steps in pursuing a diagnosis are a thorough review of systems and physical exam. What signs or symptoms will you assess for in your examination?**

Return to Fig. 27.1 *and write down the important signs and symptoms as they are suggested.*

Teaching points

- Vital sign abnormalities: hypotension, tachycardia, tachypnea, hypoxia.
- Physical exam findings: altered mental status, rhonchi/rales, new cardiac murmur, abdominal tenderness, asymmetric lower extremity swelling, joint swelling or erythema, skin rashes or breakdown, erythema or purulence around incisions, indwelling lines, tubes, or drains.
- Symptoms: dyspnea, productive cough, dysuria, joint pain.

F. **Our patient is tachycardic and tachypneic. On physical exam, he is confused and lethargic. Ronchi are auscultated in his left lower lung field. His surgical incision site is clean and dry, and does not have any surrounding erythema, although his right leg appears more swollen than his left leg. Based on exam findings and the most likely causes of fever, additional diagnostic testing should be considered. What are some chemistry, microbiology, or imaging studies you would order for our patient? Are there any other studies you might obtain for a patient in the hospital with a fever?**

Write down appropriate labs and studies as they are suggested.

Teaching points

- Chemistry: CBC w/differential, urinalysis.
- Micro: sputum, urine, blood cultures (remember to obtain blood cultures from indwelling lines in addition to a peripheral sample).
- Imaging: chest x-ray; venous ultrasound, CT PE (based on signs/symptoms of DVT or PE).
- Additional studies that could be considered based on a patient's presentation or symptoms include lipase, LFTs, *C. diff* stool testing, CT abdomen, or soft tissue ultrasound.

G. **Our patient's labs and imaging demonstrate a leukocytosis and left lower lobe consolidation. Management of fever should be targeted to the most likely cause based on the workup. What next steps would you take to manage his fever? Would you start any medications?**

Write down the key management steps as shown in the figure.

Teaching points

- If infection is suspected, consider whether the patient is stable enough to obtain culture data prior to starting antibiotics. If able, it is best to obtain cultures prior to starting empiric antibiotics to help guide therapy.
- Choose empiric broad-spectrum antibiotics based on a patient's individual risk factors (e.g. prior MRSA infection or antibiotic exposure) and most likely source of infection.
- Consider removal of indwelling lines if there is a high suspicion for catheter-related infection.
- If non-infectious fever is suspected or diagnosed, treat the underlying cause (e.g., discontinue potential offending medications, treat PE).

- Consider antipyretics to relieve discomfort from fever, but they are not routinely necessary.
- Based on his time in the hospital, our patient meets criteria for a hospital-acquired pneumonia. Next steps would include obtaining blood and sputum cultures if they have not yet been obtained and starting broad-spectrum antibiotics to cover nosocomial organisms.

Return to objectives and emphasize key points

1. Develop a differential diagnosis for infectious and non-infectious causes of fever in a hospitalized patient (*circle or underline each of the following common causes on your diagram*).
    - Hospital-acquired pneumonia
    - Ventilator-associated pneumonia
    - Catheter-associated urinary tract infection
    - Central line-associated bloodstream infection
    - Surgical site infection
    - *C. diff* colitis
    - DVT/PE
    - Medications
    - Transfusion reactions
2. Describe the diagnostic approach to determining the cause of fever in the hospital.
    - Review the patient's history and clinical context.
    - Perform a thorough review of systems and physical exam.
    - Evaluate any indwelling lines, tubes, drains, and surgical sites.
    - Pursue diagnostic testing (chemistry, microbiology, imaging) based on the history and exam findings.
3. Explain the initial management of fever in a hospitalized patient.
    - Treat the most likely underlying cause, based on workup.
    - Start antibiotics if infection is suspected, especially if the patient is clinically unstable.
    - Try to get cultures before starting antibiotics.

Resources

1. O'Grady NP, Barie PS, Bartlett JG, Bleck T, Carroll K, Kalil AC, et al. Guidelines for evaluation of new fever in critically ill adult patients: 2008 update from the American College of Critical Care Medicine and the Infectious Diseases Society of America. Crit Care Med. 2008;36(4):1330–49.
2. Centers for Disease Control and Prevention. Heathcare-associated infections [Internet]. Atlanta: CDC; 2016. Available from: https://www.cdc.gov/hai/surveillance/index.html.

3. Kalil AC, Metersky ML, Klompas M, Muscedere J, Sweeney DA, Palmer LB, et al. Management of adults with hospital-acquired and ventilator-associated pneumonia: 2016 clinical practice guidelines by the infectious disease Society of America and the American Thoracic Society. Clin Infect Dis. 2016;63(5):e61–111.
4. Patel RA, Gallagher JC. Drug Fever. Pharmacotherapy. 2010;30(1):57–69.

Chapter 28
Approach to Genital Lesions

Toby Sinton and Joyce Wipf

Learning Objectives
1. Generate a systematic approach to the various causes of genital lesions.
2. Differentiate between ulcerated and non-ulcerated infectious lesions.
3. Appreciate the essentials of testing for sexually transmitted infections leading to genital lesions.
4. Consider the common causes of noninfectious lesions and features that suggest multisystem disease or malignancy.

Clinical Vignette: Mr. Jones is a 30-year-old man with a history of post-traumatic stress disorder (PTSD) and chronic right knee pain who comes to clinic to establish primary care. He reports that a "spot" appeared on his penis about 1 week ago. This is the first time he has had something like this.

A. **Genital lesions cover a wide spectrum of etiologies. When thinking through the potential differential diagnosis, it can be helpful to first think about the infectious vs non-infectious potential causes. What questions would you want to ask to help you identify the patient's risk of a sexually transmitted infection (STI)?**

Ask learners to list specific sexual history questions they would ask the patient.

Teaching points
- It is imperative to take a detailed sexual history including if the patient has sex with men, women, or both, and their sexual practices.
- Also consider getting a travel history, including asking about sex tourism.
- Inquire regarding if they have a history of sexually transmitted infections.

T. Sinton (✉) · J. Wipf
VA Puget Sound Health Care System, Department of Medicine, Division of General Internal Medicine, University of Washington, Seattle, WA, USA
e-mail: tsinton@uw.edu

S. Mookherjee et al. (eds.), *Chalk Talks in Internal Medicine*,
https://doi.org/10.1007/978-3-030-34814-4_28

B. **He has had three new sexual partners in the past 4 months, one male and two females. He engages in oral, vaginal, and anal insertive sex, and uses condoms 50% of the time. He has not travelled outside the United States. On physical examination, he appears well and has a single ulcer on the anterior shaft of the penis. It measures 1 × 1.5 cm and is well demarcated. His history makes a sexually transmitted infection most likely (but be mindful that even in the setting of a high-risk sexual history, your patient's skin findings could be due to a non-infectious etiology). Infectious genital lesions can be further divided into groups based on if they are ulcerated or non-ulcerated. Ulcerated lesions can be further classified as painful or painless. What are the two most common infectious causes of ulcerated genital lesions? Which one is painful and which one is painless?**

Write out headings for "infectious," "non-infectious," "ulcerated," "non-ulcerated," "painful," and "non-painful," as shown in Fig. 28.1. *Add "HSV" and "syphilis" as they are suggested by the learners.*

Teaching points

- The most common cause of ulcerated genital lesions in the United States (by far) is HSV (herpes simplex virus). The lesion is typically painful.
- The second most common STI causing ulcers in the United States is syphilis (*Treponema pallidum*), which is on the rise for both men and women. The vast majority of new cases are in men (>80%), particularly in men who have sex with men (MSM). The chancre of syphilis should be non-tender.
- Chancroid (*Haemophilus ducreyi*) classically presents as a painful ulcer. While common in the developing world, it is extremely uncommon in the developed world (with seven—7!—total cases reported to the CDC in 2016). It generally should only be considered in those from/travelled to sub-Saharan Africa, Southeast Asia, and Latin America.
- Lymphogranuloma venereum—LGV—(*Chlamydia trachomatis*) and granuloma inguinale—donovanosis—(*Klebsiella granulomatis*) present as painless ulcers. These are also very uncommon in the United States. These should be very low on the differential.

C. **What other physical exam findings point to different infectious causes of ulcerated lesions?**

Add the classic findings for HSV, syphilis, and chancroid.

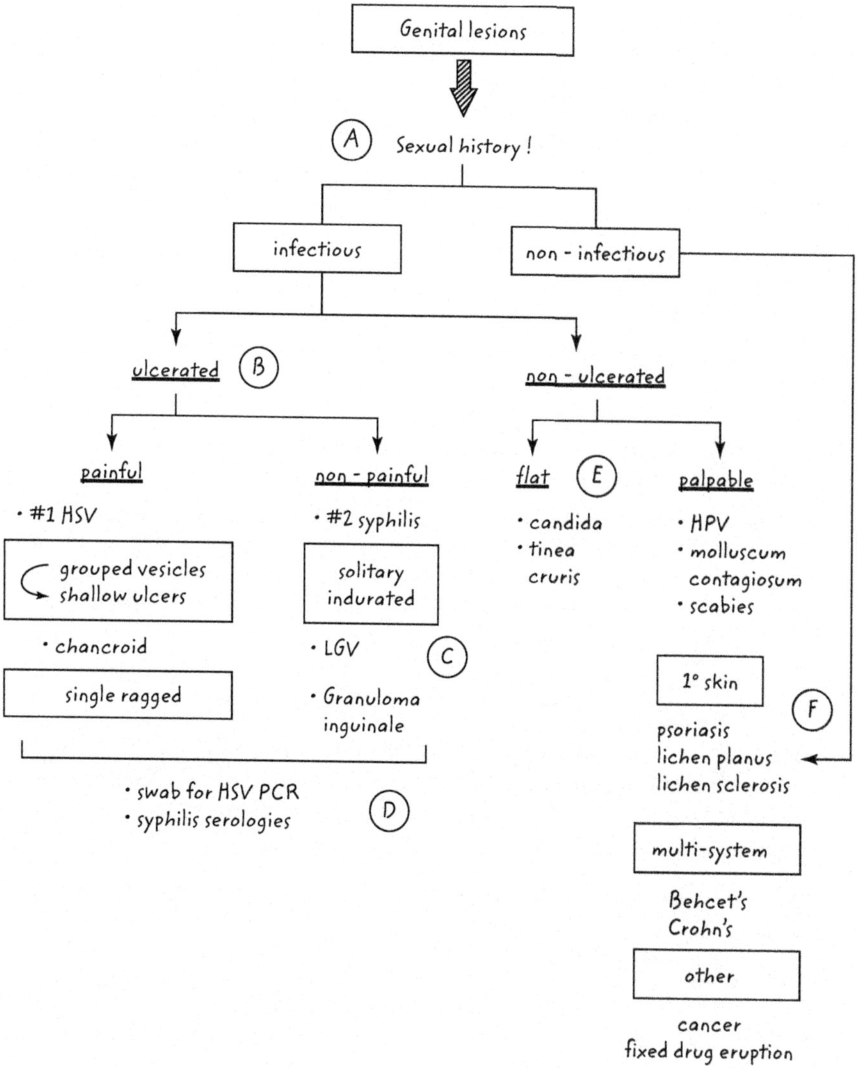

Fig. 28.1 Approach to genital lesions, A–F

Teaching points

- HSV classically presents as a grouping of vesicles that then evolve into shallow ulcerations that are typically painful (though they can be painless!).
- The chancre of syphilis should be nontender and indurated, and is usually solitary (rarely several lesions can occur at once). Nontender inguinal adenopathy may also be present.
- Chancroid classically presents as a single, painful, indurated ulcer with "ragged" borders (though multiple ulcerations can also be present). Also look out for tender, unilateral inguinal lymphadenopathy, which can become fluctuant.
- But again, keep in mind that while being familiar with the classic presentations of various genital sexually transmitted infections is helpful, there is a large amount of overlap in how different infections present.

D. **If you think the ulcer is due to an STI, what testing would you order?**

Write down tests for ulcerated lesions as shown in Fig. 28.1.

- If there is any suspicion that the lesion is or could be from an STI, obtain a swab that can be sent for HSV PCR, culture, or direct fluorescence antibody testing.
- Serology for syphilis—The interpretation can be confusing. In part, this is because labs use both treponemal antibody tests and non-treponemal tests, and different labs perform these tests in different orders.
- Nontreponemal tests have high sensitivity. These include the Rapid Plasma Reagin (RPR) and Venereal Disease Research Laboratory (VDRL) methods. These tests can be done quantitatively (serial dilutions), which informs both the extent of infection (more dilutions = more extensive infection) and the success of treatment (declining titers over time with antibiotics).
- Treponemal antibody tests have high sensitivity and specificity. Results are not quantified, but reported as reactive/nonreactive/inconclusive.

E. **Don't forget about the nonulcerated infectious lesions! These can be further characterized based on physical exam as flat or palpable. What are some of the most common nonulcerated infectious genital lesions? Which are characteristically flat, and which are typically palpable?**

Write down the causes of flat and palpable non-ulcerated lesions as suggested by learners.

Teaching points

- Both candida and tinea cruris are flat lesions. They can be pruritic or painful, and KOH preparation with microscopy confirms the diagnosis: pseudohyphae and yeast forms for candida and hyphae for tinea. Both are treated with antifungals (usually topical; oral if severe disease or immunosuppression).
- Candida has clearly demarcated, confluent, erythematous patches. Look for discrete red, flat lesions on the periphery of the rash (satellite lesions).
- Tinea cruris causes plaques that are well-demarcated, ranging in color from red to brown. Look for scale and central clearing; tinea rarely affects genital skin itself.

- The genital warts of HPV (human papilloma virus) are palpable. Typically, the diagnosis is made clinically, but they can be biopsied if questionable.
- *Molluscum contagiosum* is a common virus in children and young adults. Look for firm, flesh-colored, "pearly" papules with central umbilication (umbilication should be present on at least some lesions).
- Scabies is intensely pruritic, often worse at night. Look for small, erythematous papules and burrows.

F. **You diagnose Mr. Jones with syphilis and treat him with benzathine penicillin G 2.4 million units IM (and test him for other STIs!). He does well and comes back to see you a year later with a new "spot" on his penis that has been growing over the past few months. It is quite itchy. He has had no sexual partners since his last visit with you. On exam, you see a 1 cm scaling plaque on the dorsum of the glans without any exudate. What are some of the noninfectious causes of genital lesions?**

Write down "primary skin issues," "multi-system," and "other" as shown in Fig. 28.1, *and add diagnoses to the appropriate category as they are suggested by the learners.*

Teaching points

- This is a large, heterogeneous group that includes primary inflammatory skin conditions, cutaneous manifestations of systemic disease, and many other processes.
- Primary inflammatory skin conditions include psoriasis, lichen planus, and lichen sclerosis. Performing a full skin examination may be helpful in identifying other areas of involvement and making the diagnosis.
- Detailed past medical history and review of systems may be needed to identify multisystem disease associated with genital skin lesions such as Behçet disease, and Crohn's disease.
- Make sure to ask about medications (including over-the-counter) to rule out a fixed-drug eruption (look for erythema and blistering).
- The vast majority of genital malignancies are squamous cell carcinoma, which can be nonspecific in appearance and mimic other conditions (e.g., psoriasis). If the lesion looks questionable, is growing quickly, or is not responding to treatment, it should be biopsied.

Return to objectives

1. Differentiate between ulcerated and nonulcerated infectious lesions:

    - HSV: most common ulcerated lesion in the United States.
    - Syphilis: second most common ulcerated lesion in the United States.
    - Chancroid, LGV, granuloma inguinale: extremely uncommon in the United States.
    - Candida and tinea have overlapping features on exam, and are treated similarly
    - HPV and *Molluscum contagiosum* can be diagnosed clinically

2. Appreciate the essentials of testing for STIs:
   - Genital ulcers should be swabbed to be tested for HSV.
   - Testing for syphilis is based on a combination of serologic tests including treponemal and non-treponemal tests.
3. Consider common causes of noninfectious lesions and features that suggest multisystem disease or malignancy:
   - Inflammatory: psoriasis and lichen planus
   - Multisystem disease: Behçet (oral ulcers), Crohn's disease (GI involvement)
   - Other: drug eruptions (blisters), rapid growth/unusual appearance (malignancy)

Resources

1. Augenbraun, Michael. Syphilis and the nonvenereal treponematoses. Infectious Diseases: The Clinicians' Guide to Diagnosis, Treatment, and Prevention, 2017.
2. Centers for Disease Control and Prevention. 2016 sexually transmitted diseases surveillance. Atlanta: CDC; 2010.
3. Klausner JD, Hook EW. Current diagnosis & treatment. Sex Transm Dis. 2007;
4. Roett MA, Mayor MT, Uduhiri KA. Diagnosis and management of genital ulcers. AAFP. 2012;85(3):254–62.
5. Rosen T. Update on genital lesions. JAMA. 2003;290(8):1001–5.
6. Wolff K, Johnson RA, Saavedra AP. Fitzpatrick's color atlas and synopsis of clinical dermatology. 7th ed. New York: McGraw-Hill; 2013.

Chapter 29
Approach to Pulmonary Embolism

Mellena Giday and Traci Takahashi

Learning Objectives
1. Describe pulmonary embolism and the risk factors for PE (Virchow's Triad).
2. Recognize the common signs and symptoms of PE.
3. Utilize a systematic approach to evaluate a suspected PE based on its pre-test probability.
4. Selectively use D-dimer testing in the diagnosis of PE.

Clinical Vignette: A 35-year-old woman presents to the emergency department with difficulty breathing and chest pain after returning from vacation in Europe. She states that she takes no medications apart from birth control pills. She recalls a distant relative had "clots in his legs" once, but she has no other family history. On physical exam, she was found to have a heart rate of 110, blood pressure of 110/85, and oxygen saturation of 89% on ambient air. Cardiopulmonary exam was unremarkable. Bilateral lower extremities were normal on physical exam.

A. **What is a pulmonary embolism?**

Write down the definition and types of PE as shown in Fig. 29.1.

Teaching points
- Definition: Obstruction of a pulmonary artery or its branches by material traveling from somewhere else in the body.
- A thromboembolism or blood clot is the most common type of pulmonary embolism; rarer causes include air, fat, and tumor.

M. Giday (✉)
Harborview Medical Center, Department of Medicine, Division of General Internal Medicine, University of Washington, Seattle, WA, USA
e-mail: mellenag@uw.edu

T. Takahashi
VA Puget Sound Health Care System, Department of Medicine, Division of General Internal Medicine, University of Washington, Seattle, WA, USA

S. Mookherjee et al. (eds.), *Chalk Talks in Internal Medicine*,
https://doi.org/10.1007/978-3-030-34814-4_29

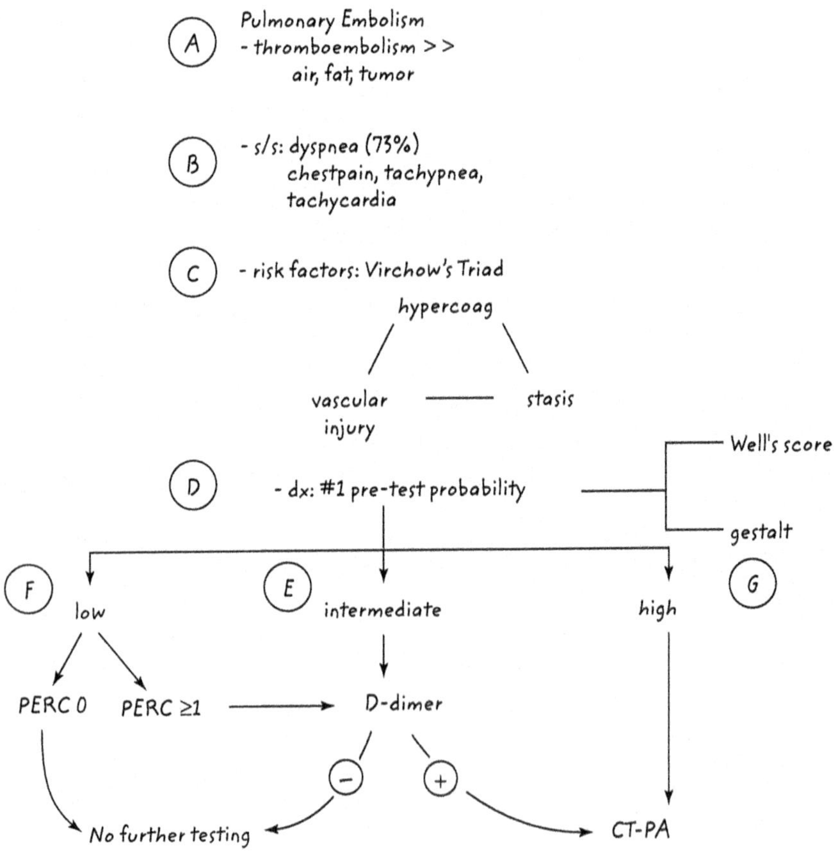

Fig. 29.1 Approach to pulmonary embolism: A–G

- For purposes of this talk, PE = pulmonary thromboembolism (blockage of a pulmonary artery or its branches from a blood clot traveling from somewhere else in the body).

B. **What signs and symptoms of pulmonary embolism does this patient have?**

Write down the key signs and symptoms as suggested by learners.

Teaching points

- Dyspnea and pleuritic chest pain, which are the most common symptoms with estimated frequency of 73% and 66%, respectively.
- Other signs and symptoms can include tachypnea (70%), cough (37%), tachycardia (30%), lower extremity swelling (28%), hemoptysis (13%), hypotension, and elevated jugular venous pressure (JVD) (see Chest, 1991—full reference below).
- This patient's signs and symptoms are consistent with PE: difficulty breathing, pleuritic chest pain, tachycardia, hypoxia.
- It can be difficult to diagnose PE because the signs and symptoms can be non-specific and not always present.

C. **Venous thromboembolism is thought to originate from alterations in blood flow, vascular injury, or hypercoagulable states. These factors are referred to as Virchow's triad. What risk factors for pulmonary embolism does this patient have? What other risk factors would you want to ask patients about?**

Write down the risk factors as suggested by the learners.

Teaching points

- The patient has several risk factors, including estrogen/oral contraceptive therapy and recent long-distance travel (defined as flights over 4 h).
- Additional factors that can lead to hypercoagulability include malignancy, sepsis, nephrotic syndrome, or genetic hypercoagulable state.
- Additional factors that can lead to stasis include paralysis and prolonged immobility.
- Additional factors that can lead to vascular wall injury include surgery, trauma, and intravascular catheters.
- But of course, a person can still have a PE without any identifiable risk factors.

D. **What is the first step in deciding which tests or studies to use to diagnose pulmonary embolism?**

Write down "pre-test probability." Poll the learners regarding their clinical gestalt regarding the probability the patient has a PE and then compare this to her Well's Score. Re-creating the Well's Score on the board is an option.

Teaching points

- The first step is to determine the pretest probability of the patient having a PE by using a decision tool or clinical gestalt.
- Well's Score and Geneva Score are scoring systems used to risk stratify patients suspected of pulmonary embolism into low, moderate/intermediate, or high using various clinical criteria.

- Clinical gestalt of an experienced clinician has similar accuracy to that of the decision tools.

Well's score: Low risk <2 points, moderate (intermediate) risk 2–6 points, high risk >6 points		
Clinical signs and symptoms of DVT	No	Yes (+3)
PE is #1 diagnosis or equally likely	No	Yes (+3)
Heart rate >100	No	Yes (+1.5)
Immobilization at least 3 days or surgery in the previous 4 weeks	No	Yes (+1.5)
Previous, objectively diagnosed PE or DVT	No	Yes (1.5)
Hemoptysis	No	Yes (1+)
Malignancy w/treatment with in 6 months or palliative	No	Yes (1+)

E. **Our patient has an "intermediate" probability of having a PE based on her Well's Score. What test should we order next?**

Continue the algorithm as shown in Fig. 29.1 *for intermediate probability.*

- The intermediate probability group should next undergo D-dimer testing using a high sensitivity D-dimer test.
- D-dimer is a degradation product of fibrin, used in the clotting process.
- D-dimer testing is very useful in ruling out PE in low and intermediate probability groups (highly sensitive for venous thromboembolism but not very specific).
- Normal D-dimer is <500 ng/mL or an age-adjusted value of < (age ×10 ng/mL) for pts >50 years.
- D-dimer testing should be used with caution in patients that have a malignancy, are hospitalized, elderly, or pregnant.
- No further testing is needed if the D-dimer is normal in the low or intermediate probability group.
- If D-dimer is elevated, then proceed to CT-Pulmonary Angiogram.

F. **What would your next step be if she had a low probability of PE based on the Well's score?**

Continue the algorithm as shown in Fig. 29.1 *for low probability.*

Teaching points

- The pulmonary embolism rule-out criteria (PERC) identify patients with low clinical probability, in which case the risk of unnecessary testing outweighs the risk of PE.
- PERC is validated in clinical settings that have a low prevalence of PE.
- PERC scoring has eight criteria: age ≥50, SPO2 <95% on room air, heart rate ≥100, prior DVT/PE, hemoptysis, unilateral leg swelling, recent surgery/trauma, or exogenous estrogen use.
- All eight criteria must be negative to warrant no further testing. If any of the criteria are positive, additional workup is needed with D-dimer testing.

G. **And finally, what lab/study is indicated for patients with a high probability of PE?**

Complete the algorithm as shown in Fig. 29.1 *for high probability of PE.*

- Proceed directly to a CT-angiogram. There is no need to get a D-dimer first.
- For patients who have contrast dye contraindications, such as renal insufficiency or allergic reactions, a ventilation-perfusion (VQ) scan can be used.

Return to objectives

1. Describe pulmonary embolism and the risk factors for PE (Virchow's Triad).
2. Recognize the common signs and symptoms of PE.
3. Use a systematic approach to evaluate a suspected PE
    - Determine if a patient is low probability, intermediate probability, or high probability for PE using clinical gestalt or a decision tool.
    - Low probability group➔use the PERC scoring.
    - If any PERC criteria are positive➔proceed to D-dimer testing. If D-dimer is normal, no further testing is required. If it is abnormal, then move to chest imaging.
    - Intermediate group➔go directly to D-dimer testing. If it is normal, no further testing is required. If it is positive, obtain chest imaging.
    - High probability group➔go directly to chest imaging.
4. Understand the D-dimer test and its role in the diagnosis of PE.
    - Review that D-dimer testing is highly sensitive for venous thromboembolism.
    - Reiterate that D-dimer testing might not be a useful test in hospitalized, elderly, pregnant, or patients with malignancy.

Resources

1. Giordano N, Jansson P, Young M, Hagan K, Kabrhel C. Epidemiology, pathophysiology, stratification, and natural history of pulmonary embolism. Tech Vasc Interv Radiol. 2017;20(3):135–40.
2. Agnelli G, Becattini C. Acute pulmonary embolism. N Engl J Med. 2010;363:266–74. https://doi.org/10.1056/NEJMra0907731.
3. Stein P, Terrin M, Hales C, Palevsky H, Saltzman H, Thompson T, et al. Clinical, laboratory, roentgenographic, and electrographic findings in patients with acute pulmonary embolism and no preexisting cardiac or pulmonary disease. Chest. 1991;100(3):598–603.
4. Raja AS, Greenberg JO, Qaseem A, Denberg TD, Fitterman N, Schuur JD, et al. Evaluation of patients with suspected acute pulmonary embolism: best practice advice from the Clinical Guidelines Committee of the American College of Physicians. Ann Intern Med. 2015;163:701–11. https://doi.org/10.7326/M14-1772.
5. Thompson BT, Kabrhel C. Overview of acute pulmonary embolism in adults. In: Post TW, editor. Up to date [Internet]. Waltham: Up To Date; 2016. Available from: www.uptodate.com Subscription required.
6. Konstantinides S. Acute pulmonary embolism. N Engl J Med. 2008;359(26):2804–13.

Chapter 30
Management of Pneumonia

Lindee M. Strizich and John H. Choe

Learning Objectives

1. Differentiate between types of pneumonia and management strategies.
2. Describe the basic microbiology of pneumonias.
3. Develop a framework for treating pneumonia based on objectives 1 and 2.

Clinical Vignette: A 65-year-old man presents to the ED with 2 days of shortness of breath, productive cough, malaise, and subjective fevers. He is febrile with a temperature of 38.7 °C, his respiratory rate is 18, his SpO2 on room air is 94%, his HR is 95, and his blood pressure is 127/78. He has rhonchi and bronchial breath sounds over his left lower lung field. His CXR shows a left lower lobe infiltrate. You diagnose him with pneumonia.

A. **Based on his clinical presentation, in combination with his diagnostic chest x-ray, you diagnose him with community-acquired pneumonia (CAP). How do we define CAP?**

Write down the headings "CAP," "hospital acquired pneumonia (HAP)," and "Ventilator associated pneumonia (VAP),"—add the definition of CAP as shown in Fig. 30.1.

Teaching point

- CAP is an infection of the pulmonary parenchyma that occurred in a patient living outside of the healthcare setting.

L. M. Strizich (✉)
University of Washington Medical Center, Department of Medicine, Division of General Internal Medicine, University of Washington, Seattle, WA, USA
e-mail: lstrizic@uw.edu

J. H. Choe
Harborview Medical Center, Department of Medicine, Division of General Internal Medicine, University of Washington, Seattle, WA, USA

S. Mookherjee et al. (eds.), *Chalk Talks in Internal Medicine*,
https://doi.org/10.1007/978-3-030-34814-4_30

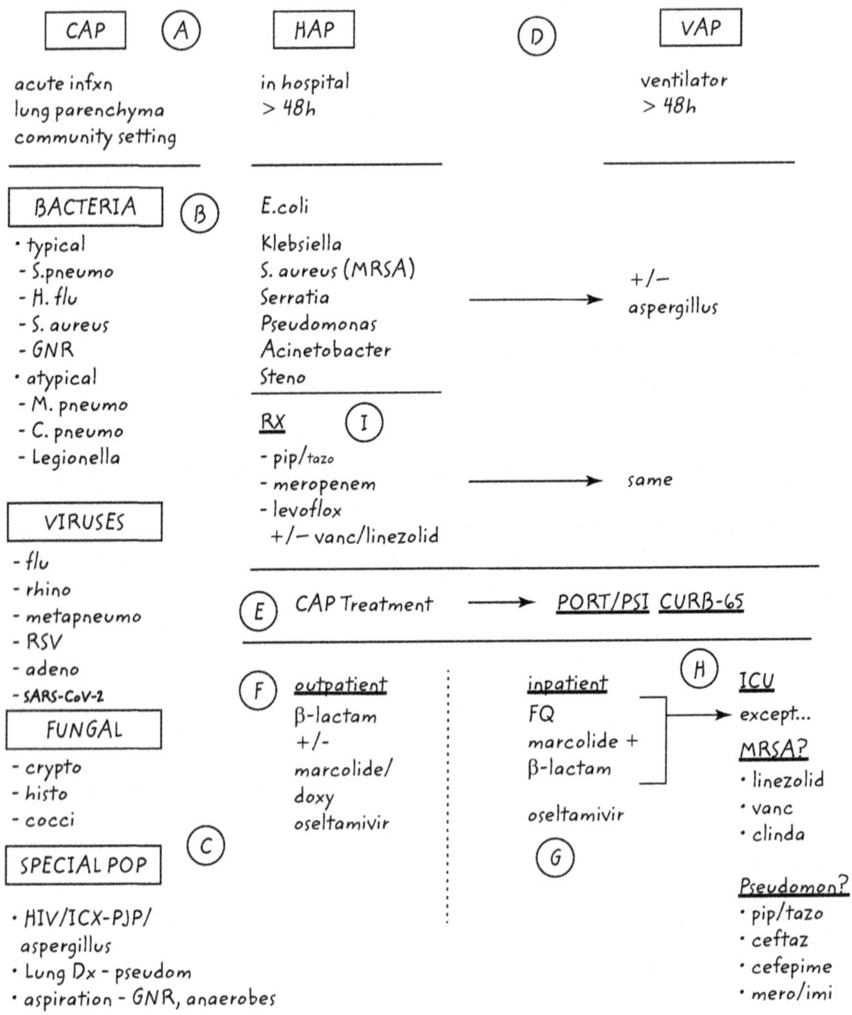

Fig. 30.1 Management of pneumonia, A–I

B. **What pathogens are the most likely cause of our patient's pneumonia?**

Make headings for "bacteria," "viruses," and "fungal," and add organisms as listed by the learners.

Teaching points

- Typical bacteria—*S. pneumoniae* (25–30% of cases), *H. influenza*, S. *aureus*, gram negative rods (GNRs) such as Klebsiella and Pseudomonas spp.
- Atypical bacteria—*Mycoplasma pneumonia, Chlamydophila pneumoniae, Legionella pneumophila.*
- Viruses—influenza, SARS-CoV-2 rhinovirus, metapneumovirus, respiratory syncytial virus, adenovirus.
- Fungal—Note that typically those at risk for fungal pneumonia are immunocompromised, but immunocompetent patients can also get *Cryptococcus neoformans, Histoplasma capsulatum, Coccidioides spp.*

C. **Some historical elements can suggest other pathogens. What pathogens would you add to your differential in patients with the following risk factors or comorbidities?**

Ask for pathogens associated in the following scenarios:

- HIV or immunosuppression?—all of the above, plus, *Pneumocystis jiroveci, Aspergillus fumigatus*, mycobacteria spp.
- Structural lung disease?—Pseudomonas spp., *Burkholderia cepacia*
- High aspiration risk?—GNRs, anaerobes if poor dentition
- Animal exposures?—bat or bird droppings—*Histoplasma*, Rabbits—*Francisella tularensis,* Birds—*Chlamydophila psittaci*
- Recent hotel stay or cruise ship trip?—Legionella

D. **If your patient were already admitted to the hospital for greater than 48 h (HAP) or had been on a ventilator for greater than 48 h (VAP), what pathogens would you have to worry about?**

List the pathogens under HAP and VAP as shown in Fig. 30.1.

Teaching points

- Hospital-acquired pneumonia (HAP): *E coli, Klebsiella, Enterobacter, S aureus (MRSA), Serratia, Pseudomonas, Acinetobacter, Stenotrophomonas*
- Ventilator-associated pneumonia (VAP): same as HAP; consider Aspergillus if immunocompromised
- Note that for HAP and VAP, you must consider multi-drug resistant (MDR) organisms such as MRSA and GNR like Pseudomonas or E coli that have multidrug resistance patterns, as clinical concern for these should inform empiric antibiotic selection.

E. **Your patient has no other medical problems, has not been recently hospitalized, nor has been treated with antibiotics in the past 6 months. Other than a WBC of 17 k, the rest of his CBC and Chem 7 are normal. Should he be admitted to the hospital? How would you decide?**

Write down PORT/PSI and CURB-65, highlighting the importance of objective risk stratification.

Teaching points

- Several tools are available to risk-stratify the patient and aid in management decisions.
- Commonly used tools include the PSI/PORT score, which includes age, sex, nursing home residency, medical comorbidities, vital sign abnormalities, laboratory data, and imaging findings.
- The CURB-65 score is easy to remember (confusion, BUN > 20, RR > 30, SBP < 90 or DBP < 60, and age >65)—hospital admission should be considered for anyone with two or more features.
- Low-risk patients (those who are less sick), such as our patient, can be treated an outpatient.

F. **You decide that your patient is low risk and can be treated as an outpatient. What antibiotics would you send him home with?**

Write down antibiotics under "outpatient."

Teaching points

- Consult local antibiotic susceptibility and practice patterns for specific antibiotic recommendations—general guidelines are given here.
- Beta-lactam (amoxicillin or amox/clav) +/- a macrolide or doxycycline, oseltamivir if concerned for influenza (*note that adding oseltamivir is true for all the categories of pneumonia and treatment settings discussed).*

G. **What if our patient's labs came back with a creatinine of 2, BUN of 40, and was requiring 2 L nasal cannula oxygen to maintain his oxygen saturation at 95%, had a respiratory rate of 20, was tachycardic to 105, and his BP was 127/78?**

Write down antibiotics under "inpatient."

Teaching points

- Higher risk patients (i.e., those who are more sick) should be admitted and further stratified to floor or ICU level care based on hemodynamic stability.
- This patient sounds stable for the acute care floor—macrolide and beta-lactam are preferred, may consider fluoroquinolone.

H. **As we are putting in admission orders, we hear that our patient is now requiring 8 L nasal cannula oxygen to maintain his oxygen saturation at 95%, his respiratory rate has increased to 32, his heart rate is now 127, and**

his blood pressure is now 95/60. Where does this patient get admitted to the hospital and what antibiotics would you choose?

Write down antibiotics under "ICU."

Teaching points

- This patient should be admitted to the ICU but the antibiotic recommendations are the same as for floor patients, unless there is concern for MRSA or *Pseudomonas spp.*
- For which patients would you worry about MRSA?—ESRD, IVDU, recent influenza-like illness, fluoroquinolone therapy in the past 3 months, necrotizing or cavitary pneumonia on imaging.
- Which antibiotics would cover MRSA?—vancomycin, linezolid, clindamycin.
- For which patients would you worry about Pseudomonas?—Patients with cystic fibrosis or other structural lung disease, a tracheostomy, neutropenia, or otherwise immunocompromised.
- Which antibiotics would you use to empirically cover Pseudomonas while awaiting culture data?—Piperacillin-tazobactam, ceftazidime, cefepime, meropenem, or imipenem if worried about extended spectrum beta lactamases.

I. **What is different about HAP and VAP treatments?**

Write down the antibiotics that you would consider for patients with VAP or HAP.

Teaching points

- S. aureus and pseudomonas must be considered and covered for, and MRSA should be covered with vancomycin or linezolid if there is a >20% prevalence based on local sensitivity patterns.
- Antibiotics to use empirically if no MDR risk factors include cefepime, piperacillin-tazobactam, meropenem may consider levofloxacin if no MDR.
- Antibiotics to consider for empiric treatment for VAP are the same as HAP—aspergillus can be considered as a potential pathogen in patients with VAP.

Return to Objectives and Emphasize Key Points

1. Understand how to categorize pneumonia and how this affects decisions for patient care. First categorize based on the type of pneumonia.
    - CAP
    - HAP
    - VAP
2. Further categorize CAP based on severity.
    - Severity scores → treatment in either outpatient or inpatient setting with inpatient further stratified to acute care floor vs. ICU

3. Describe the basic microbiology of pneumonias.
   - Note that this varies depending on if you are treating CAP, HAP, or VAP, and resistance patterns. Refer back to the most common organisms learners should be concerned about for each type of pneumonia
   - Must take into account exposures and patient characteristics.
4. Develop a framework for treating pneumonia.
   - Remind learners that their antibiotic selection should cover the organisms that they are concerned for, taking into account local antibiotic susceptibilities.

Resources

1. Wunderink RG, Waterer GW. Clinical practice. Community-acquired pneumonia. N Engl J Med. 2014;370(6):543–51, full-text, commentary can be found in N Engl J Med 2014 May 8;370(19):1861.
2. Mandell LA, Wunderink RG, Anzueto A, et al. Infectious Diseases Society of America/American Thoracic Society consensus guidelines on the management of community-acquired pneumonia in adults. Clin Infect Dis. 2007;44(Suppl 2):S27–72, full-text, commentary can be found in Clin Infect Dis 2007 Jul 1;45(1):133.
3. File TM. Community-acquired pneumonia. Lancet. 2003;362(9400):1991–2001.
4. Watkins RR, Lemonovich TL. Diagnosis and management of community-acquired pneumonia in adults. Am Fam Physician. 2011;83(11):1299–306, full-text.
5. Kalil AC, Metersky ML, Klompas M, et al. Management of Adults with Hospital-acquired and Ventilator-associated Pneumonia: 2016 clinical practice guidelines by the Infectious Diseases Society of America and the American Thoracic Society. Clin Infect Dis. 2016;63(5):e61–e111, full-text.
6. American Thoracic Society, Infectious Diseases Society of America. Guidelines for the management of adults with hospital-acquired, ventilator-associated, and healthcare-associated pneumonia. Am J RespirCrit Care Med. 2005;171(4):388–416, commentary can be found in Am J RespirCrit Care Med 2006 Jan 1;173(1):131.
7. Morrow LE, Kollef MH. Recognition and prevention of nosocomial pneumonia in the intensive care unit and infection control in mechanical ventilation. Crit Care Med. 2010;38(8 Suppl):S352–62.
8. Nair GB, Niederman MS. Nosocomial pneumonia: lessons learned. Crit Care Clin. 2013;29(3):521–46.
9. Kass SM, Williams PM, Reamy BV. Pleurisy. Am Fam Physician. 2007;75(9):1357–64.
10. Hunter JD. Ventilator associated pneumonia. BMJ. 2012;344:e3325.
11. Muscedere J, Dodek P, Keenan S, Fowler R, Cook D, Heyland D, VAP Guidelines Committee and the Canadian Critical Care Trials Group. Comprehensive evidence-based clinical practice guidelines for ventilator-associated pneumonia: prevention. J Crit Care. 2008;23(1):126–37, commentary can be found in J Crit Care 2009 Mar;24(1):149.

Chapter 31
Approach to Dyspnea

Jeffrey Redinger and Tyler Albert

Learning Objectives
1. Describe the pathophysiologic mechanisms of dyspnea.
2. Develop a differential diagnosis for dyspnea based on the pathway of an oxygen molecule through the cardiorespiratory system.

Clinical Vignette: A 43-year-old woman with hypertension and tobacco use comes to see you with 3 weeks of progressive shortness of breath and fatigue. You note that she has mildly labored breathing after walking into the exam room but is speaking in full sentences.

A. **Define dyspnea. What are the basic mechanisms that might cause our patient to feel short of breath?**

Draw the outline of the top part of Fig. 31.1 *and then write in the details as outlined in the teaching script.*

Teaching points
- Dyspnea is a subjective sensation of abnormal or uncomfortable breathing.
- Mechanisms of dyspnea include decreased arterial O_2 levels, increased CO_2 levels, or low blood pH.
- "Neuromechanical dissociation" describes the mismatch between respiratory effort and ventilation and elicits dyspnea in cases of abnormal chest wall compliance or airway resistance.

J. Redinger (✉) · T. Albert
VA Puget Sound Health Care System, Department of Medicine, Division of General Internal Medicine, University of Washington, Seattle, WA, USA
e-mail: Jeffrey.Redinger@va.gov

S. Mookherjee et al. (eds.), *Chalk Talks in Internal Medicine*,
https://doi.org/10.1007/978-3-030-34814-4_31

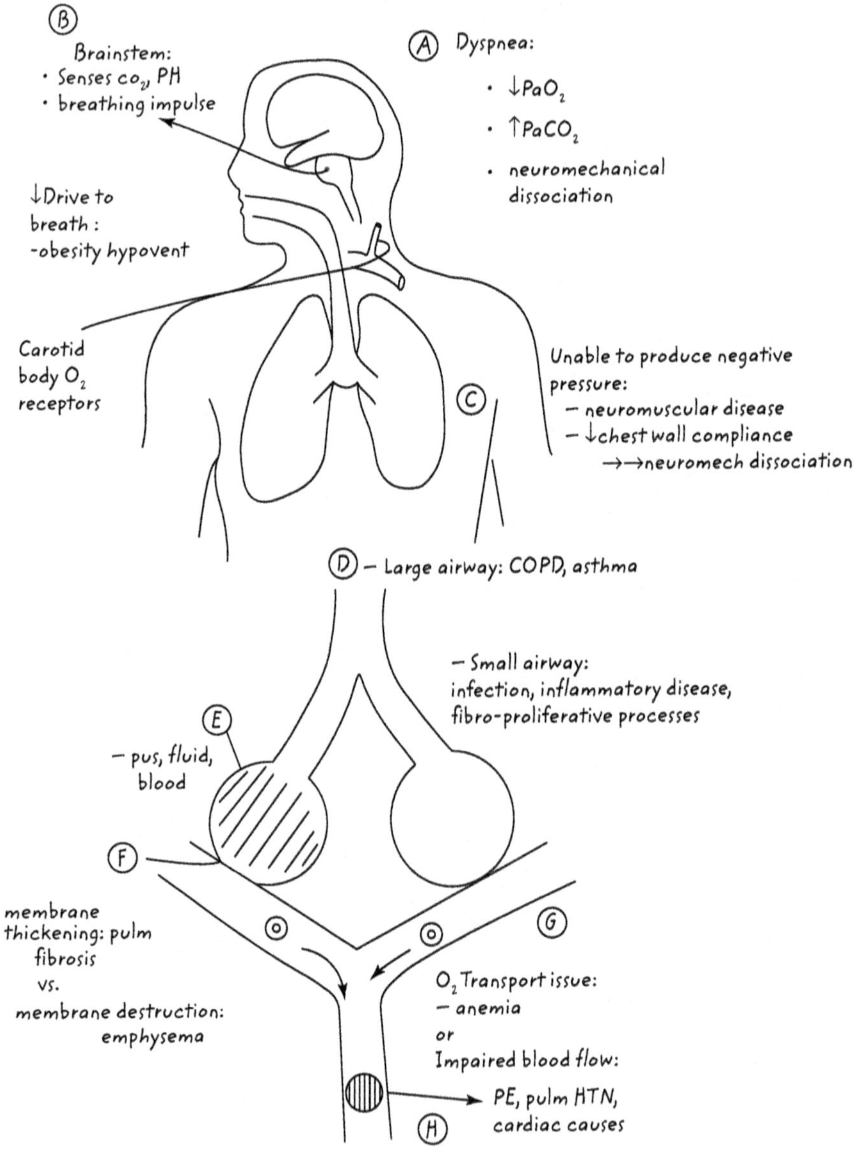

Fig. 31.1 Approach to dyspnea, A–H

B. **One way to think through possible etiologies of dyspnea is to "follow the oxygen molecule" as we breathe. What are the important first steps in initiating a breath, and where could problems arise?**

Highlight the role of vascular chemoreceptors and the midbrain in initiating a breath.

Teaching points

- The impulse to breathe is generated in the brainstem (medulla and pons) via mechanical and chemical stimuli.
- O_2 is sensed by peripheral chemoreceptors in the carotid and aortic bodies, whereas CO_2 and pH are sensed primarily in the brain by medullary chemoreceptors.
- Together with pulmonary and skeletal muscle stretch receptors, these are the major contributors to the complex feedback control system of basic breathing. Muted or absent responses can lead to a decreased "drive" to breathe, as in obesity hypoventilation.

C. **Air travels down pressure gradients, and thus in order to move oxygen from the atmosphere into the lungs, we must generate negative pressure. What specific disorders can lead to poor generation of negative pressure?**

Write down reasons for poor generation of negative pressure as suggested by learners.

Teaching points

- Abnormal neuromuscular function: diaphragmatic paralysis, myasthenia gravis, Guillain–Barré syndrome.
- Poor respiratory system compliance: fibrosis, pleural effusion, obesity, ascites, pregnancy.
- Both can impede generation of negative pressure and lead to neuromechanical dissociation.
- Remember that these disorders often cause CO_2 retention as an additional contributor to dyspnea.

D. **Oxygen first travels through the respiratory system into the large and small airways. What are some common disorders affecting airways that may cause dyspnea?**

Draw the outline of the bottom half of Fig. 31.1 *and then write in the details as learners respond to the questions.*

Teaching points

- Common large airway offenders: chronic obstructive pulmonary disease (COPD), asthma, bronchospasm, or obstructing tumor or foreign body.
- If associated with hypoxemia, the underlying mechanism is most commonly due to V_A/Q mismatch, although these diseases often cause CO_2 retention, as well.
- There are many small airway diseases, collectively termed bronchiolitis and appearing as "tree-in-bud" opacities on computed tomographic (CT) imaging.
- One framework for small airway disease is to differentiate types into infectious (viral, bacterial, mycobacterial), inflammatory (rheumatoid arthritis (RA), systemic lupus erythematosus (SLE), vasculitis), fibroproliferative (lung transplantation), or inhalational (tobacco, toxic fumes, mineral dusts) exposures.

E. **Alveolar filling processes cause dyspnea by way of impaired gas exchange from shunt resulting in decreased PaO_2. In broad terms, what are the common causes of alveolar shunt?**

Write down suggestions from the learners as shown in Fig. 31.1.

Teaching points

- The most common etiologies are pus (pneumonia), water (pulmonary edema), and blood (alveolar hemorrhage).
- Remember that atelectasis, while not a filling process, can cause shunt due to complete collapse of alveoli.

F. **Several causes of dyspnea result from pathology beyond the level of the alveoli. What processes can alter the alveolar–capillary membrane?**

Highlight the alveolar–capillary membrane as shown in Fig. 31.1.

Teaching points

- Efficient gas exchange depends on a thin alveolar–capillary membrane and a large surface area for exchange.
- Diseases that destroy (emphysema) or thicken (pulmonary fibrosis) the alveolar–capillary membrane can decrease total membrane surface area and slow the rate of diffusion.
- However, membrane abnormalities are rarely a cause of dyspnea in themselves. Rather, these disorders have other features as a source of dyspnea, as in COPD (hyperinflation, air trapping) or fibrosis (decreased compliance, increased work of breathing).
- One exception: alveolar–capillary membrane diseases can result in dyspnea during exercise due to shortened capillary transit time, decreasing the effective time for gas exchange and equilibration.

G. **How is O_2 transported in the blood, and what abnormalities with this process can cause dyspnea?**

Draw in the red blood cells and potential oxygen transportation issues as shown in Fig. 31.1.

Teaching points

- O_2 is either bound to hemoglobin or dissolved in blood, with the bound portion making up the vast majority of oxygen content.
- Low O_2 content can result from either decreased total hemoglobin or functional alterations of hemoglobin leading to impaired O_2 binding.
- The two main causes of dyspnea to consider at this level are thus anemia or dyshemoglobinemias such as CO poisoning or methemoglobinemia.

H. **Inefficient blood flow can also lead to impaired gas exchange. What disorders affect blood flow resulting in dyspnea?**

Draw in the pulmonary embolism as shown in Fig. 31.1 *and list other reasons for impaired blood flow as suggested by learners.*

- Like small airway diseases, this list is long—emphasize common disorders.
- The two main categories to include are pulmonary vascular diseases (pulmonary hypertension, pulmonary embolism (PE)) and cardiac disorders (systolic or diastolic heart failure, myocardial infarction (MI), arrhythmia, tamponade).

Back to the case: the patient notes that she can only walk 1–2 blocks before becoming dyspneic. She has significant fatigue and periodic lightheadedness, but has had no cough, wheezing, fevers, chills, weight loss, or hemoptysis. S_pO_2 is 97% on ambient air. She is pale with significant pallor of conjunctiva and mucous membranes. She has scleral icterus and you can palpate her spleen 2 cm below the left costal margin. Laboratory tests reveal a hemoglobin of 4 g/dL and a total bilirubin of 4.5, and peripheral smear shows spherocytosis. You diagnose her with hemolytic anemia and triage the patient to the emergency department.

Return to objectives and emphasize key points

1. Describe the pathophysiologic mechanisms of dyspnea.
   - Decreased arterial O_2 levels
   - Increased blood CO_2 levels
   - Neuromechanical dissociation
2. Develop a differential diagnosis for dyspnea based on the pathway of an oxygen molecule through the cardiorespiratory system.
   - Initiation of breath ➔ obesity hypoventilation
   - Generation of negative pressure ➔ neuromuscular disorders, decreased compliance
   - Large airways ➔ COPD, asthma, obstructing tumor
   - Small airways ➔ infectious, inflammatory, or toxic bronchiolitis
   - Alveolus ➔ pus, water, or blood
   - Alveolar–capillary membrane ➔ fibrosis or emphysema
   - Hemoglobin ➔ anemia, dyshemoglobinemia
   - Blood flow ➔ PE, pulmonary hypertension, cardiac disorders

Resources

1. Banzett RB, Schwartzstein RM. Dyspnea: don't just look, ask! Am J Respir Crit Care Med. 2015;192:1404.
2. Laviolette L, Laveneziana P. Dyspnoea: a multidimensional and multidisciplinary approach. Eur Respir J. 2014;43:1750–62.
3. Manning HL, Schwartzstein RM. Pathophysiology of dyspnea. N Engl J Med. 1995;333:1547.
4. Parshall MB, et al. An official American Thoracic Society statement: update on the mechanisms, assessment, and management of dyspnea. Am J Respir Crit Care Med. 2012;185(4):435–52.
5. Scano G, Ambrosino N. Pathophysiology of dyspnea. Lung. 2002;180:131.
6. Schwartzstein RM. The language of dyspnea. In: Mahler DA, O'Donnell DE, editors. Dyspnea: mechanisms, measurement, and management. New York: Marcel Dekker; 2005. p. 115.
7. Schwartzstein RM, Dyspnea AL. In: Broaddus VC, Murray JF, Nadel JA, editors. Murray and Nadel's textbook of respiratory medicine. 6th ed. Philadelphia: Elsevier Saunders; 2016. p. 485–96.

Chapter 32
Interpretation of Pulmonary Function Tests

Scott Hagan and Tyler Albert

Learning Objectives
1. Define the key components of pulmonary function testing (PFT).
2. Use flow-volume loops to aid in the interpretation of PFTs.
3. Recognize common patterns of pulmonary disease seen on PFTs.

Clinical Vignette: A 50-year-old woman with a 20-pack-a-year smoking history presents to clinic with chronic dyspnea.

A. **As part of a basic evaluation you decide to order pulmonary function tests (PFTs). What are the main components of pulmonary function tests? What are their normal values?**

Create the spirometry, lung volume, and DLCO table. Label the first column "normal" and leave the second and third columns blank. Fill in the normal values for each measurement.

Teaching points
- Spirometry, lung volumes, and DLCO are the three main parts of PFTs.
- Spirometry: assesses for airflow obstruction by measuring FEV1 (forced expiratory volume in 1 s), FVC (forced vital capacity), and the FEV1/FVC ratio. This can be performed in clinic and can assess for reversibility of obstruction through bronchodilator responsiveness.

S. Hagan (✉) · T. Albert
VA Puget Sound Health Care System, Department of Medicine, Division of General Internal Medicine, University of Washington, Seattle, WA, USA
e-mail: Scott.Hagan1@va.gov

S. Mookherjee et al. (eds.), *Chalk Talks in Internal Medicine*,
https://doi.org/10.1007/978-3-030-34814-4_32

- Lung volumes: usually performed using a plethysmograph, measures TLC (total volume at full inhalation), RV (residual volume after full exhalation), VC (vital capacity, often greater than FVC in patients with obstructive lung disease), and FRC (functional residual capacity, volume remaining at the end of tidal exhalation).
- DLCO (diffusion capacity for carbon dioxide): measurement of gas crossing the alveolar–capillary barrier, a marker of surface area for gas exchange, however, can also be decreased with pulmonary vascular diseases; should be corrected for anemia.

B. **How is spirometry represented on a flow-volume loop?**

Draw and label the axes. Depending on the audience, consider asking a learner to draw a representative flow volume loop for a normal patient; redraw or correct it if necessary.

Teaching points

- Flow-volume loops represent the appropriateness of airflow for given lung volumes, and have characteristic shapes for each disease processes.
- A common point of confusion is that the inspiratory flow curve begins descending from the far-right side of the *x*-axis.
- Remember that FEV1 is not represented on a flow-volume loop as time is not represented on the curve.

C. **You order spirometry for our patient. What do you notice is different about this patient's flow loop? What would the corresponding values be for their spirometry and lung volumes?**

Draw out the patient's flow-volume loop, labeled C on Fig. 32.1. *Ask learners to fill in the FEV1, FVC, and FEV1/FVC ratio loop in comparison to normal loop as increased (↑), decreased (↓), or unchanged (−).*

Teaching points

- The "scooped out" expiratory curve indicates airflow obstruction, which is confirmed by the reduced FEV1/FVC ratio.
- Additionally, the curve is shifted to the left, suggesting hyperinflation (increased TLC) and air trapping (increased RV).

D. **Which diseases cause airflow obstruction and how might you distinguish them with PFTs?**

Write asthma and COPD as the main diagnoses, provide the negative bronchodilator response, and make the point that this does not reliably differentiate between the two.

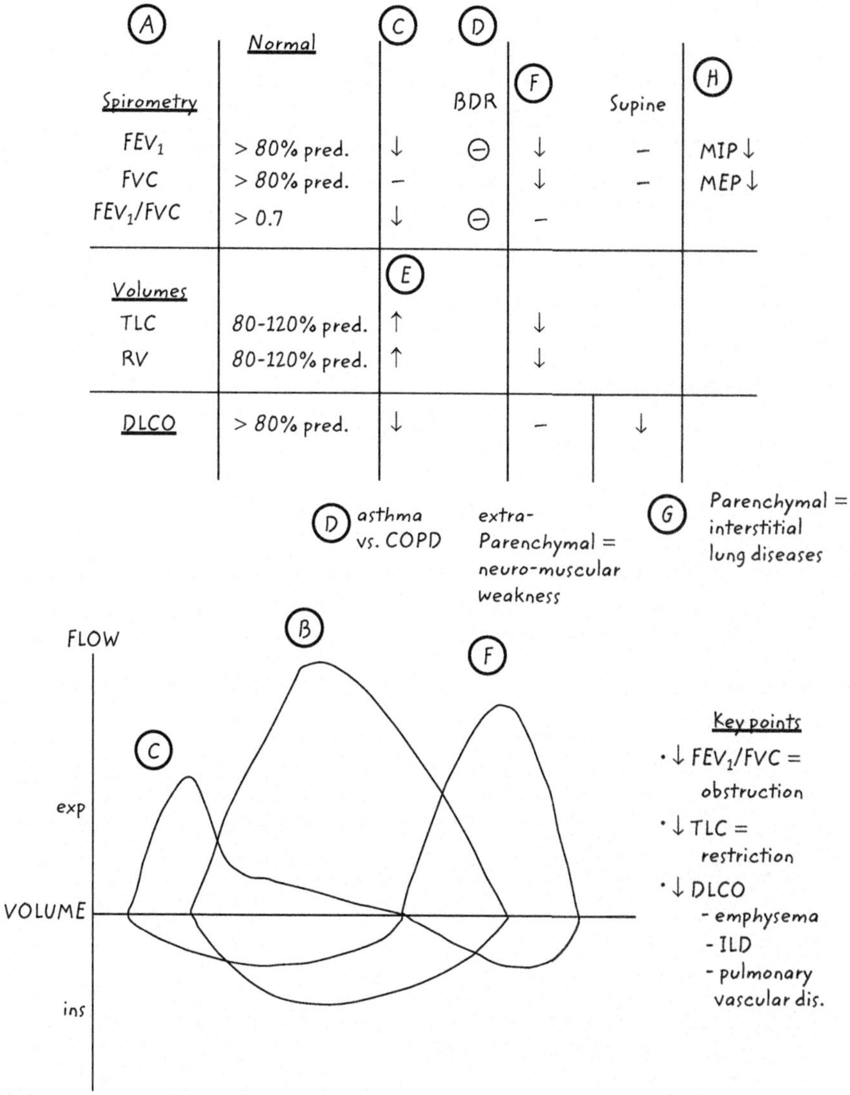

Fig. 32.1 Interpretation of pulmonary function tests, A–H

Teaching points

- Asthma and COPD (a syndrome resulting from chronic bronchitis and emphysema) are the two main obstructive lung diseases.
- Bronchodilator responsiveness (BDR, an increase of 12% *and* 200 cc of FVC *or* FEV1) measures the reversibility of airflow obstruction; however, this does NOT reliably distinguish asthma from COPD.
- The most important distinguishing feature of asthma versus COPD is clinical history: age of onset, smoking history, family history, and related diagnosis (e.g., other atopic diseases), productive cough, etc.

E. **You obtain lung volumes and a DLCO on our patient. How does this help?**

Write in the increased TLC and RV and reduced DLCO for our patient, underline COPD as the more likely diagnosis in this patient.

Teaching points

- An increased total lung capacity (hyperinflation) and/or residual volume (air trapping) are both more common with emphysema, and COPD, however, can be seen with severe, chronic asthma.
- A reduced DLCO (a decrease in the surface area for gas exchange) is suggestive of emphysema as opposed to asthma.
- Our patient developed dyspnea later in life, with a reduced DLCO, an elevated RV, and a negative BDR. She likely has emphysema, which is diagnosed anatomically (histology or radiographically).

F. **Imagine a different flow-volume loop for this patient. What do you notice has changed?**

Draw out the final flow-volume loop, labeled F on Fig. 32.1. *Fill in the third column of the chart as learners identify a reduced TLC, RV, and FVC. Give them the rest of the values (low FEV1, normal FEV1/FVC, normal DLCO).*

Teaching points

- We notice that her flow rates are preserved, and her FEV1/FVC is preserved, ruling out obstruction.
- All of her volumes have declined, indicating restriction.

G. **The patient's DLCO is preserved. What does this tell us about the differential for her restrictive lung disease (RLD)?**

Write out the key considerations for reduced and unchanged DLCO as shown in Fig. 32.1.

Teaching points

- DLCO helps to distinguish parenchymal (low DLCO, e.g., interstitial lung diseases) from extra-parenchymal (normal DLCO) RLD.
- Differential for extra-parenchymal RLD: diaphragmatic paralysis, pleural diseases (scarring, effusions), neuromuscular weakness (myasthenia gravis, amyo-

trophic lateral sclerosis (ALS), multiple sclerosis (MS)), chest wall disorders (obesity, scoliosis), extrathoracic disorders (ascites).

H. **What further pulmonary function tests could help distinguish the cause of the patient's extra-parenchymal RLD?**

Write out the supine spirometry, maximum inspiratory pressure (MIP), and maximum expiratory pressure *(MEP) findings as shown in* Fig. 32.1.

Teaching points

- Supine spirometry: A decline in FVC below 20% is suggestive of diaphragmatic weakness, as a weakened diaphragm is unable to move abdominal contents without the help of gravity.
- Maximum inspiratory pressure (MIP) and maximum expiratory pressure (MEP): A reduced MIP and/or MEP can be suggestive of neuromuscular weakness and can help delineate between inspiratory and expiratory muscle involvement.
- *Write her supine spirometry, MIP, and MEP values in the chart.* The patient's supine spirometry was unchanged, while MIPs and MEPs were reduced, indicating neuromuscular disease. The patient ultimately was diagnosed with amyotrophic lateral sclerosis.

Return to objectives and key points

1. Key PFTs to focus on for interpretation: FEV1/FVC (airflow obstruction), TLC (restriction), and DLCO (emphysema, interstitial lung disease (ILD), pulmonary vascular disease).
2. Flow-loop patterns are helpful adjunct to PFT values. A "scooped out" curve suggests airflow obstruction, while a small and narrow curve suggests RLD.
3. Extra tests to order: For reduced FEV1/FVC, order BDR; for reduced TLC with normal DLCO, order supine spirometry and MIP/MEP.

Resources

1. Pellegrino R, Viegi G, et al. Series "ATS/ERS task force: standardisation of lung function testing": interpretative strategies for lung function tests. Eur Resp J. 2005;26:948–68.
2. Benditt JO. A primer on reading pulmonary function tests. Accessible at: https://courses.washington.edu/med610/pft/pft_primer.html.
3. Bays AM, Luks AM. A tutorial in pulmonary function test interpretation. Accessible at: https://depts.washington.edu/uwmedres/Library/eLearning/Pulmonary/.

Chapter 33
Management of Chronic Obstructive Pulmonary Disease

Neil Argyle and William Weppner

Learning Objectives

1. Describe a systematic approach for taking a history and physical in patients with suspected chronic obstructive pulmonary disease (COPD).
2. Interpret diagnostic tests to make the diagnosis of COPD.
3. Describe a stepwise approach to the treatment of COPD.

Clinical Vignette: A 65-year-old man presents to the clinic with progressive shortness of breath with exertion, occurring daily over the last year. He has chronic cough with sputum production that is more prominent in the morning. He is a one-pack-per-day smoker, with a 45-pack-year history. His physical exam shows he is afebrile, with a heart rate of 90 beats per minute, blood pressure of 135/85 mmHg, a respiratory rate of 22 per minute, saturation of 90% on room air. He is tachypneic, with a notable prolonged expiratory phase with faint end-expiratory wheezing. No crackles, no dullness to percussion, and no egophony were observed. Diminished breath sounds throughout.

A. **What presenting symptoms would make you consider a workup for COPD?**

Write out the headings "history / symptoms," "diagnosis," and "imaging" on the white board. Add appropriate presenting symptoms as suggested by learners.

Teaching points

- Patients who present with dyspnea on exertion (or at rest) that is progressively worsening over time are more likely to be suffering from COPD. Additional questions could be asked about:
- Weight loss: Patients with end-stage COPD often present with weight loss.

N. Argyle (✉) · W. Weppner
Boise VA Medical Center, Department of Medicine, Division of General Internal Medicine, University of Washington, Seattle, WA, USA
e-mail: Neil.Argyle@va.gov

S. Mookherjee et al. (eds.), *Chalk Talks in Internal Medicine*,
https://doi.org/10.1007/978-3-030-34814-4_33

- Morning headaches: Nighttime hypoxia leads to morning headaches that resolve after being awake and improving their saturations.
- Chronic cough is associated with COPD, with or without sputum production.
- Environmental exposures: including but not limited to tobacco, occupational hazards (such as mining), and biomass fuel exhaust.
- Other underlying lung pathology: Patients are at increased risk if they have a history of asthma, repeated lung infections as a child, or premature birth.

B. **You suspect that your patient may have COPD. What should your next diagnostic test be?**

Write down the key points under "diagnosis" as shown in Fig. 33.1.

Teaching points

- Pulmonary function testing (PFT) is done to make a formal diagnosis of COPD. PFTs measure the patient's FEV1 (forced expiratory volume in 1 s) and FVC (forced vital capacity). These values are measured before and after the administration of bronchodilator therapy to determine the reversibility of the obstruction.
- In the setting of an obstructive airway disease pattern, FEV1/FVC < 0.7, a patient history consistent with COPD, and a lack of reversibility, then a diagnosis of COPD is made.
- FEV1 is then used to determine the severity of obstruction.
- (>80 = mild, 50–80% = moderate, 30–50% = severe, <30% very severe).
- If FEV1 and FVC are partially reversible, then an asthmatic component is present (i.e., asthma-COPD overlap syndrome).
- If administration of a bronchodilator shows significant reversibility, then it is more consistent with asthma.

C. **Should we get imaging for this patient? When would you want to get imaging in a patient with COPD?**

Write down the key points under imaging as shown in Fig. 33.1.

Teaching points

- Imaging is not routinely required.
- If a patient presents during an acute exacerbation, then imaging should be done to exclude an alternative diagnosis for their dyspnea, such as:
  - Underlying pneumonia
  - Pulmonary embolism
  - Pneumothorax

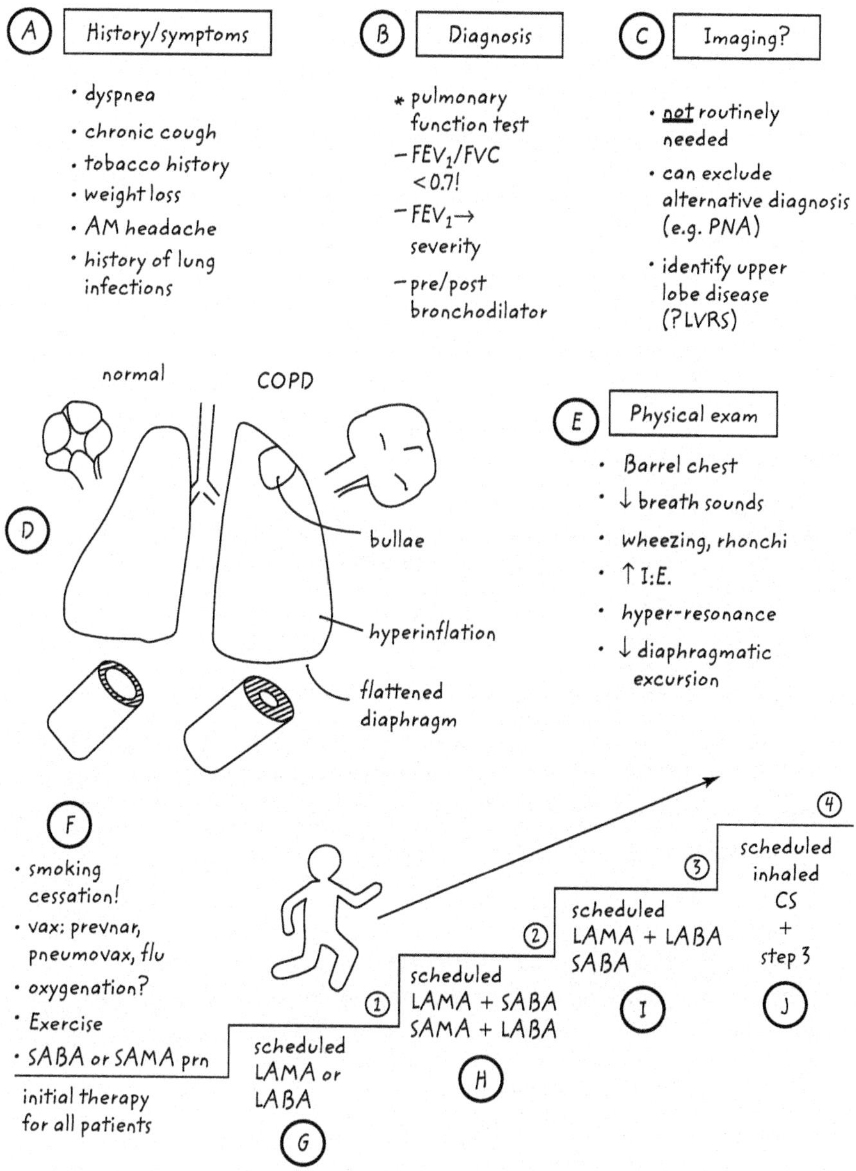

Fig. 33.1 Management of chronic obstructive pulmonary disease, A–J

- To rule out other comorbidities:
  - Lung cancer
  - Bronchiectasis
  - Pleural disease
  - Interstitial lung disease
  - Heart failure
- Imaging can further support the diagnosis if the cause remains unclear from history and physical.
- Imaging can identify predominantly upper lobe disease that may benefit from lung volume reduction surgery.

D. **COPD is characterized by thickened, inflamed airways and enlarged, destroyed alveolar airspaces. What might be seen on his chest X-ray that would support a diagnosis of COPD?**

Draw the outlines of the normal lung, alveolus, and airway. Also draw a lung, alveolus, and airway affected by COPD. Ask the learners for features that might be seen on imaging in a lung with COPD and add them as suggested.

Teaching points

- While the chest X-ray can be useful, it is not sufficient to rule in or rule out COPD—spirometry is always needed if COPD is suspected.
- Hyperinflated lungs.
- Flattened diaphragms.
- Bullae.
- Centrilobular emphysema (alpha-1-antitrypsin deficiency affects the bases).

E. **The changes in the lungs due to COPD can often be detected on physical examination. When you examine our patient, what findings might be present? What physical exam findings would suggest an acute exacerbation?**

Relate the physical exam findings to the drawing of the lungs, as they are suggested by learners.

Teaching points

- Increased anterior–posterior (AP) diameter ("barrel-chest")
- Diminished breath sounds with wheezing, rhonchi, and a prolonged expiratory phase
- Hyperresonance on percussion
- Decreased diaphragmatic excursion
- During an acute exacerbation you can see:
  - Tachypnea
  - Inability to speak full sentences
  - Accessory muscle use

- Increased work of breathing
- Cyanosis
- Pulses paradoxus (a systolic blood pressure decrease of greater than 20 mmHg with inspiration)

F. **Evidence-based treatment of stable COPD is approached in a stepwise fashion, and patients move up the "steps" based on severity of disease and response to treatments. What treatment recommendations are appropriate for all COPD patients?**

Draw the outline of the five steps as shown in Fig. 33.1 *and start at the lowest step.*

Teaching points

- Smoking cessation reduces the rate of decline in lung function—most important!
- Prevention of infection: Prevnar 13, Pneumovax, and influenza vaccinations.
- Adequate oxygenation: Oxygen may be used to target goal levels of PaO_2 55–65 mmHg or SpO_2 of 88–92%. For patients below these levels (at rest, during exercise, and during sleep), oxygen should be administered to prevent cor pulmonale and decrease mortality. Recent evidence suggests that although patients with $SpO_2 < 89\%$ at rest will benefit from long-term oxygen, patients with temporary desaturations due to exercise did not benefit from long-term oxygen therapy (NEJM 2016, see the reference below).
- Increased exercise! Consider formal referral for pulmonary rehabilitation for patients with more severe COPD, frequent flares, or those with persistent functional limitations; in such patients, this has been shown to improve exercise capacity, decrease dyspnea, and improve quality of life.
- Short-acting bronchodilators: short-acting beta-2 agonists (SABAs), e.g., albuterol, or short-acting muscarinic antagonists (SAMAs), e.g., ipratropium.

G. **If not responding to initial treatment, you should "step up" therapy, moving up to Step 1. What is the key component of the first step-up?**

Add the key component of each step as shown in Fig. 33.1.

Teaching points

- Instead of a SABA or SAMA as needed, provide a scheduled long-acting muscarinic antagonist (LAMA) such as tiotropium or long-acting beta agonist (LABA) such as formoterol.
- Practice pearl—most people functionally "jump over" this step, as they are often already on a SABA from Step 1, and a LAMA or LABA is added (so they are already up to Step 2!).
- In general, long-acting medications are preferred over short-acting medications because of decreased exacerbations, increased quality of life, and less decline in FEV1.

H. **If not responding to Step 1 treatment, you should step up therapy further. How does the therapy change with Step 2?**

Add the key component of each step as shown in Fig. 33.1.

Teaching points

- Change to a scheduled combination of a short-acting and long-acting regimen, either LAMA and SABA or SAMA and LABA (1 long and 1 short).
- Practice pearl—a common "trip up" on this step is inadvertently continuing ipratropium (SAMA) when adding tiotropium (LAMA). Ipratropium competitively binds to the same receptor, making tiotropium much less effective, and functionally bringing the patient back to "ground level."

I. **If not responding to Step 2 treatment, you should step up therapy yet again. How does treatment change with the next step?**

Add the key component of each step as shown in Fig. 33.1.

Teaching point

- Change to scheduled combination of two long-acting medications LABA and LAMA, with short- acting (SABA) rescue inhaler (2 long and 1 short).

J. **If not responding to Step 3 treatment, you should step up therapy to the last step. What medication is added at the last step?**

Add the key component of each step as shown in Fig. 33.1.

Teaching points

- Continue the 2 long and 1 short regimen in Step 3, with the addition of an inhaled corticosteroid (ICS). This provides a triple long-acting therapy, in addition to rescue SABA.
- Another "trip up" on this step is some (conflicting) evidence suggesting that ICS may increase risk of associated pneumonia.
- While this step can be useful for stabilizing patients with severe COPD and recent exacerbations, there is some evidence that patients can be safely tapered off ICS, to just a LAMA/LABA combination.

Return to Objectives and Emphasize Key Points

1. Describe a systematic approach for taking a history and physical in patients with suspected chronic obstructive pulmonary disease (COPD).
2. Interpret diagnostic tests to make the diagnosis of COPD.

   - Imaging: not routinely needed
   - Pulmonary function testing:

     – FEV1 to determine the severity of disease.
     – FEV1/FVC ratio <0.7 to make the diagnosis of COPD.
     – Response to bronchodilators will demonstrate if has an asthma component as well.

3. Describe a stepwise approach to the treatment of COPD.

   - Initial treatment: smoking cessation, vaccinations, oxygen levels, exercise, short-acting rescue inhaler (SABA)
   - Step-up therapy with combinations: short- and long-acting bronchodilators, potentially with inhaled corticosteroids

Resources

1. Vogelmeier CF, Criner GJ, Martinez FJ, et al. Global strategy for the diagnosis, management, and prevention of chronic obstructive lung disease 2017 report: GOLD executive summary. Eur Respir J. 2017;49:1700214.
2. RK Albert DHA, Blackford AL, et al. A randomized trial of long-term oxygen for COPD with moderate desaturation. N Engl J Med. 2016;375:1617–27.
3. Kew KM, Seniukovich A. Inhaled steroids and risk of pneumonia for chronic obstructive pulmonary disease. Cochrane Database Syst Rev. 2014;3:CD010115.

Chapter 34
Approach to Sleep-Disordered Breathing

Ken He and Grady Paden

Learning Objectives
1. Distinguish between different types of sleep-disordered breathing.
2. Identify common symptoms and risk factors for obstructive sleep apnea.
3. Describe STOP-Bang tool and diagnostic sleep study methods for obstructive sleep apnea.
4. Identify basic treatment options for obstructive sleep apnea.

Clinical Vignette: A 52-year-old man complains of daytime sleepiness despite obtaining what he feels is an adequate amount of sleep each night. He denies difficulty falling asleep at night. He also reports snoring, apneas witnessed by his wife, and unrefreshing sleep. He finds it difficult to stay awake during sedentary activities. Medical history is notable for coronary artery disease with prior stents, and poorly controlled hypertension. He is a shift worker, falls asleep on the job, and in his car while stopped in traffic. Body mass index (BMI) is 32 and his neck size is 16 inches. Remainder of his physical exam is unremarkable.

A. What is considered to be "excessive daytime sleepiness"?

Write down ideas as suggested by learners—emphasize that there isn't a standard definition.

Teaching points
- Standard definition for excessive daytime sleepiness is lacking.

K. He (✉)
VA Pittsburgh Health Care System, Pittsburgh, PA, USA
e-mail: Ken.He@va.gov

G. Paden
VA Puget Sound Health Care System, Department of Medicine, Division of General Internal Medicine, University of Washington, Seattle, WA, USA
e-mail: Grady.Paden@va.gov

S. Mookherjee et al. (eds.), *Chalk Talks in Internal Medicine*,
https://doi.org/10.1007/978-3-030-34814-4_34

- Acceptable definitions include persistent sleepiness after apparently adequate or even prolonged nighttime sleep, the inability to stay awake and alert during the day when the circadian drive to sleep is low, or inadvertently falling asleep in undesirable situations that impacts daytime function and quality of life.
- Some patients may describe sleepiness as "fatigue" or "lack of energy."
- There are questionnaires that can help quantify a patient's sleepiness; the most commonly used is the Epworth Sleepiness Scale. The patient is asked how likely they are to fall asleep in several scenarios, including watching TV, stopped in traffic while driving a car, while lying down to rest during the day.

B. **What are some general causes of excessive daytime sleepiness or fatigue?**

Write down suggestions from learners as shown in Fig. 34.1.

Teaching points

- Before jumping to the diagnosis of sleep-disordered breathing, alternative etiologies should be considered. These include:

  - Insufficient sleep: For adults aged 18–64 years, expert consensus recommends 7–9 hours of sleep each day, and more if chronically sleep deprived.
  - Medical disorders: May disturb sleep, diminish sleep quality, and cause fatigue. Examples are heart failure, stroke, and liver disease.
  - Mood disorders: If uncontrolled may disrupt sleep quality and manifest as sleepiness or fatigue. Examples are depression and posttraumatic stress disorder (PTSD).
  - Medications and substances: e.g., alcohol, opioids, benzodiazepines, and antihistamines.
  - Nonrespiratory sleep disorder may disrupt and diminish sleep quality or independently cause excessive sleepiness. Categories and examples include hypersomnia disorder (narcolepsy), restless legs syndrome, and circadian rhythm disorder (shift work).

C. **Based on this patient's complaints of snoring, witnessed apneas, and unrefreshing sleep, you suspect sleep-disordered breathing as a cause of excessive daytime sleepiness. What are the different types of sleep-disordered breathing and what risk factors are they associated with?**

First prompt the learners to name the types of sleep-disordered breathing as you outline the Venn diagram, and then ask the learners to volunteer associated risk factors.

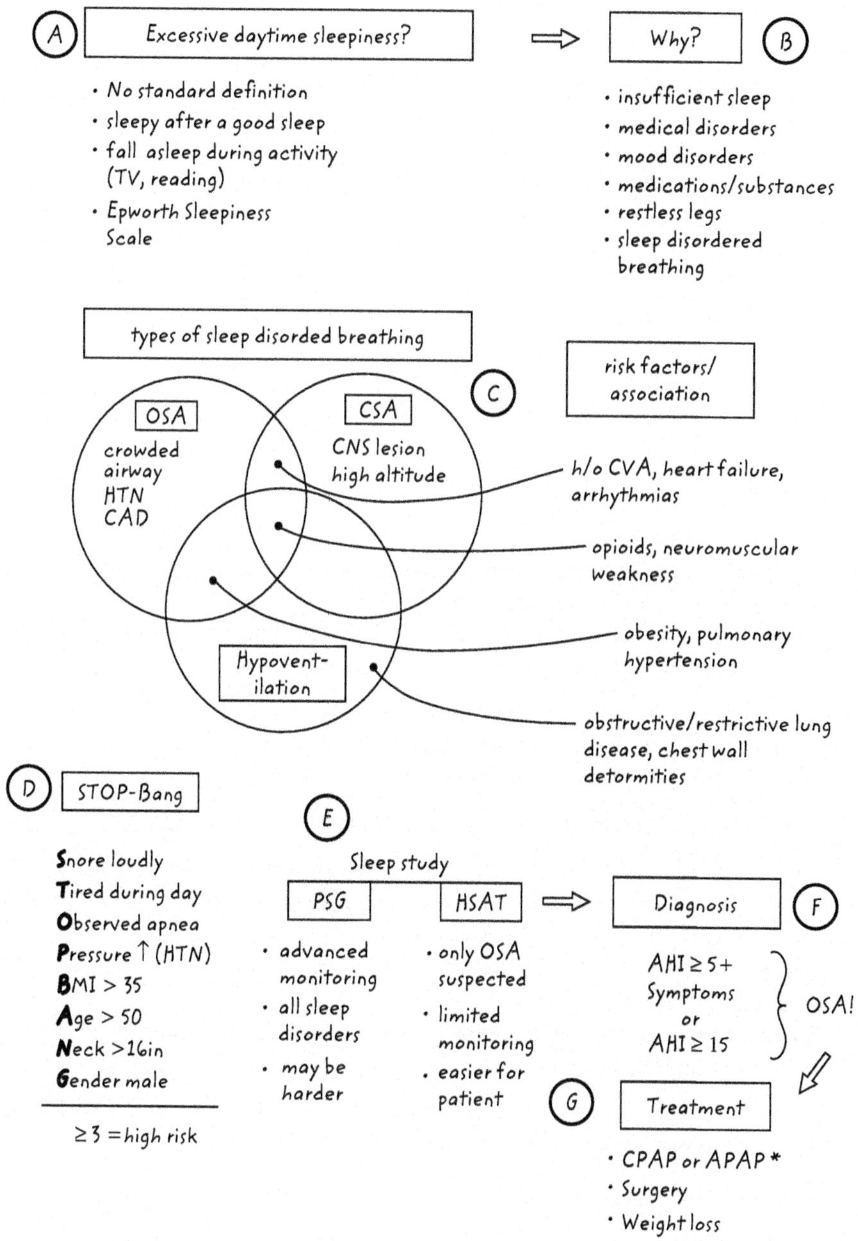

Fig. 34.1 Approach to sleep-disordered breathing: A–G

Teaching points

- Pathologic forms of sleep-disordered breathing that result in disturbed sleep and additional health risks include:
  - Obstructive sleep apnea. Characterized by upper airway narrowing or collapse during sleep while respiratory effort continues.
  - Central sleep apnea. Characterized by reduction or cessation of airflow due to reduced or absent respiratory effort.
  - Sleep-related hypoventilation. Characterized by an abnormal increase of arterial CO_2 ($PaCO_2$) during sleep.
- Risk factors/disease associations include:
  - Obstructive sleep apnea (OSA): crowded airway, refractory hypertension (HTN), coronary artery disease (CAD).
  - Central sleep apnea (CSA): central nervous system (CNS) lesions, travel to high altitude.
  - Hypoventilation: obstructive and restrictive lung disease, thoracic/chest wall deformities.
  - Obesity and pulmonary HTN are associated with both OSA and hypoventilation.
  - History of (H/O), cerebrovascular accident (CVA), heart failure, and arrhythmia are associated with both OSA and CSA.
  - Opioids and neuromuscular weakness can contribute to all forms of sleep-disordered breathing.

D. **On the basis of symptoms and risk factors, you strongly suspect that the patient has OSA. Before sending him for a sleep study, how would you estimate the pretest probability of OSA?**

Write down the STOP-Bang tool as shown in Fig. 34.1.

Teaching points

- There are several screening tools (e.g., STOP-Bang Questionnaire, Berlin Questionnaire, Preoperative Questionnaire).
- The most widely used is the STOP-Bang based on ease of use and available evidence.
- There are different ways to interpret the score. Based on the original study, ≥3 is considered high risk for OSA. Specificity increases with higher score.

E. **In order to diagnose OSA, the patient needs to have a sleep study. What are the main types of sleep studies and how are they different?**

Write down the key features of each form of sleep study.

Teaching points

- Laboratory-based sleep study, also called polysomnography (PSG).
  - Completed overnight in a sleep center: gold standard sleep test.

- Monitoring includes but is not limited to brain activity electroencephalogram (EEG), eye movements (to discern rapid eye movement (REM) sleep), airflow, respiratory movement, muscle tone electromyogram (EMG), heart rate (or electrocardiography (ECG)), pulse oximetry, and audiovisual recording of the patient.
- Useful for assessment of various sleep disorders, not just OSA.
- A sleep technologist who is present ensures adequate data collection. In certain situations, the tech can also initiate therapy for OSA.

- Home sleep apnea test (HSAT) or portable monitoring is the other type.
  - Most often done in the patient's usual sleep environment.
  - There is no attendant.
  - Data acquisition is typically limited to airflow, respiratory movement, heart rate, and pulse oximetry.
  - Should only be utilized to diagnose patients with high likelihood of OSA, without concern for other sleep disorders.
- This patient is a good candidate for home sleep apnea testing due to classic symptoms of OSA, and no major risk factors for CSA or hypoventilation.

F. **He is found to have an apnea-hypopnea index (AHI) of 12. How do you define the AHI and what does this mean? Does this patient have OSA?**

Add the key points under "diagnosis."

Teaching points

- Apnea-hypopnea index is defined as the number of apneas or hypopneas that occurs per hour of sleep study.
  - Apnea is ≥90% drop in baseline airflow lasting ≥10 s.
  - Hypopnea is ≥30% drop in baseline airflow lasting ≥10 s associated with arousal from sleep and/or ≥3% oxygen desaturation.
- Diagnosis of OSA is based on attributable symptoms and AHI.
  - Symptoms + AHI ≥5
  - AHI ≥15 if no symptoms
- AHI is also used to stratify OSA severity.
  - Mild = AHI ≥5 to <15
  - Moderate = AHI ≥15 to <30
  - Severe = AHI ≥30

G. **This patient can now formally be diagnosed with OSA. What are his treatment options?**

Write down the main treatment options, putting an asterisk by CPAP or APAP.

Teaching points

- Even though he has mild OSA, he has OSA attributable symptoms; thus, treatment is indicated. The goal of treatment is to improve symptom burden.
- Treatment is recommended for mild OSA if symptomatic or presence of comorbidities associated with OSA.
- Treatment is recommended for moderate or worse OSA severity regardless of symptoms to mitigate associated health risks (e.g., vascular disease).
- Positive airway pressure (PAP) is first-line therapy. This works by splinting open the airway, and is highly effective for all OSA severities. Typically, continuous (CPAP) or autotitrating (APAP) devices are recommended. APAP devices can self-adjust to achieve pressure requirements. Therapy adherence is the biggest issue.
- Alternatives to PAP. These are all considered as second-line or adjunct therapies.
  - Oral appliances are second line. Good for less severe OSA as they are less effective than PAP, but adherence is generally better. Also called dental appliance or mandibular advancement/repositioning devices.
  - Positional therapy. Typically, a mechanical barrier (e.g., wedge) to prevent sleeping in the supine position. Only effective for patients with OSA isolated to this position.
  - Weight loss. Any weight reduction is helpful.
  - Sleep surgery. Consists of soft tissue or bony modification to decrease upper airway collapsibility and/or increase airway volume/patency.

Return to Objectives and Emphasize Key Points

1. Distinguish between different types of sleep-disordered breathing: obstructive sleep apnea, central sleep apnea, sleep-related hypoventilation.
2. Identify hallmark symptoms and risk factors for obstructive sleep apnea.
   - Snoring, witnessed apneas
   - Daytime sleepiness or fatigue
   - Anatomically crowded airway, refractory hypertension, coronary artery disease, obesity, and stroke
3. Describe different sleep study methods and when to refer for sleep testing.
   - Point out the utility of STOP-Bang and OSA risk assessment.
   - Point out there are two different formats of sleep studies.
4. Identify basic treatment options for obstructive sleep apnea.
   - Highlight that PAP is the most effective form of therapy.

Resources

1. American Academy of Sleep Medicine. International classification of sleep disorders. 3rd ed. Darien: American Academy of Sleep Medicine; 2014.
2. Kapur VK, Auckley DH, Chowdhuri S, et al. Clinical practice guideline for diagnostic testing for adult obstructive sleep apnea: an American Academy of Sleep Medicine clinical practice guideline. J Clin Sleep Med. 2017;13(3):479–504.
3. Epstein LJ, Kristo D, Strollo PJ, et al. Clinical guideline for the evaluation, management and long-term care of obstructive sleep apnea in adults. J Clin Sleep Med. 2009;5(3):263–76.
4. Chung F, Subramanyam R, Liao P, et al. High STOP-Bang score indicates a high probability of obstructive sleep apnoea. Br J Anaesth. 2012;108(5):768–75.
5. Johns MW. A new method for measuring daytime sleepiness: the Epworth sleepiness scale. Sleep. 1991;14(6):540–5.

Chapter 35
Approach to Acute Kidney Injury

Andrea S. Christopher and Melissa M. Hagman

Learning Objective
1. Define acute kidney injury.
2. Outline a systematic approach to evaluate acute kidney injury.
3. Identify common causes of acute kidney injury.

Clinical Vignette: A 69-year-old man with history of osteoarthritis and benign prostatic hypertrophy presents with 24 h of nausea and vomiting. He takes ibuprofen and tamsulosin. His lab results today show a creatinine of 1.9 mg/dL. At his annual exam 2 days ago, his creatinine was 1.1 mg/dL.

A. **What is the definition of acute kidney injury (AKI)? Does this patient have AKI?**

   Write down the definition of AKI above of the urinary tract Fig. 35.1.

Teaching points
- Definition: an abrupt (<48 h) increase in creatinine by 0.3 mg/dL from baseline, an increase in creatinine by 50% from baseline, or urine output less than 0.5 mL/kg/h for 6 h or more.
- Cannot estimate glomerular filtration rate (GFR) using the serum creatinine in AKI because GFR calculation requires a steady state.
- Given that this patient had a 0.8 mg/dL increase in creatinine within 48 h, he has AKI.

A. S. Christopher (✉) · M. M. Hagman
Boise VA Medical Center, Department of Medicine, Division of General Internal Medicine, University of Washington, Seattle, WA, USA
e-mail: andrea.christopher@va.gov

S. Mookherjee et al. (eds.), *Chalk Talks in Internal Medicine*,
https://doi.org/10.1007/978-3-030-34814-4_35

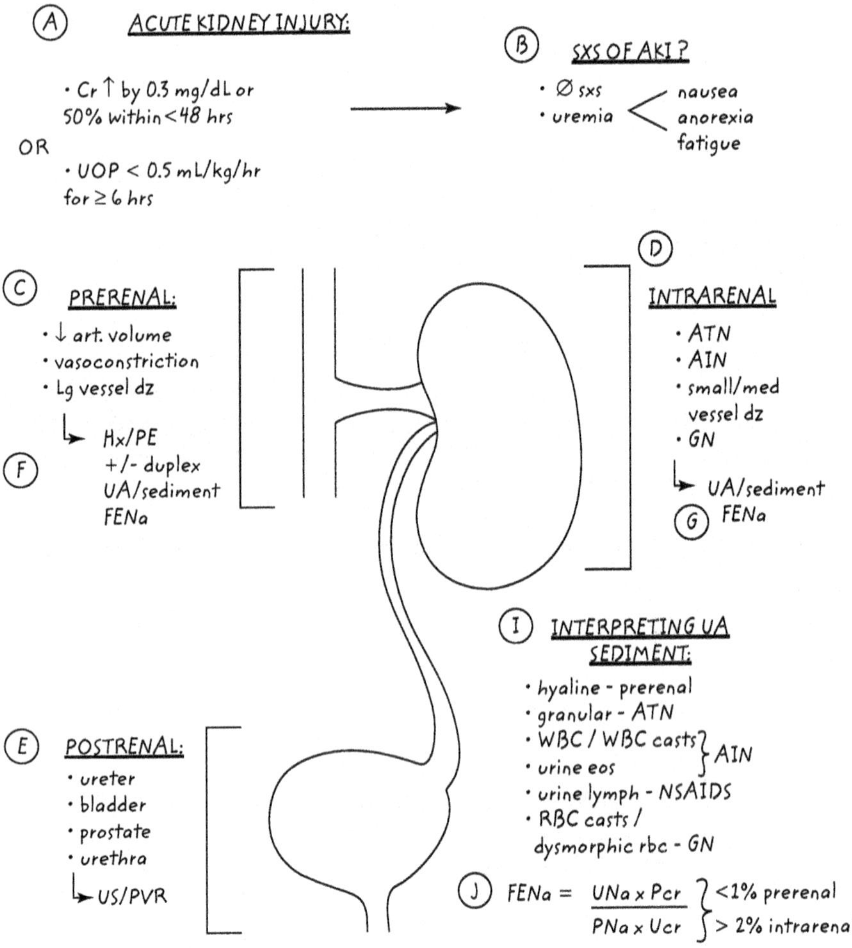

Fig. 35.1 Approach to acute kidney injury, A–F, G, I, J

B. **What are the symptoms of AKI?**

Write down the symptoms of AKI as they are suggested by the learners.

- May be asymptomatic.
- Symptoms of uremia: nausea, anorexia, fatigue.
- In this patient, it is hard to tell if nausea is from a different cause and preceded AKI or whether it is a side effect from the AKI.

C. **The common causes of AKI fall into three categories: prerenal, intrarenal, and postrenal. In this patient, what are the most likely prerenal causes of his AKI? Looking at the urinary tract, what are possible prerenal causes of his AKI?**

Write down categories of prerenal causes on the urinary tract figure as potential etiologies are mentioned, adding any key etiologies that are missed.

Teaching points

- Decreased arterial volume
  - Hypovolemia (tank)
  - Reduced cardiac output (pump)
  - Systemic vasodilation (pipes)
- Renal vasoconstriction
  - Nonsteroidal anti-inflammatory drugs (NSAIDs)
  - Angiotensin-converting enzyme inhibitors (ACEi)/angiotensin receptor blockers (ARBs)
  - Hypercalcemia
  - Hepatorenal syndrome
- Large vessel disease
  - Renal artery stenosis (+ACEi or ARB)
  - Vasculitis
  - Dissection
  - Abdominal compartment syndrome
  - Venothromboembolism (VTE)
- In this patient, most likely causes are hypovolemia from nausea and vomiting or medication side effect from ibuprofen.

D. **What are common intrarenal causes of AKI? In this patient, what is the most likely intrarenal cause of AKI?**

Write down categories of intrarenal causes of AKI on the urinary tract figure as potential etiologies are mentioned, adding any key etiologies that are missed.

Teaching points

- Acute tubular necrosis (ATN).
  - Drugs (aminoglycosides, amphotericin, cisplatin)
  - Pigments (rhabdomyolysis)
  - Crystals (uric acid, methotrexate, indinavir, oral sodium phosphate)
  - Monoclonal (immunoglobulin light chains)
  - Intravenous contrast
  - Ischemia (progression of prerenal disease)
- Acute interstitial nephritis (AIN).
  - Allergic (drugs, including antibiotics, NSAIDs, proton pump inhibitors)
  - Infection (bacteria, mycobacteria, viruses, fungi)
  - Infiltrative disease (sarcoid)
  - Autoimmune (Sjögren's syndrome, systemic lupus erythematosus)
- Small and medium vessel disease.
  - Thrombotic thrombocytopenia purpura (TTP)/hemolytic uremic syndrome (HUS)
  - Disseminated intravascular coagulopathy (DIC)
  - Preeclampsia
  - Malignant hypertension
  - Cholesterol emboli
- Glomerulonephritis (GN).
- In this patient, the most likely intrarenal causes of AKI are allergic (e.g., AIN from NSAIDs) or infection (e.g., *Legionella*, *Escherichia coli*).

E. **What are common post-renal causes of AKI? In this patient, what is the most likely postrenal cause of AKI?**

Write down postrenal causes of AKI on the urinary tract as potential etiologies are mentioned, adding any key etiologies that are missed.

- Ureteral obstruction (nephrolithiasis, GU malignancy, ureteral stenosis, retroperitoneal fibrosis)
- Bladder obstruction (benign prostatic hypertrophy, prostate cancer, neurogenic bladder, anticholinergic medications, and urethral stricture)
- In this patient, the most likely postrenal cause of AKI is bladder obstruction (benign prostatic hypertrophy).

F. **What are the key physical exam findings, labs, and studies to evaluate for prerenal causes of AKI?**

Write down key components as suggested by learners.

Teaching points

- History and exam
  - Tachycardia—hypovolemia

  - Axillary dryness—hypovolemia
  - Warm, clammy skin—peripheral vasodilation (sepsis)

- Imaging such renal or urinary tract ultrasound, post-void residual (PVR) or Renal duplex
- Urine studies - including urinalysis with urine sediment microscopy, fractional excretion of sodium (FENa) or fractional excretion of urea (FEUrea)

G. **How would you evaluate this patient for intrarenal causes of AKI?**

Write down key components as suggested by learners.

Teaching points
- Urinalysis with urine sediment microscopy
- Fractional excretion of sodium (FENa) or fractional excretion of urea (FEUrea)

H. **How would you evaluate this patient for postrenal causes of AKI?**

Write down key components as suggested by learners.

Teaching points
- Postvoid residual (PVR)
- Renal/urinary tract ultrasound (US)

I. **The patient's urine sediment reveals hyaline casts and granular casts. How do you interpret this result?**

Summarize the significance of sediment findings on Fig. 35.1 *as they are mentioned.*

Teaching points
- For this patient:
  - Hyaline casts—prerenal
  - Granular casts—ATN
  - Most likely dehydration from vomiting and component of ATN from taking ibuprofen for osteoarthritis
- Other considerations:
  - White blood cell (WBC) and WBC casts—AIN
  - Urine eosinophils—AIN
  - Urine lymphocytes—NSAIDs
  - Red blood cell (RBC) casts and dysmorphic RBC—glomerulonephritis

J. **What is the significance of the FENa? What clinical scenarios disrupt interpreting the FENa and what alternative options exist?**

Add the formula to calculate FENa and FEUrea.

Teaching points
- FENa = (urine sodium × plasma creatinine)/(plasma sodium × urine creatinine).
  - FENa <1%—prerenal, also blood urea nitrogen (BUN)/creatinine >20 and urine osmolality (Uosm) > 500 mOsm/kg

  - FENa >2%—intrarenal

- Use the FEUrea for patients who have taken loop diuretics
  - FEUrea = (urine urea × plasma creatinine)/(plasma BUN × urine creatinine)
  - FEUrea <35%—prerenal
  - FEUrea >50%—intrarenal

Return to Objectives and Emphasize Key Points

1. Define acute kidney injury.
   - An abrupt (<48 h) increase in creatinine by 0.3 mg/dL from baseline, an increase in creatinine by 50% from baseline, or urine output less than 0.5 mL/kg/h for 6 h or more
   - Cannot estimate GFR using the serum creatinine in AKI because GFR calculation requires a steady state
2. Outline a systematic approach to evaluate acute kidney injury.
   - Start by categorizing into prerenal, intrarenal, and postrenal etiologies.
   - Target history and physical exam toward identifying potential triggers for AKI and volume status to investigate prerenal etiologies.
   - Examine urine sediment for evidence of intrarenal etiologies.
   - Image the urinary tract for obstruction for postrenal etiologies.
3. Identify common causes of acute kidney injury.
   - Prerenal: decreased arterial volume, renal vasoconstriction, and large vessel disease
   - Intrarenal: acute tubular necrosis, acute interstitial nephritis, small and medium vessel disease, and glomerulonephritis
   - Postrenal: ureteral obstruction, bladder obstruction

Resources

1. KDIGO. Clinical practice guideline for acute kidney injury. Kidney Int Suppl. 2012;2:124–38.
2. McGee SR. Evidence-based physical diagnosis. 3rd ed. Philadelphia, PA: Elsevier; 2012.
3. Simerville JA, Maxted WC, Pahira JJ. Urinalysis: a comprehensive review. Am Fam Physician. 2005;71:1153–62.
4. KDIGO. Clinical practice guideline for acute kidney injury. Kidney Int Suppl. 2012;2:124–38.
5. Simerville JA, Maxted WC, Pahira JJ. Urinalysis: a comprehensive review. Am Fam Physician. 2005;71:1153–62.

Chapter 36
Approach to Hyponatremia

Kelly Nakamura and Doug Paauw

Learning Objectives
1. Determine how quickly to correct hyponatremia.
2. Use volume status to create a differential diagnosis for hyponatremia.
3. Use urine studies to evaluate the cause of hyponatremia.

Clinical Vignette: A 78-year-old woman with a history of congestive heart failure, hypertension, insulin-dependent diabetes, and depression presents to the emergency department with abdominal pain and nausea. She reports eating and drinking well despite her symptoms. She shows you a record of her daily morning weights and there has been no change. Her serum sodium is 125 mEq/L.

A. **What is the definition of hyponatremia?**

   Write the definition as shown in Fig. 36.1.

B. **How quickly should this patient's hyponatremia be corrected?**

   Continue the algorithm as shown in Fig. 36.1.

Teaching points
- This patient has a normal mental status. Serum sodium should be increased slowly: less than 0.5 mEq/L per hour *and* less than 8 mEq/L in the first 24 h.
- Why do we correct sodium slowly? A rapid increase in serum sodium can cause osmotic demyelination, a type of severe brain damage that occurs when water shifts out of brain cells.

K. Nakamura (✉)
Harborview Medical Center, Department of Medicine, Division of General Internal Medicine, University of Washington, Seattle, WA, USA
e-mail: kmn15@uw.edu

D. Paauw
University of Washington Medical Center, Department of Medicine, Division of General Internal Medicine, University of Washington, Seattle, WA, USA

S. Mookherjee et al. (eds.), *Chalk Talks in Internal Medicine*,
https://doi.org/10.1007/978-3-030-34814-4_36

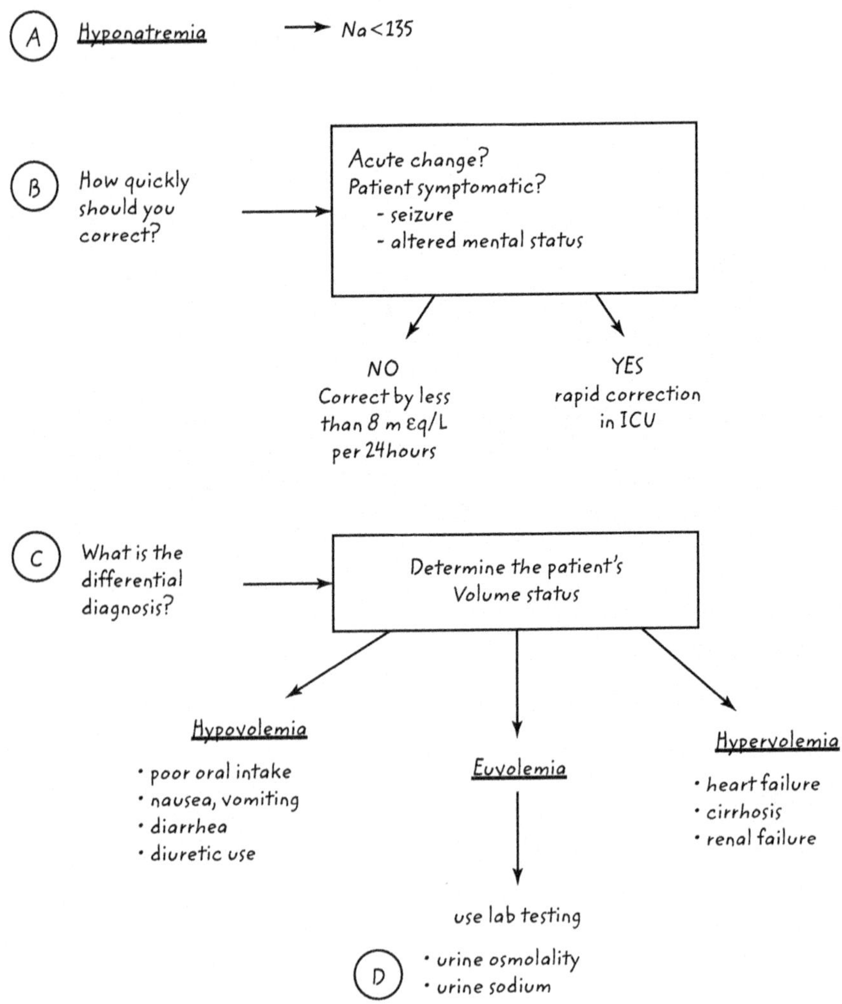

Fig. 36.1 Approach to hyponatremia: A–D

- Acute or symptomatic hyponatremia, identified by seizure or altered mental status, may require rapid correction in an intensive care unit (ICU) setting.

C. **On physical exam, the patient has a normal heart rate and blood pressure, moist mucous membranes, clear lung fields, and no lower extremity edema. A differential diagnosis for hyponatremia can be generated on the basis of a patient's volume status: hypovolemic, euvolemic, or hypervolemic. What are some common causes of hypovolemic and hypervolemic hyponatremia?**

Create the headings for the three categories, and write down causes as suggested by learners as shown in Fig. 36.1.

Teaching points
- Causes of hypovolemic hyponatremia include poor oral intake, vomiting, diarrhea, and diuretic use.
- Causes of hypervolemic hyponatremia include renal failure, congestive heart failure, and cirrhosis. In these conditions, the patient's total body volume is increased but their effective arterial volume is low. These conditions are usually identified during the medical history.
- Causes of euvolemic hyponatremia are determined by urine studies.

D. **What are the two urine studies that you should send to evaluate euvolemic hyponatremia? How do you interpret the results?**

*Create a table with columns for urine osmolality and urine sodium (*Fig. 36.2*). Write in the three sets of values given, and ask learners for the differential diagnosis in each case.*

Teaching points
- If a patient is hyponatremic, the kidneys should excrete normally water and produce maximally dilute urine, with urine osmolality less than 100 mEq/L.
- If urine osmolality is less than 100 mEq/L, either the patient has primary polydipsia (the kidneys cannot excrete water as fast as it is consumed), or the patient has low solute intake ("beer drinker's potomania" or "tea and toast diet") and there is not enough solute in the blood to excrete water normally.
- If urine osmolality is greater than 100 mEq/L with a high urine sodium, the most likely diagnosis is syndrome of inappropriate antidiuretic hormone secretion (SIADH).
- If urine osmolality is greater than 100 mEq/L and urine sodium is less than 20 mEq/L, consider low effective arterial blood volume due to hypovolemia or hypervolemia (i.e., heart failure).

E. **Our patient's urine osmolality is 421 mEq/L and urine sodium is 50 mEq/L. She is not taking a diuretic. Thyroid stimulating hormone (TSH) and morning (AM) cortisol are normal. What are your diagnosis and treatment plan?**

Draw a circle around SIADH, the most likely diagnosis in this case.

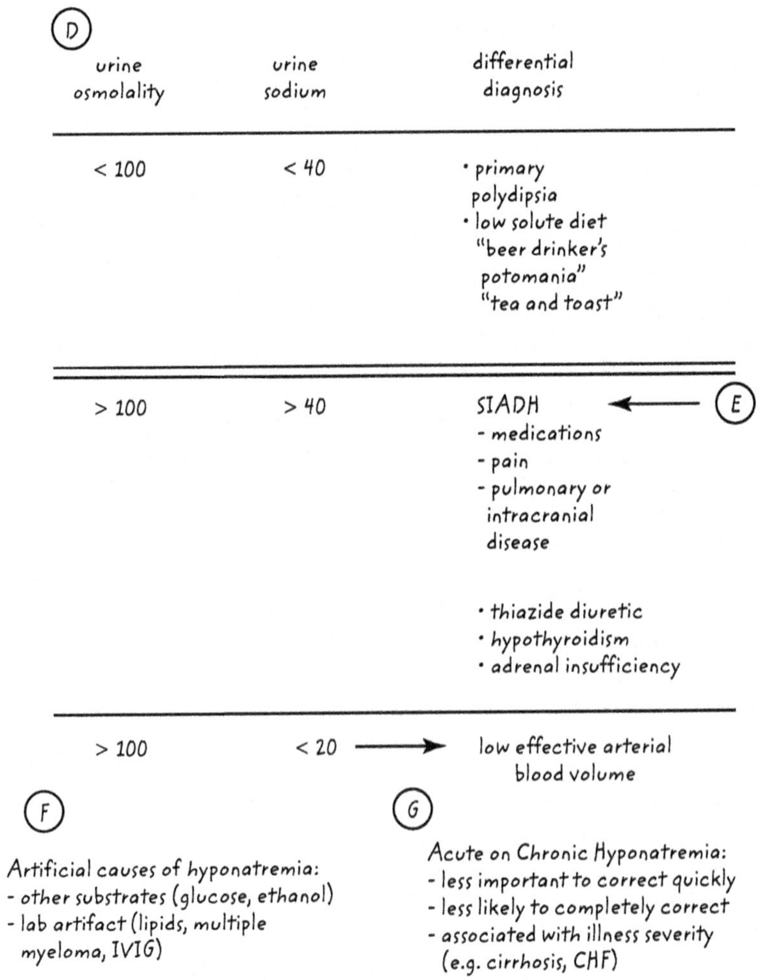

Fig. 36.2 Approach to hyponatremia: D–G

Teaching points

- Our patient has SIADH: her urine is not maximally dilute despite low serum sodium levels. Further history is needed to determine the cause of SIADH. Potential secondary causes of excess ADH are pain, medications (including selective serotonin reuptake inhibitors (SSRIs), serotonin-norepinephrine reuptake inhibitor (SNRIs), anticonvulsants, and antipsychotics), pulmonary processes, and intracranial processes.
- Hyponatremia caused by thiazide diuretics causes an identical picture with an inappropriately high urine osmolality. Other less common possibilities are adrenal insufficiency and severe hypothyroidism.
- The treatment of SIADH is fluid restriction, usually 1.5–2 L per day.

F. **The serum concentration of other substances can affect the serum sodium concentration. Can you think of examples of this effect?**

Write down "artificial" causes of hyponatremia as suggested.

Teaching points

- High serum concentrations of glucose, urea, or ethanol cause the serum sodium concentration to decrease.
- "Pseudohyponatremia" occurs with high serum concentrations of lipids or protein (e.g., hypertriglyceridemia, intravenous immunoglobulin (IVIG) therapy, or multiple myeloma). This is a lab artifact, not an actual change in serum sodium concentration.
- In the scenarios listed earlier, serum osmolality is normal (around 286 mEq/L) or high. You can measure serum osmolality directly, but it is usually not necessary in the appropriate clinical context.

G. **Records show that the patient's serum sodium has been 128–131 mEq/L over the past year. How does this information influence your assessment?**

Write down key points for acute or chronic hyponatremia.

Teaching points

- In this case, the patient has acute or chronic hyponatremia. Chronic hyponatremia is common among elderly patients.
- It is generally less urgent to correct acute or chronic hyponatremia than severe acute hyponatremia, unless the patient is symptomatic. Patients with chronic hyponatremia are unlikely to reach normal sodium levels even with treatment.
- Both chronic and acute hyponatremia are associated with increased morbidity and mortality, and are markers of illness severity in conditions such as congestive heart failure and cirrhosis.

Return to Objectives and Emphasize Key Points

1. Determine how quickly to correct hyponatremia.
   - Use symptoms (mental status, seizures) to determine speed with which to correct hyponatremia.
   - If rapid correction is needed, this should be accomplished in the ICU.
2. Use volume status to create a differential diagnosis for hyponatremia.
   - Hypovolemic hyponatremia can be due to vomiting, poor intake, diarrhea, or excessive diuretic use.
   - Hypervolemic hyponatremia is commonly seen in kidney failure, heart failure, or cirrhosis.
   - Euvolemic hyponatremia requires urine testing to determine potential causes.
3. Use urine studies to evaluate the cause of hyponatremia,
   - Dilute urine (urine osmolality <100) with low urine sodium implies excessive intake of hypotonic fluids (primary polydipsia or "tea and toast" diet).
   - Concentrated urine (urine osmolality >100) with high urine sodium implies inappropriate ADH secretion (SIADH), which can be caused by medications, pain, and intracranial or pulmonary etiologies.

Resources

1. Adrogué HJ, Madias NE. Hyponatremia. N Engl J Med. 2000;342(21):1581.
2. Sterns RH. Treatment of severe hyponatremia. Clin J Am Soc Nephrol. 2018;13(4):641.
3. Spasovski G, Vanholder R, Allolio B, et al. Clinical practice guideline on diagnosis and treatment of hyponatraemia. Nephrol Dial Transplant. 2014;29(Suppl 2):i1.

Chapter 37
Workup of Chronic Kidney Disease

Naomi Shike and Somnath Mookherjee

Learning Objectives
1. Use an anatomical framework to build a differential for causes of chronic kidney disease.
2. Choose appropriate tests to workup chronic kidney disease.

Clinical Vignette: A 58-year-old man establishes care in your clinic. You notice that his creatinine is 1.8 mg/dL and eGFR is 40. In looking through records, you see that 6 months ago his creatinine was 1.7 and 2 years ago it was 1.4. His past medical history lists hypertension, type 2 diabetes mellitus, and low back pain. No other records are available.

A. **Does this patient have CKD? How is CKD defined?**

Write down the definition of CKD as shown in Fig. 37.1.

Teaching points
- CKD is defined as daily urine albumin excretion of ≥30 mg OR eGFR <60 mL/min/1.73 m^2.
- Abnormality must have been present for at least three months.
- This is a continuum: most causes of CKD also have a corresponding version of AKI; therefore, the "definition" is a somewhat arbitrary cutoff.

N. Shike (✉)
Harborview Medical Center, Department of Medicine, Division of General Internal Medicine, University of Washington, Seattle, WA, USA
e-mail: shike@uw.edu

S. Mookherjee
University of Washington Medical Center, Department of Medicine, Division of General Internal Medicine, University of Washington, Seattle, WA, USA

S. Mookherjee et al. (eds.), *Chalk Talks in Internal Medicine*,
https://doi.org/10.1007/978-3-030-34814-4_37

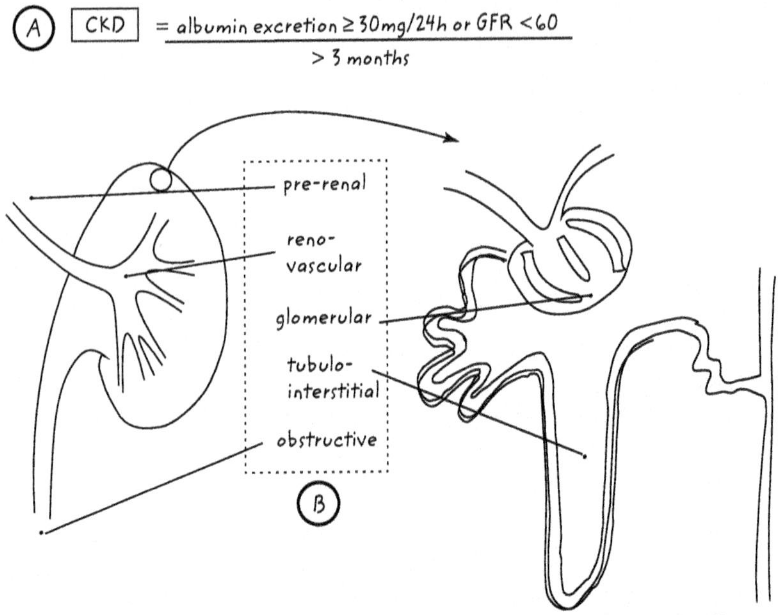

B Site	C Causes	D tests
pre-renal	CHF, cirrhosis, ATN	echo, LFT'S, (mainly history)
renal vascular	RAS/atherosclerosis, fibromusc. dysplasia	Renal US/duplex, CT angiogram
glomerular	hypertensive nephro-sclerosis, diabetic nephropathy, nephrotic/nephritic syndrome	UA, spot protein/creatinine
tubulo-interstitial	PC KD, nephrocalcinosis, autoimmune, meds/toxins	Urine micro, autoimmune serologies
obstructive	prostate, bladder, other pelvic	CT, US

Fig. 37.1 Workup of chronic kidney disease: A–D

B. **It is useful to consider the potential causes of his CKD by taking an anatomical approach. What are the five major anatomical sites that we should be familiar with in considering the cause of his CKD?**

Draw the schematic of the kidney and the nephron as shown in Fig. 37.1. *Label the sites as the learners list them, and list them in the table at the same time.*

C. **What are some specific causes of CKD that correspond to each anatomical site?**

List causes as suggested by the learner.

Teaching points
- Acute tubular necrosis (ATN) can resolve versus progress to CKD.
- Nephritic and nephrotic syndromes start as AKI; some can resolve versus progress to CKD.
- While many of these etiologies have acute correlates, some are truly chronic—such as hypertensive nephrosclerosis, polycystic kidney disease.

D. **The patient's history will usually guide the work-up for CKD. What initial work-up would you do for this patient? What if the other anatomical sites were suspected?**

List the tests under "glomerular," and then fill out the rest of the table as tests and studies are suggested by the learners.

Teaching points
- The history is the primary guide for the work-up of the patient.
- If after an initial work-up the etiology is unclear, and especially if the renal dysfunction is worsening, renal biopsy may be needed (as well as nephrology consultation).

Return to Objectives and Emphasize Key Points
1. Use an anatomical framework to build a differential for causes of chronic kidney disease.
    - Return to the diagrams and circle pre-renal, reno-vascular, glomerular, tubulointerstitial, and obstructive.
2. Choose appropriate tests to work up chronic kidney disease.
    - Highlight the common initial tests: urine protein/albumin, UA, abdominal computed tomography (CT) or US, assessment of renal arteries.
    - Renal biopsy may be needed if these tests do not provide a diagnosis or renal failure progresses.

Resources

1. Visconti L, Cernaro V, Ricciardi CA, et al. Renal biopsy: still a landmark for the nephrologist. World J Nephrol. 2016;5(4):321–7. https://doi.org/10.5527/wjn.v5.i4.321.
2. Fraser SD, Blakeman T. Chronic kidney disease: identification and management in primary care. Pragmat Obs Res. 2016;7:21–32. https://doi.org/10.2147/POR.S97310.
3. Kidney Disease: Improving Global Outcomes (KDIGO) CKD Work Group. KDIGO 2012 clinical practice guideline for the evaluation and management of chronic kidney disease. Kidney Int Suppl. 2013;3:1–150.

Chapter 38
Approach to Microscopic Hematuria

Somnath Mookherjee, Lauren A. Beste, Jared W. Klein, and Jennifer Wright

Learning Objectives

1. Use a systematic approach to evaluation of microscopic hematuria.
2. Describe common causes of microscopic hematuria.
3. Distinguish between "glomerular" and "nonglomerular" sources of microscopic hematuria.
4. Identify risk factors for genitourinary (GU) malignancy.

Clinical Vignette: A 62-year-old man comes to see you because he received notification that his insurance examination urine dipstick had shown "blood." He is confused by these results as he has never seen blood in his urine.

A. **How do we define hematuria—do we know that he really has it?**

Write the definition as shown in Fig. 38.1.

Teaching points

- The term "gross hematuria" is used to describe visible blood in the urine. The term "microscopic hematuria" is used when blood is not visible to the naked eye, only noted upon microscopic examination.

S. Mookherjee (✉) · J. Wright
University of Washington Medical Center, Department of Medicine, Division of General Internal Medicine, University of Washington, Seattle, WA, USA
e-mail: smookh@u.washington.edu

L. A. Beste
VA Puget Sound Health Care System, Department of Medicine, Division of General Internal Medicine, University of Washington, Seattle, WA, USA

J. W. Klein
Harborview Medical Center, Department of Medicine, Division of General Internal Medicine, University of Washington, Seattle, WA, USA

S. Mookherjee et al. (eds.), *Chalk Talks in Internal Medicine*,
https://doi.org/10.1007/978-3-030-34814-4_38

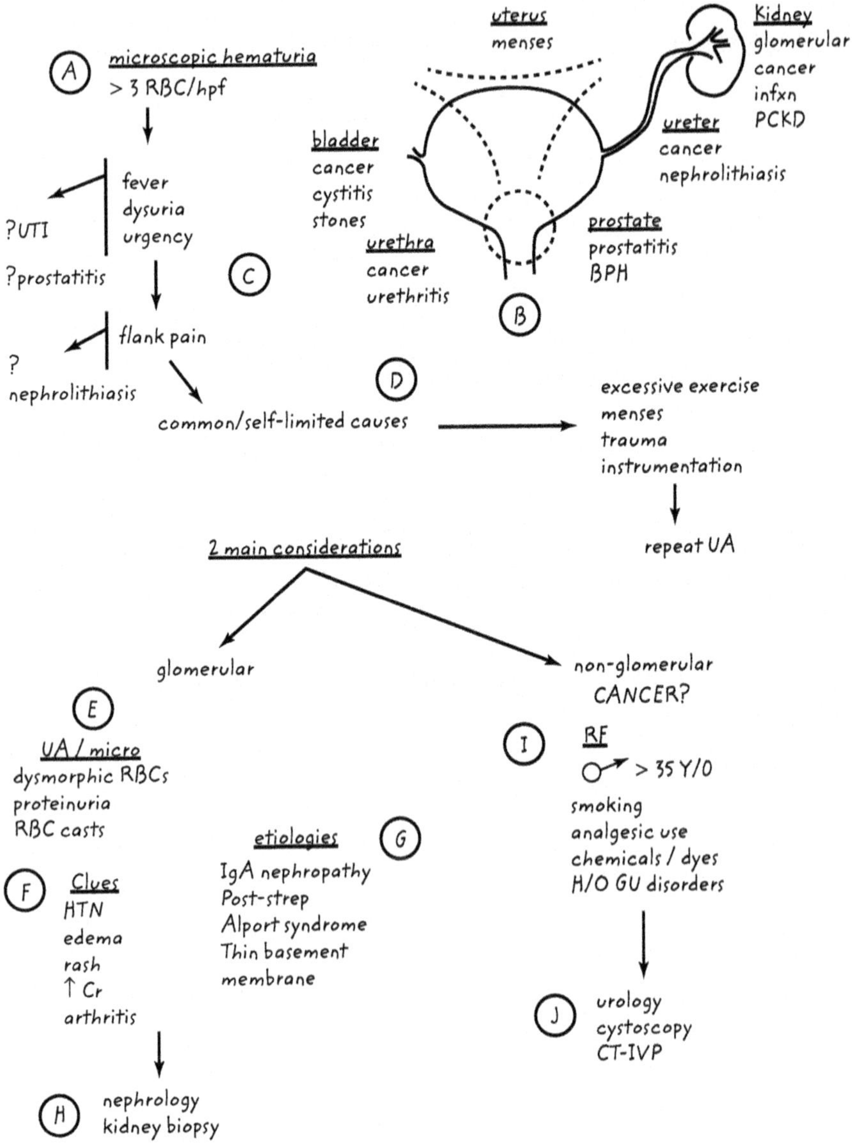

Fig. 38.1 Approach to asymptomatic hematuria: A–J

- Positive blood on urine dipstick is not sufficient to diagnose microscopic hematuria, as this is a very sensitive test with frequent false positives.
- Instead, microscopic urine analysis must be performed to assess for red blood cells in the urine.
- Greater than 3 red blood cells per high-powered field (RBC/hpf) is generally considered to be hematuria.

B. **You order a microscopic urinalysis (UA). The UA shows six red blood cells per high-powered field (RBC/hpf) and is otherwise normal. Based on this definition, this patient has microscopic hematuria. Looking at this outline of the GU tract, what are some possible causes of his hematuria?**

Write down causes on the figure of the urinary tract as potential etiologies are mentioned, adding any key etiologies that are missed.

Teaching points

- The source of red blood cells can be from anywhere in the urinary tract.
- It is useful to use anatomy as a framework to build the differential diagnosis; in addition, it is useful to reflect on the benign (cystitis) versus concerning etiologies (malignancy) and to consider potential nonurinary sources of red blood cells (e.g., menses).

C. **Some of the etiologies that were mentioned can be quite symptomatic. It is important to confirm that our patient isn't having any symptoms consistent with nephrolithiasis, urinary tract infection, or prostatitis. What are some key questions about symptoms to ask the patient?**

Write down key symptoms as suggested by learners.

Teaching points

- Ask about fevers, chills, dysuria, urgency, abdominal pain, and flank pain.
- If these symptoms are present, then further evaluation and treatment should be pursued.
- For hematuria in the setting of a GU infection or nephrolithiasis, unless the etiology is clearly uncomplicated urinary tract infection (UTI), repeat the UA 6 weeks after treatment to ensure the hematuria resolves.
- Further evaluation should be pursued if hematuria persists.

D. **Our patient isn't having any symptoms—we can describe him as having asymptomatic microscopic hematuria. What are some potential benign or self-limited causes of asymptomatic microscopic hematuria?**

Write down common benign causes and the follow-up as shown in Fig. 38.1.

Teaching points

- Recent menses, excessive exercise (running, biking), trauma to the GU tract (such as a Foley catheter or other instrumentation)
- In these cases it is critical to recheck a UA (American Urological Association [AUA] guidelines recommends after 6 weeks) to ensure that the hematuria has resolved.
- If hematuria persists, then further evaluation should be pursued.

E. **Our patient is asymptomatic and doesn't have any of the common causes of benign hematuria. A useful way to organize his workup is to consider "glomerular" and "nonglomerular" etiologies. This is helpful in reaching the correct diagnosis and will guide the evaluation. What findings on the UA indicate a glomerular source of bleeding?**

Write down UA findings as shown in the figure.

Teaching points

- See the figure—key findings include dysmorphic red blood cells (acanthocytes), RBC casts on microscopic exam and proteinuria

F. **Our patient is asymptomatic, but sometimes signs and symptoms of disease can develop insidiously. What are the key clues on history, physical examination, and labs that might suggest a glomerular source of bleeding?**

Write down important clues as suggested by learners.

G. **What are some common causes of asymptomatic glomerular hematuria?**

The list of etiologies is long—emphasize common and asymptomatic etiologies.

- IgA nephropathy—often presents post-URI.
- Poststreptococcal—caused by Group A strep, 2 weeks after pharyngitis, 6 weeks after skin infection.
- Alport syndrome—X-linked, associated with hearing loss, ocular changes.
- Thin basement membrane syndrome—usually nonprogressive, "maybe not a disease."

H. **If you did suspect a glomerular source of hematuria in this patient, what would be your next step?**

Emphasize the two key next steps as shown in Fig. 38.1.

Teaching points

- Refer to nephrology, may proceed to renal biopsy.
- Guidelines differ in their recommendations regarding the appropriate evaluation of patients with signs of a glomerular source of microscopic hematuria.
- The AUA recommends concurrent nephrology and urology evaluations, whereas some other groups recommend starting with a referral to nephrology.

I. **Our patient doesn't have any characteristics of glomerular bleeding. The most concerning etiology of asymptomatic nonglomerular bleeding is cancer. What risk factors for GU tract cancer does this patient have?**

Write down key risk factors, emphasizing those listed in Fig. 38.1.

Teaching points

- Male
- Age >35 years
- History of smoking
- Chemicals or dyes (benzenes or aromatic amines)
- Analgesic abuse
- History of gross hematuria
- History of urologic disorder or disease
- History of irritative voiding symptoms
- History of pelvic irradiation
- History of chronic urinary tract infection
- History of exposure to known carcinogenic agents or chemotherapy such as alkylating agents
- History of chronic indwelling foreign body

J. **What will be your next step for this patient?**

Continue the algorithm as shown.

Teaching points

- Imaging of the GU tract should be performed. The preferred study is a CT urography, which is a multiphase contrast study with high sensitivity for detecting renal parenchymal masses in addition to other GU tract abnormalities.
- Patients over age 35 years need to have a cystoscopy to evaluate for malignancy. Patients under age 35 years may need to have cystoscopy, depending on their other risk factors for malignancy.

Return to Objectives and Emphasize Key Points

1. Recognize common causes of microscopic hematuria—circle these in the figure.
   - Cancer
   - Infection (e.g., bladder, kidney, prostate)
   - Stones
   - IgA nephropathy
   - Poststreptococcal
   - Benign (e.g., menses, exercise)
2. Distinguish between "glomerular" and "nonglomerular" sources of asymptomatic microscopic hematuria—circle these in Fig. 38.1.
   - UA—glomerular with dysmorphic RBCs, RBC casts, protein
   - Other clues—glomerular with hypertension, fluid overload, elevated creatinine

3. Identify risk factors for GU malignancy—circle/asterisk these in the figure.
   - Male
   - Age >35 years
   - History of smoking
   - Chemicals or dyes (benzenes or aromatic amines)
   - Analgesic overuse
   - History of gross hematuria
   - History of urologic disorder or disease

Resources

1. Nielsen M, Quaseem A. Hematuria as a marker of occult urinary tract cancer: advice for high-value care from the American College of Physicians. Ann Intern Med. 2016;164(7):488–97.
2. Niemi MA, Cohen RA. Evaluation of microscopic hematuria: a critical review and proposed algorithm. Adv Chronic Kidney Dis. 2015;22(4):289–96. https://doi.org/10.1053/j.ackd.2015.04.006.
3. Davis R, Jones JS, Barocas DA, et al. Diagnosis, evaluation and follow-up of asymptomatic microhematuria (AMH) in adults: AUA guideline. J Urol. 2012;188(6 Suppl):2473–81.
4. Sharp VJ, Barnes KT, Erickson BA. University of Iowa Hospitals and Clinics, Iowa City, Iowa. Assessment of Asymptomatic Microscopic Hematuria in Adults. Am Fam Physician. 2013;88(11):747–54.
5. Davis R, Jones S, Barocas DA, Castle EP, Lang EK, Leveillee RJ, Messing EM, Miller SD, Peterson AC, TMT T, Weitzel W, Urol J. Diagnosis, evaluation and follow-up of asymptomatic microhematuria (AMH) in adults: AUA guideline. 2012;188(6 Suppl):2473–81. Accessible at: http://www.auanet.org/education/guidelines/asymptomatic-microhematuria.cfm.

Chapter 39
Prevention and Management of Gout

James Darnton and Christopher Knight

Learning Objectives
1. Provide lifestyle modification recommendations to prevent gout flares.
2. Treat a gout flare with the appropriate medication(s).
3. Identify suitable candidates for urate-lowering therapy (ULT).
4. Provide appropriate ULT and concurrent anti-inflammatory prophylaxis.

Clinical Vignette: A 62-year-old man with congestive heart failure (CHF) and diabetes mellitus is seen in your primary care clinic for recurrent painful swelling of the right knee. He was seen in the emergency department for an episode of painful swelling of the right knee 6 months ago. At that time, analysis of the synovial fluid revealed intracellular negatively birefringent needle-shaped crystals.

A. **For this talk, we are assuming the diagnosis of gouty arthritis has already been made—the differential for monoarticular arthritis is broad. In this instance, the patient has crystal proven gout, and monoarticular arthritis in the same joint which can reasonably be assumed to be another gout attack.**

   Write "acute gouty arthritis" on the white board.

B. **Diet can provoke gout and gout flares. What would you advise this patient to avoid in his diet?**

   Write down foods and beverages as suggested by learners.

J. Darnton (✉)
Harborview Medical Center, Department of Medicine, Division of General Internal Medicine, University of Washington, Seattle, WA, USA
e-mail: jdarnton@uw.edu

C. Knight
University of Washington Medical Center, Department of Medicine, Division of General Internal Medicine, University of Washington, Seattle, WA, USA

S. Mookherjee et al. (eds.), *Chalk Talks in Internal Medicine*,
https://doi.org/10.1007/978-3-030-34814-4_39

Teaching points
- Organ meats with high purine content (e.g., liver, kidney)
- High-fructose corn syrup
- Alcohol (particularly beer)

C. **What medications would you review and, if possible, discontinue?**

Write down appropriate medications as suggested by learners.

Teaching points
- Thiazide and loop diuretics
- Niacin
- Calcineurin inhibitors

D. **Primary gout refers to the occurrence of gout without a clear reason for overproduction or undersecretion of uric acid—but primary gout can accompany common comorbidities such as obesity, hypertension, or diabetes. In secondary gout, a reason for elevated uric acid can be identified, such as the medications noted earlier. What are some other causes of secondary gout?**

List causes as suggested by learners.

Teaching points
- There are MANY causes, including renal failure, lead intoxication, renal failure, medullary cystic kidney disease.

E. **Should you check a serum uric acid level in this patient? When should you measure uric acid levels?**

Write down indications for checking a serum uric acid level.

- The serum uric acid level during a flare is not helpful for making the diagnosis or guiding treatment.
- Measure a serum uric acid level once flare resolves if considering secondary causes of hyperuricemia.
- Screen for uric acid overproduction by urine uric acid evaluation in patient subsets with gout onset before age 25 or a history of urolithiasis.
- Serum uric acid level would need to be checked if chronic urate-lowering therapy is started.
- For this patient, the flare should resolve before a uric acid level is obtained.

F. **How will you treat your patient's gout flare?**

Write down the treatment options as shown in Fig. 39.1.

Teaching points
- Nonsteroidal anti-inflammatory drugs (NSAIDs):
  - Maximum dose until the acute flare has completely resolved.
  - Naproxen and indomethacin are approved by the Food and Drug Administration (FDA) for use in gout, but others in the class may be as effective.

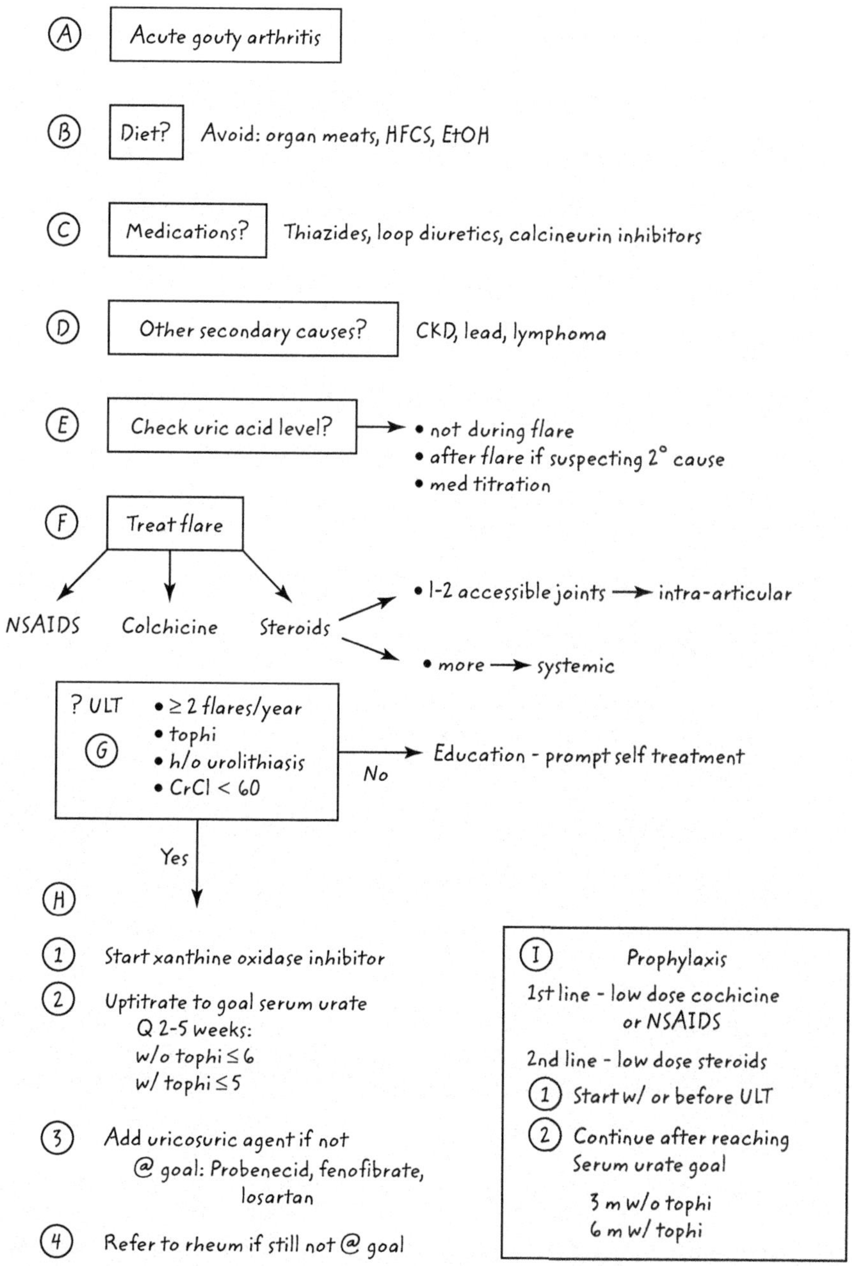

Fig. 39.1 Prevention and management of gout, A–I

  - Celecoxib (Cox-2 inhibitor) or NSAID + PPI could be considered in patients with GI contraindication to NSAID.

- Colchicine: 1.2 mg loading dose, followed by 0.6 mg 1 h later, and then 0.6 mg once-twice daily until attack resolves.
- Steroids.
  - Dosing strategies vary. Many clinicians use prednisone 40 mg daily until flare starts to resolve, followed by a 7- to 10-day taper.
  - If only 1–2 joints are involved, can consider intra-articular (possibly in combination with one of the other first-line oral treatments).
- Refractory cases: consider switching to an alternate monotherapy, combining two of the above, or referring to rheumatology for consideration of an IL-1 receptor antagonist (Anakinra).
- For our patient, heart failure is a relative contraindication for high-dose NSAIDs, and his diabetes management may be complicated by steroid use, so colchicine +/– intra-articular steroids may be the best treatment option.

G. **What reasons would prompt you to start urate-lowering therapy (ULT) for your patient?**

Write down reasons as suggested by learners.

Teaching points

- Criteria are:
  - Tophus or tophi by clinical examination or imaging
  - Frequent attacks of acute gouty arthritis (≥2 a year)
  - Past urolithiasis
  - Gout with stage 3 or worse chronic kidney disease (CKD) (creatinine clearance <60 mL/min/1.73 m^2)
- In the case, this is the patient's second attack in 6 months, so ULT is indicated.

H. **What ULT would you prescribe? How do you find the right dose?**

Write out algorithm for ULT as shown.

Teaching points

- Allopurinol is the cheaper of the xanthine oxidase inhibitors (XOIs).
- Patients are at risk for allopurinol hypersensitivity syndrome (AHS), which can lead to Stevens Johnson syndrome (SJS), toxic epidermal necrolysis (TEN), and drug reaction with eosinophilia and systemic symptoms (DRESS).
- To minimize the risk, start at a dose of 100 mg/day (50 mg/day in stage 4 or worse CKD) and uptitrate gradually every 2–5 weeks.
- Prior to initiation, consider testing for HLA-B∗5801 in populations at higher risk for severe AHS (Koreans with stage 3 or worse CKD, and Han Chinese and Thai, irrespective of renal function).
- Continue up-titration until uric acid is below goal (<6 for patients without tophi, <5 for patients with tophi). If the goal is not achieved with maximum allopurinol, add on a uricosuric agent, most commonly probenecid.

- If still not at goal, consider pegloticase (usually prescribed by a rheumatologist). Febuxostat is an alternative XOI, which is more expensive but does not cause AHS. It should be used in patients at high risk of AHS.

I. **Initiation of ULT can cause a gout flare. How can this be prevented?**

Complete the prophylaxis box as shown in Fig. 39.1.

- Any treatment for acute gout (NSAIDs, colchicine, systemic steroids) can be used for prophylaxis against ULT-induced flares at low doses. NSAIDs or colchicine are first-line choices.
- Start when initiating ULT. Continue until reaching serum uric acid goal, and then for an additional:
  - Three months if no tophi
  - Six months if tophi present

Return to Objectives and Emphasize Key Points

1. Provide lifestyle modification recommendations to prevent gout flares.
   - Avoid the following foods/drinks:
   - Organ meats with high purine content (e.g., liver, kidney).
   - High-fructose corn syrup.
   - Alcohol (particularly beer).
   - Avoid the following medications: thiazide and loop diuretics, niacin, calcineurin inhibitors
2. Treat a gout flare with the appropriate medication(s):
   - NSAIDs, colchicine, or steroids (systemic or intra-articular)
3. Identify suitable candidates for urate-lowering therapy (ULT).
   - Tophus or tophi by clinical examination or imaging
   - Frequent attacks of acute gouty arthritis (>2 a year)
   - Past urolithiasis
   - Gout with stage 3 or worse CKD (creatinine clearance <60 mL/min/1.73 m^2)
4. Provide appropriate ULT and concurrent anti-inflammatory prophylaxis.
   - Allopurinol is first line with target uric acid <6 in patients without tophi and <5 in patients with tophi.
   - Add uricosuric agent once at max dose, if not at goal.

Resources

1. Khanna D, Puja P, Fitzgerald J, Signh M, Bae S, Neogi T, et al. 2012 American College of Rheumatology Guidelines for Management of Gout. Part 1: systemic nonpharmacologic and pharmacologic therapeutic approaches to hyperuricemia. Arthritis Care Res. 2012;64(10):1431–46.
2. Khanna D, Puja P, Fitzgerald J, Signh M, Bae S, Neogi T, et al. 2012 American College of Rheumatology Guidelines for Management of Gout. Part 2: therapy and antiinflammatory prophylaxis of acute gouty arthritis. Arthritis Care Res. 2012;64(10):1447–61.

Chapter 40
Approach to Monoarticular Arthritis

Gabrielle Berger and Thomas Payne

Learning Objectives

1. Describe a diagnostic framework for monoarticular arthritis.
2. Identify features of the history and physical examination that help differentiate causes of monoarticular arthritis.
3. Explain the indications for arthrocentesis.
4. Interpret key findings in synovial fluid analysis.

Clinical Vignette: A 63-year-old man with Crohn's disease, on infliximab, and osteoarthritis presents to the emergency room with 2 days of increasing right knee pain associated with swelling and redness. He felt warm at home but hasn't taken his temperature. He plays tennis and golf regularly, despite osteoarthritis in both hips and knees. He thinks his current knee pain is different from his chronic pain.

A. **How should we characterize this patient's knee pain?**

Ask learners to describe the arthritis in terms of the number of joints affected.

Teaching points

- The term "arthralgia" refers to pain in a joint. The term "arthritis" is used to describe *inflammation* in a joint.
- Arthritis can be described according to the number of joints involved. "Monoarticular arthritis" refers to involvement of one joint.
- When a few joints are involved, we use the term "oligoarticular arthritis"; widespread joint involvement is "polyarticular arthritis."

G. Berger (✉) · T. Payne
University of Washington Medical Center, Department of Medicine, Division of General Internal Medicine, University of Washington, Seattle, WA, USA
e-mail: gberger@uw.edu

S. Mookherjee et al. (eds.), *Chalk Talks in Internal Medicine*,
https://doi.org/10.1007/978-3-030-34814-4_40

B. **What are the two broad categories of arthritis?**

Write the two category headings on the board. Under "Inflammatory," fill in "septic," "crystalline," and "autoimmune disease" on top of the boxes on the left side of the board. Under "Non-inflammatory," write "trauma" and "tumors" on top of the boxes on the right side of the board (Fig. 40.1).

Teaching points

- Arthritis can be divided into two broad categories: inflammatory and noninflammatory.
- Synovial fluid with ≥2000 white blood cells (WBCs)/mm^3 is diagnostic of inflammatory arthritis. We will talk more about synovial fluid analysis in a few minutes.
- The three major subcategories of inflammatory arthritis are infectious/septic, crystalline arthropathies, and arthropathy caused by autoimmune disease. The major causes of noninflammatory arthritis include trauma, hemarthrosis, tumors, and osteoarthritis.

C. **Our patient is complaining of 2 days of increasing pain that feels different from his baseline. How does the time course help create a framework for thinking about specific causes of monoarticular arthritis?**

Write "acute, subacute, and chronic" in a vertical line on the far left side of the board.

Teaching points

- Symptom onset can be acute, subacute, or chronic. The timing of symptoms helps differentiate causes of monoarticular arthritis.
- For example, bacterial septic arthritis is acute in onset, can cause rapid joint destruction, and requires urgent diagnosis and management.

D. **Let's start with acute monoarticular arthritis. What are the most common bacterial causes of acute septic arthritis? What are the major causes of crystalline arthropathies?**

Add suggestions from the learners to the appropriate categories.

Teaching points

- Staphylococcal species causes greater than 80 percent of cases of septic arthritis, with Streptococcal species as the next most common etiology.
- Gram-negative rods (GNRs), such as *Escherichia coli*, comprise a smaller percentage.
- Gonococcal arthritis is even less common, though it remains an important cause in patients with high-risk sexual practices.

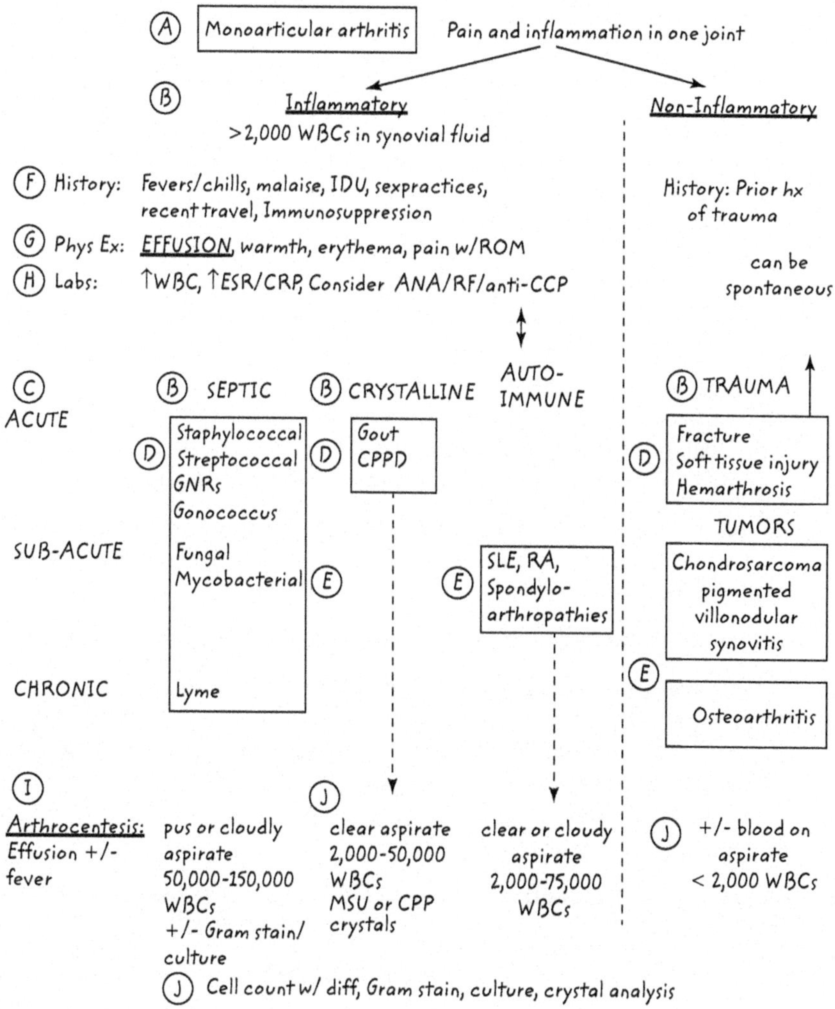

Fig. 40.1 Approach to monoarticular arthritis, A–J

- Septic arthritis is usually monoarticular and monomicrobial.
- The major causes of crystalline arthropathies are gout and calcium pyrophosphate crystal deposition (CPPD) disease (a.k.a. "pseudogout").
- Causes of traumatic arthritis include fracture, soft tissue injury, and hemarthrosis.

E. **What are the diagnoses that fall into the subacute and chronic categories?**

Add suggestions from the learners to the appropriate categories.

Teaching points

- Fungal and mycobacterial infections usually have a subacute course. Lyme disease (*Borrelia burgdorferi*) and syphilis (*Treponema pallidum*) can cause a chronic infectious arthritis.
- Certain autoimmune illnesses can cause a monoarticular arthritis, including systemic lupus erythematosus (SLE), rheumatoid arthritis (RA), and the seronegative spondyloarthropathies (inflammatory bowel disease, ankylosing spondylitis, psoriatic arthritis, and reactive arthritis).
- These diseases may present as a mono- or polyarticular arthritis, and usually with a subacute time course (though acute onset is possible).
- On the noninflammatory side, tumors can cause subacute monoarticular arthritis, while osteoarthritis is the most common cause of chronic arthritis.

F. **Our patient is on infliximab for Crohn's disease and has osteoarthritis. What other history should we ask our patient to help differentiate causes of monoarticular arthritis?**

Ask learners for important history elements and add them to the white board.

- Systemic symptoms including fevers, chills, fatigue, and malaise.
- Recent or prior trauma or joint instrumentation.
- Risk factors for septic arthritis including injection drug use (IDU), high-risk sexual practices, travel history, and history of immunosuppression.
- Other risk factors include age >80 years, prosthetic joints, diabetes, rheumatologic diseases, and hemophilia.

G. **What physical examination findings could help narrow the initial differential diagnosis?**

Add physical examination features below the history.

- Presence of a joint effusion on examination in the absence of recent trauma strongly points toward an inflammatory arthritis.
- Warmth, erythema, and exquisite tenderness with range of motion (ROM) also raise concern for septic arthritis, particularly in the presence of systemic symptoms such as fever. However, these examination findings alone cannot rule out other causes of inflammatory monoarticular arthritis.

H. **Can blood tests help differentiate causes of monoarticular arthritis? Which labs would you send for this patient?**

Write down appropriate labs on the whiteboard.

- Blood tests may point toward an inflammatory process; however, no blood test can diagnose the cause of monoarticular arthritis.
  - Complete blood cell (CBC) count: Leukocytosis is concerning for septic arthritis; however, a mild elevation in the WBC count can also be seen with crystalline arthropathies.
  - Erythrocyte sedimentation rate (ESR)/C-reactive protein (CRP): sensitive but not specific for inflammatory processes.
  - Uric acid is *not* helpful in the acute setting.
- Consider sending an antinuclear antibodies (ANA), rheumatoid factor (RF), and anti-cyclic citrullinated peptide (CCP) antibody if there is a high index of suspicion for SLE or RA.

I. **On examination, our patient's temperature was 101.2 °F. His knee was warm to the touch with a moderate effusion. There was tenderness to palpation of the knee joint and passive range of motion elicited extreme pain at 30 degrees flexion. CBC revealed WBC 15.5 with 90% neutrophils. ESR was 50, and CRP 95. What are these findings most concerning for and what is your next step in workup?**

Emphasize the need for arthrocentesis in this situation.

Teaching points

- Fever, leukocytosis, elevated inflammatory markers, the presence of an effusion, and marked tenderness with range of motion strongly suggest septic arthritis.
- Crystalline arthropathies could present similarly; however, fever is less common.
- Monoarticular arthritis due to fungal or mycobacterial infection is unlikely to develop over 2 days. Arthritis due to autoimmune disease is unlikely to be this painful on examination.
- The patient should have an arthrocentesis to analyze the synovial fluid.
- Arthrocentesis should be considered whenever an effusion is present to differentiate between inflammatory and noninflammatory causes of arthritis.
- If fever is present, arthrocentesis should always be performed to rule out septic arthritis. Consider consulting your orthopedic or rheumatology colleagues if you are unable to safely obtain synovial fluid.

J. **What tests should you send on the synovial fluid to help make a diagnosis?**

Write down the tests that should be sent, then write down the typical values for each type of arthritis.

- Send synovial fluid for cell count with differential, gram stain, culture, and crystal analysis.

- Appearance: aspiration of pus strongly suggests septic arthritis. The presence of blood indicates hemarthrosis, often due to trauma, tumor, or hemophilia.
- Cell count:
  - Septic arthritis generally has 50,000–150,000 WBCs/mm^3 with a neutrophilic predominance.
  - Cell count in crystalline arthropathies typically ranges from 2000 to 50,000 WBCs/mm^3; however, it can be as high as 100,000 WBCs/mm^3.
  - Cell count in autoimmune arthritis ranges from 2000 to 75,000 WBCs/mm^3.
- Gram stain: positive in some but not all cases of septic arthritis (sensitivity 30–50%).
- Culture: positive in the majority of nongonococcal bacterial arthritis.
- Crystal analysis: the most common are monosodium urate (MSU) crystals (diagnostic of gout) and calcium pyrophosphate crystals (diagnostic of CPPD disease).

Our patient's synovial fluid analysis revealed 140,000 WBCs/mm^3 with 85% neutrophils. Gram stain revealed gram-positive cocci in clusters; culture grew *Staphylococcus* *aureus*. He was admitted to the hospital and treated with intravenous antibiotics and surgical washout. He completed 2 weeks of antibiotics in the hospital with a plan to continue oral antibiotics and rehabilitation after discharge.

Return to Objectives and Emphasize Key Points

1. Describe a diagnostic framework for monoarticular arthritis
   - Monoarticular arthritis can be categorized as inflammatory or noninflammatory.
   - Use the timing of symptom onset (acute, subacute, chronic) to guide the differential diagnosis.
   - Major subcategories of inflammatory arthritis include septic, crystalline, and arthritis due to autoimmune disease.
2. Identify features of the history and physical examination that help differentiate causes of monoarticular arthritis
   - Maintain a high index of suspicion for septic arthritis as rapid diagnosis and treatment are essential to avoid joint destruction.
   - Key risk factors for septic arthritis include the presence of systemic symptoms including fevers, age >80, injection drug use, high-risk sexual practices, relevant travel history, and prosthetic joints.
   - Presence of a joint effusion on examination in the absence of recent trauma strongly points toward an inflammatory arthritis.
3. Explain the indications for arthrocentesis
   - Consider arthrocentesis whenever an effusion is present to differentiate causes of arthritis.

- Arthrocentesis is particularly important when there a patient presents with fever and a joint effusion.

4. Interpret key findings in synovial fluid analysis

- Inflammatory arthritis: >2000 WBCs/mm^3
- Septic arthritis: 50,000–150,000 WBCs/mm^3
- Crystalline arthropathies: 2000–50,000 WBCs/mm^3 + MSU crystals (gout) or calcium pyrophosphate crystals (CPPD)

Resources

1. Becker J, et al. Acute monoarthritis: diagnosis in adults. Am Fam Physician. 2016;94(10):810–6.
2. Chokkalingam S, et al. Diagnosing acute monoarthritis in adults: a practical approach for the family physician. Am Fam Physician. 2003;68(1):83–90.
3. Margaretten M, et al. Does this adult patient have septic arthritis? JAMA. 2007;297(13):1478–88.
4. Lingling M, et al. Acute monoarthritis: what is the cause of my patient's painful swollen joint? CMAJ. 2009;180(1):59–65.
5. Aderinto J, et al. Early syphilis: a cause of mono-arthritis of the knee. Ann R Coll Surg Engl. 2008;90(5):W1–3.

Chapter 41
Management of Fibromyalgia

Anna Hagan and Jennifer Wright

Learning Objectives
1. Recognize signs and symptoms of fibromyalgia.
2. Complete the workup, including ordering appropriate tests, to establish the diagnosis of fibromyalgia.
3. Manage fibromyalgia in the primary care setting through both nonpharmacologic and pharmacologic strategies.
4. Determine when to refer patients with fibromyalgia to a specialist for further management.

Clinical Vignette: A 33-year-old woman comes to your primary care clinic for evaluation of fatigue and back pain. For the past 4 months she has had difficulty sleeping, an upset stomach with occasional diarrhea, and pain in her back, arms, and legs. For the past several years she has had fatigue and waxing and waning pain, and she is worried that there is "something really wrong." A friend suggested that she be evaluated for fibromyalgia.

A. **In what patient population should you suspect fibromyalgia?**

Write down the key demographic characteristics as shown in Fig. 41.1.

Teaching points
- Can affect any patient, regardless of sex or age, but affects women more than men.
- Fibromyalgia is the most common cause of musculoskeletal pain in women of ages 20–55 years.

A. Hagan (✉)
Harborview Medical Center, Department of Medicine, Division of General Internal Medicine, University of Washington, Seattle, WA, USA
e-mail: annafahy@uw.edu

J. Wright
University of Washington Medical Center, Department of Medicine, Division of General Internal Medicine, University of Washington, Seattle, WA, USA

S. Mookherjee et al. (eds.), *Chalk Talks in Internal Medicine*,
https://doi.org/10.1007/978-3-030-34814-4_41

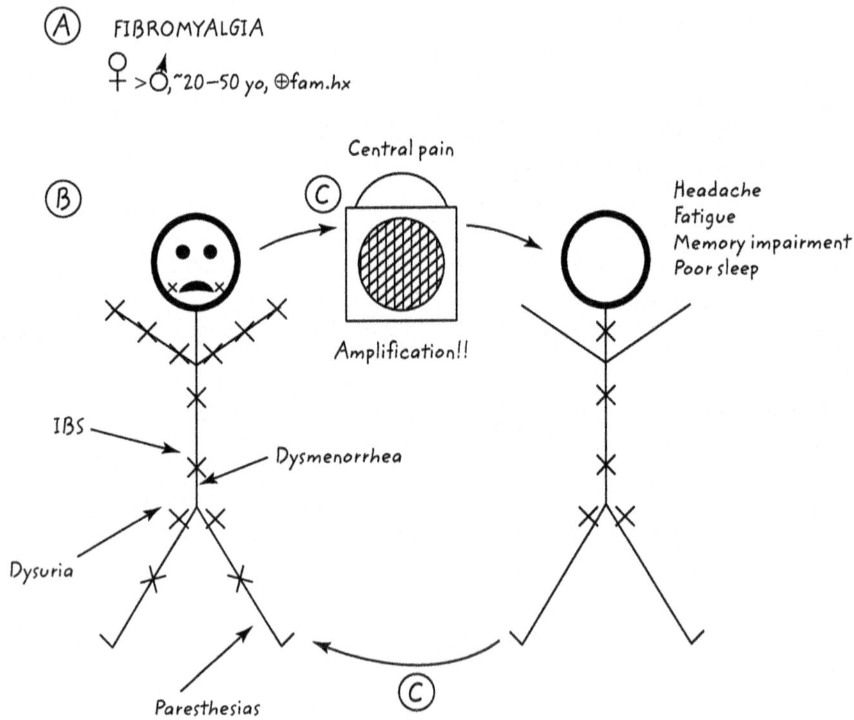

Fig. 41.1 Management of fibromyalgia, A–C

- It is suspected to potentially have a genetic component, as fibromyalgia is more common in individuals with a family history of fibromyalgia.
- Occurs more commonly in patients who already have a diagnosis of osteoarthritis, rheumatoid arthritis, or other autoimmune disease.

B. **Your patient's symptoms include difficulty sleeping, occasional diarrhea, as well as pain in her back, arms, and legs. Are these symptoms consistent with fibromyalgia? What other signs and symptoms should you ask about when you suspect this diagnosis?**

Write down key additional signs and symptoms as suggested by learners.

Teaching points

- Diffuse pain (see below) + other somatic symptoms (such as those described by our patient) and no other more likely etiology is consistent with fibromyalgia.
- Widespread Pain Index and Symptom Severity Scale (both easy to access and available online, www.arthritis-research.org) are specific resources used to definitively make the diagnosis; these tools allow the patient to self-report where they have pain and the severity of other associated symptoms.
- Commonly affected pain regions include bilateral jaw, bilateral shoulder girdle, bilateral upper arms, bilateral lower arms, chest, abdomen, neck, upper back, lower back, bilateral hips/buttocks, bilateral upper legs, and bilateral lower legs.
  - Pearl: These pain regions are different from the "tender points" that were previously used to define fibromyalgia. Tender points are no longer part of the diagnostic criteria.
  - Patients often describe this pain as a deep muscular pain.
- Patients also have other somatic symptoms: fatigue, memory impairment, unrefreshing sleep, cramping abdominal pain/diarrhea (irritable bowel syndrome (IBS)-like symptoms), dysuria, dysmenorrhea, depression, headache, and paresthesias.
- Symptoms must be present for at least 3 months.

C. **Fibromyalgia is a centralized pain syndrome, in contrast to osteoarthritis or rheumatoid arthritis, which are common peripheral pain syndromes. Peripheral stimuli—pain, menstrual cramps, stomach upset—are amplified because of abnormal central pain processing.**

Draw the amplification loop as shown in Fig. 41.1.

Teaching point

- The pathways that process pain centrally overlap with pathways involved in mood, sleep, memory—this is likely in part why fibromyalgia symptoms can involve fatigue, poor sleep, memory problems, etc.

D. **You move on to your physical examination. What findings would point toward or against a diagnosis of fibromyalgia?**

From this point on you will work your way through Fig. 41.2, *adding in information as you move through the case.*

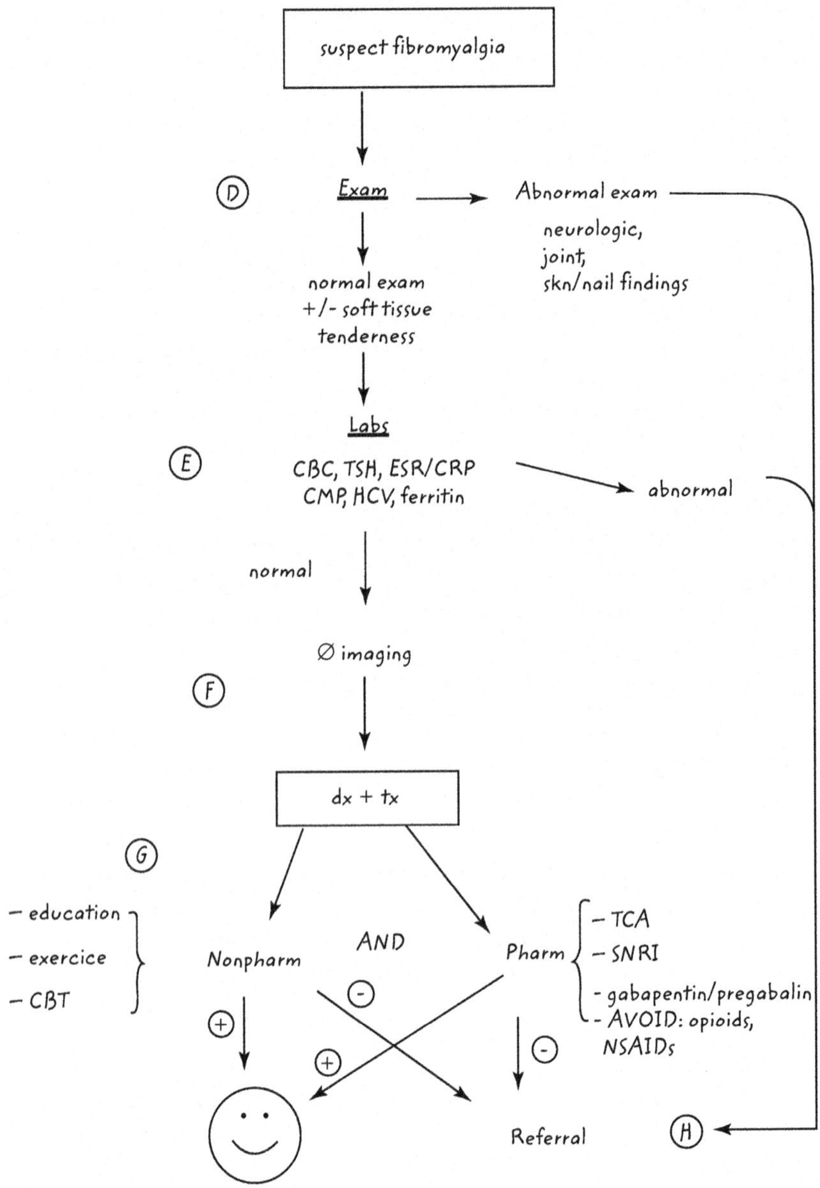

Fig. 41.2 Management of fibromyalgia, D–H

- Examination should be essentially normal, with exception of tenderness of some soft tissues.
- Patients with fibromyalgia commonly describe pain with inflation of the blood pressure cuff.
- Important to evaluate for evidence of alternative etiologies of their diffuse pain symptoms: joint redness or swelling, muscle weakness, neurological abnormalities, and/or skin or nail changes that could suggest a systemic autoimmune disease.
- Abnormal physical examination findings are a red flag and should raise concern for a different diagnosis.

E. **Her physical examination is normal. What labs would you order to complete your workup, and what results would you expect?**

List labs as suggested by learners.

Teaching points

- The labs you obtain may vary based on patient symptoms. Testing performed to rule out alternative etiologies, no definitive test diagnoses fibromyalgia. Consider evaluation for:
- Anemia—complete blood cell (CBC) count
- Hypothyroidism—thyroid stimulating hormone (TSH)
- Inflammatory conditions—erythrocyte sedimentation rate (ESR), C-reactive protein (CRP)
- Hepatitis C—hepatitis C virus (HCV) antibody
- Low ferritin (in premenopausal women)—Iron panel
- Occult liver disease—liver function tests (LFTs)
- Occult renal disease—basic metabolic panel (BMP)
- Abstain from ordering more specific rheumatologic labs (antinuclear antibodies (ANA), rheumatoid factor, anti-cyclic citrullinated peptide (anti-CCP)) unless there is objective evidence of autoimmune disease.

F. **The patient wonders if X-ray films would be helpful to determine the cause of her pain. What additional diagnostic testing would you suggest performing?**

Write down any imaging studies suggested by learners and then cross them out.

Teaching point

- Imaging is generally not needed, unless there are concerning localizing findings on examination.

G. **Based on her history, physical, and normal labs, you make the diagnosis of fibromyalgia for your patient. What options do you have to manage her diagnosis in the primary care setting?**

Write down pharmacologic and nonpharmacologic treatments as suggested by learners as shown in Fig. 41.2.

Teaching points

- **Nonpharmacologic therapy:**
- Patient education—center around the importance of self-management approach to treatment.
  - Pearl: Sometimes simply giving a patient the diagnosis of fibromyalgia has therapeutic benefit, because they have lived for months/years with unexplained pain.
- Exercise program—"graded exercise" program, starting with very modest amount of aerobic activity and slowly increasing. e.g. 20–30 min, 2–3 times per week.
  - Avoid doing "too much too soon," which can exacerbate pain.
  - Pearl: Providing an exercise "prescription" may improve adherence.
- Psychological therapy—specifically cognitive–behavioral therapy (CBT), stress reduction.
- Complementary and alternative medicine (CAM)—not rigorously studied; possible benefits with multiple treatment modalities including acupuncture, yoga, chiropractic care, tai chi.
- If patients have comorbid depression or obstructive sleep apnea, treatment of these conditions may offer a significant benefit to their fibromyalgia pain symptoms.
- **Pharmacologic therapy:**
- Although medication can be helpful with specific pain symptoms, it is very unlikely to achieve substantial overall improvement without concurrent nonpharmacologic strategies.
- Tricyclic antidepressants (TCA): e.g. nortriptyline and cyclobenzaprine—this is classically considered a muscle relaxant, but its mechanism of action is essentially the same as a TCA.
  - Pearl: good for patients with comorbid insomnia.
- Serotonin and norepinephrine reuptake inhibitors (SNRI): e.g. duloxetine, milnacipran (specific Food and Drug Administration [FDA] indications for fibromyalgia).
  - Pearl: good for patients with comorbid depression
- Gabapentin (off-label use)/pregabalin (specific FDA indication).
  - Pearl: good for patients with anxiety, problems with sleep
- Opioids and nonsteroidal anti-inflammatory drugs (NSAIDs) are largely ineffective and generally should be avoided. This reflects the fact that fibromyalgia pain is related to abnormal central pain processing rather than nociceptive pain.
  - Exception: If patients have comorbid peripheral pain conditions such as osteoarthritis, treatment such as NSAIDs may be appropriate.

H. **You provided education on nonpharmacologic approaches, as well as prescribed an SNRI. She returns to your clinic several times over the next few months without any improvement in her symptoms. At what point would you refer her to a specialist?**

Draw "negative" arrows from pharmacologic and nonpharmacologic treatments to "referral" as shown in Fig. 41.2.

Teaching points

- Atypical symptoms, lab abnormalities—based on symptoms could consider rheumatology or neurology referral.
- Challenging pain management—consider referral to pain specialist.
- Significant comorbid psychiatric disease—referral to psychiatry or psychology.
- Concern for sleep apnea—referral to sleep medicine specialist.
- Failure to respond to appropriate treatments—referral to rheumatology.

Return to Objectives and Emphasize Key Points

1. Recognize signs and symptoms of fibromyalgia
   - Widespread pain
   - Other somatic complaints
   - No other explanation for symptoms
2. Complete the workup, including ordering appropriate tests, to establish the diagnosis of fibromyalgia
   - Basic labs (CBC, BMP, LFTs, TSH, ESR/CRP, HCV antibody, iron studies)
   - Autoimmune serologies and imaging are generally not needed.
3. Manage fibromyalgia in the primary care clinic setting through both nonpharmacologic and pharmacologic strategies
   - Nonpharmacologic measures include patient education, graduated exercise, and counseling.
   - Pharmacologic strategies include tricyclic antidepressants, SNRIs, and gabapentin/pregabalin. NSAIDs and opioids should be avoided.
4. Determine when to refer patients with fibromyalgia to a specialist for further management
   - Atypical symptoms, failure to respond to treatment, comorbid illness (sleep apnea, mental health disorders).

Resources

1. Clauw DJ. Fibromyalgia: a clinical review. JAMA. 2014;311(15):1547–55.
2. Kodner C. Common questions about the diagnosis and management of fibromyalgia. Am Fam Physician. 2015;91(7):472–8.
3. Wolfe F. The American College of Rheumatology preliminary diagnostic criteria for fibromyalgia and measurement of symptom severity. Arthritis Care Res. 2010;62:600–10.

Chapter 42
Approach to Acute Altered Mental Status

Tiffany Chen and Susan Merel

Learning Objectives

1. Describe a systematic approach to acute altered mental status (AMS) in the hospitalized patient.
2. Identify the indications for brain imaging in a patient presenting with acute altered mental status.
3. Demonstrate the use of the Confusion Assessment Method (CAM) tool for diagnosing delirium.

Clinical Vignette: A 70-year-old man with prostate cancer with bony metastases presents with acute altered mental status. His family says he seemed fine over the phone a few days ago, but when they came to see him today, he was disheveled, the house was a mess, and he seemed confused—not recognizing who they were and mumbling incoherently.

A. **What are three overarching categories for thinking about the differential diagnosis for this patient's altered mental status?**

Write AMS in a triangle with branch points out to central nervous system (CNS), delirium, and psych (Fig. 42.1).

B. **What are potential CNS causes for this patient's altered mental status?**

Write down what learners suggest, grouping into structural/pressure disorders, inflammatory/infection etiologies, and seizure.

C. **What history and physical examination findings would determine if this patient needs head imaging?**

T. Chen (✉) · S. Merel
University of Washington Medical Center, Department of Medicine, Division of General Internal Medicine, University of Washington, Seattle, WA, USA
e-mail: chentc@uw.edu

S. Mookherjee et al. (eds.), *Chalk Talks in Internal Medicine*,
https://doi.org/10.1007/978-3-030-34814-4_42

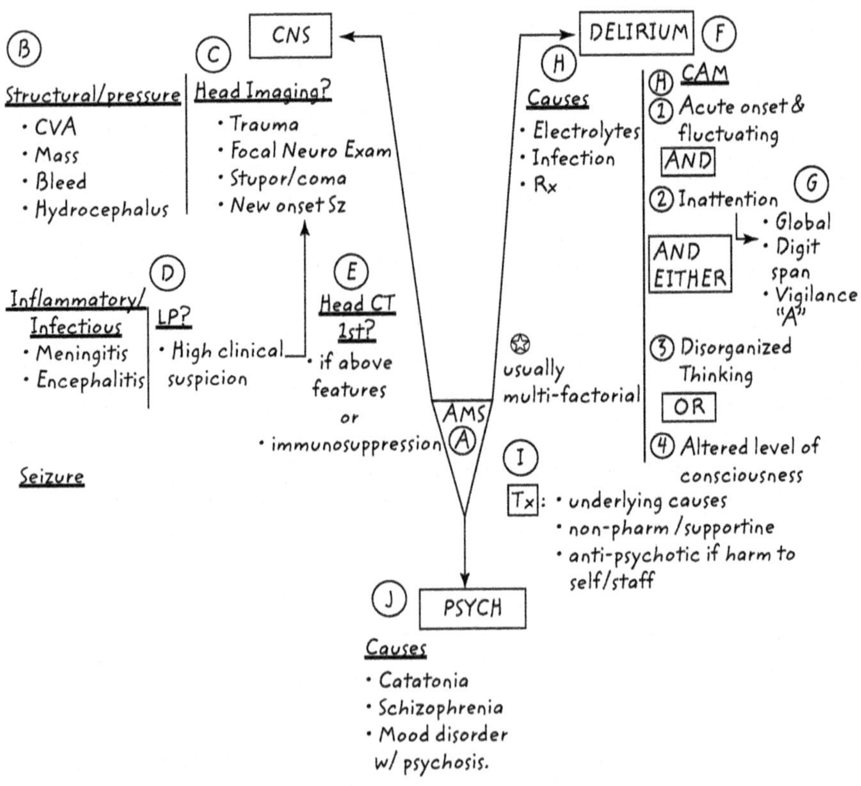

Fig. 42.1 Approach to acute altered mental status, A–J

Write down correct indications for head imaging as they are suggested by learners.

Teaching points
- Indications for head imaging are focal neurologic signs, trauma/fall, stupor/coma, and inability to do an adequate neurologic examination.

D. **This patient intermittently follows 1 step commands and appears to have a nonfocal comprehensive neurologic examination. However, you also note a large hematoma on his head and several abrasions on his extremities and decide to get a head computed tomographic (CT) scan, which is negative for bleed or metastases. Does this patient need a lumbar puncture to evaluate his altered mental status?**

Poll the learners regarding whether they would obtain a lumbar puncture (LP).

Teaching points
- The classic triad for bacterial meningitis is fever, neck stiffness, and altered mental status. However, it is important to have a high clinical suspicion even if only one of these features is present, especially if the patient is immunocompromised, has HIV infection, or if there are no alternative explanations for the mental status change.
- Less than half of adults with community-acquired bacterial meningitis have classic triad of fever, AMS, neck stiffness, and about one-fourth lack fever on presentation.
- Altered mental status that develops while the patient is hospitalized is unlikely to be nosocomial meningitis without some kind of CNS instrumentation.

E. **This patient was afebrile and had no nuchal rigidity. He hasn't had any recent chemotherapy, so LP can be deferred. If the patient had an indication for LP, would he need a head CT scan to look for signs of elevated intracranial pressure before the procedure? What are the indications for a head CT scan prior to LP?**

Indicate the same reasons for obtaining brain imaging plus immunosuppression.

F. **It seems like primary CNS causes are unlikely in this patient. On examination he is lethargic, awakens to voice but doesn't engage in the interview for more than 30 seconds at a time and often gives nonsensical answers. He is oriented only to self, incorrectly reports the year as "1980" and when asked about where he is located, he repeats "1980." What clinical syndrome does this patient seem to have? What clinical tool can you use to recognize/diagnose delirium?**

Lead learners through the CAM assessment.

Teaching points

- The Confusion Assessment Method (CAM) (see resources below for reference) is a widely used tool to asses for delirium—the components are:
- Acute onset and fluctuating course
- **AND** Inattention
- **AND EITHER** disorganized thinking
- **OR** altered level of consciousness

G. **How do you assess attention?**

Poll learners on how they would assess for attention/inattention.

Teaching points

- Observation/global: The patient is very distracted. You find yourself asking same question multiple times. The patient may keep repeating the answer to previous question.
- Digit Span: Ask the patient to repeat a series of random numbers, beginning with a string of two digits and then increasing. Inability to repeat a string of at least five digits indicates a probable impairment.
- Vigilance A Test: used mostly in ICUs for intubated patients; provider says 10 letters, 4 of which are A's (ex. SAVEHAART or CASABLANCA). Patient instructed to squeeze hand when the provider says "A." Error if patient does not squeeze on "a" *or* squeeze incorrectly with a different letter. Screening is positive if >2 error.

H. **Can you identify some possible underlying medical causes for his delirium?**

Write up learner's suggestions as appropriate.

Teaching points

- Would make sure to add infection, electrolyte disturbances, and medications if not mentioned.
- Most delirium is multifactorial.

I. **How should we treat this patient's delirium?**

Write down the key treatments for delirium.

- Treating any underlying cause, and nonpharmacologic measures such as reorientation, normalizing sleep-wake cycle, and mobilization.
- Antipsychotics sometimes used for severe delirium with harm to self/staff, but there is no evidence they help prevent or effectively treat delirium.

J. **What are some psychiatric causes of altered mental status?**

Write down common psychiatric conditions suggested by learners as shown in Fig. 42.1.

Return to Objectives and Emphasize Key Points

1. Describe a systematic approach to acute altered mental status in the hospitalized patient
   - Classify into CNS, delirium, psychiatric causes
2. Identify the indications for brain imaging in a patient presenting with acute altered mental status
   - Trauma
   - Focal neuro exam
   - Stupor/coma
   - New seizure
   - Before LP in immunocompromised patients suspected of meningitis/encephalitis
3. Demonstrate the use of the CAM tool for diagnosing delirium
   - Acute onset and fluctuating course
   - AND inattention
   - AND EITHER disorganized thinking
   - OR altered level of consciousness

Resources

1. Theisen-Toupal J, et al. Diagnostic yield of head computed tomography for the hospitalized medical patient with delirium. J Hosp Med. 2014;9(8):497–501.
2. Van de Beek D, et al. Clinical features and prognostic factors in adults with bacterial meningitis. NEJM. 2004;351:1849–59.
3. Inouye S, et al. Clarifying confusion: the confusion assessment method. Ann Intern Med. 1990;113(1):941–8.
4. Pompei P, et al. Detecting delirium among hospitalized older patients. Arch Intern Med. 1995;155(3):301–7.
5. Inouye SK, et al. Delirium in elderly people. Lancet. 2014;383(9920):911–22.
6. Flaherty JH, et al. Antipsychotics in the treatment of delirium in older hospitalized adults: a systematic review. J Am Geriatr Soc. 2011;59(Suppl 2):S269–76.

Chapter 43
Approach to Vertigo

Michael Northrop and Kim O'Connor

Learning Objectives

1. Categorize vertigo by duration (episodic versus continuous) and whether it is provoked by head movements.
2. Understand how and when to perform the Dix-Hallpike examination to evaluate for benign paroxysmal positional vertigo (BPPV).
3. Utilize the head impulse, nystagmus, test of skew (HINTS) examination to help differentiate peripheral from central etiologies of vertigo.

Clinical Vignette: A 65-year-old man with hypertension and history of a transient ischemic attack presents to the clinic for the evaluation of dizziness. He describes a sensation of spinning that is accompanied by nausea that makes him slightly unsteady on his feet that has been present daily for the past week. On examination, he has normal orthostatic vital signs, unremarkable cardiac and neurologic examinations with a normal gait.

A. **What is vertigo?**

Write down the definition as shown in Fig. 43.1.

Teaching points

- Vertigo is the illusion of movement, usually experienced as spinning dizziness, but it can also be experienced as a sensation of tilting and swaying.
- It is often accompanied by nausea and vomiting.

M. Northrop (✉)
VA Puget Sound Health Care System, Department of Medicine, Division of General Internal Medicine, University of Washington, Seattle, WA, USA

K. O'Connor
University of Washington Medical Center, Department of Medicine, Division of General Internal Medicine, University of Washington, Seattle, WA, USA

S. Mookherjee et al. (eds.), *Chalk Talks in Internal Medicine*,
https://doi.org/10.1007/978-3-030-34814-4_43

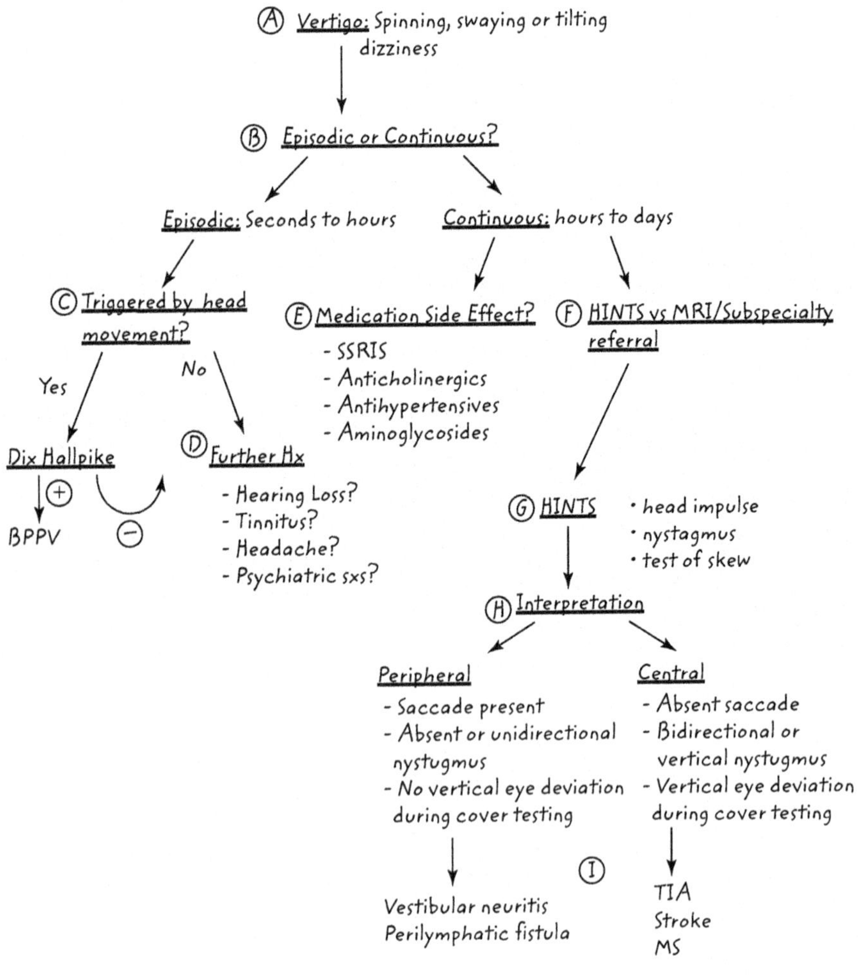

Fig. 43.1 Approach to vertigo, A–J

B. **How would you characterize the pattern of the patient's vertigo?**

Continue the algorithm as shown in Fig. 43.1.

Teaching points
- Episodic: episodes lasting seconds to hour.
- Continuous: episodes lasting hours to days.

C. **Our patient has been having vertigo for days; therefore, it is considered continuous. While there can be an overlap between episodic and continuous vertigo, an important diagnostic question is to determine if the vertigo is triggered by head movement. If our patient's vertigo were triggered by head movements, what physical examination maneuver should be considered? How is it performed?**

If possible, review New England Journal of Medicine (NEJM) video for demonstration of the Dix-Hallpike maneuver: www.youtube.com/watch?v=KLt2LtISPmQ

Teaching points
- The Dix-Hallpike maneuver can diagnose BPPV (sensitivity and specificity of about 75%).
- Emphasize that while most etiologies of vertigo are made worse by head movement, BPPV is usually triggered by a change in head position.
- To perform the Dix-Hallpike:
  - Sit the patient upright. The patient should have no nystagmus in a seated position.
  - Rotate the patient's head 30–45 degrees to the side being tested while instructing him to keep his eyes open and focused on your nose.
  - While supporting the patient's head, quickly lie him supine, allowing the neck to hyperextend slightly over the examination table.
  - Wait 20 seconds to observe for upbeat and torsional nystagmus (along with a patient complaint of vertigo), which is a positive finding for BPPV involving the posterior semicircular canal.

D. **If the patient has episodic vertigo not triggered by head movements and/or a negative Dix-Hallpike examination, what further history would you want to assess for spontaneous causes?**

Write down relevant responses as suggested by learners.

Teaching points
- Sensorineural hearing loss and tinnitus are part of the diagnostic criteria for Meniere's disease.
- Headache may suggest vestibular migraine.
- Psychiatric symptoms may suggest panic attack or other psychiatric condition.

E. **In our patient, head movements sometimes make his symptoms worse, but not always. Since he is experiencing continuous vertigo (lasting hours to days), we need to determine if a medication may be the culprit. What medication classes are associated with vertigo?**

Write down the main classes of medications.

Teaching points

- Many different classes of medications may manifest vertigo as a side effect.
- The mechanisms of vertigo include cardiac effects (alcohol, antihypertensives, narcotics), anticholinergic effects (muscle relaxants, antihistamines), cerebellar toxicity (benzodiazepines), and ototoxicity (aminoglycosides).
- Selective serotonin re-uptake inhibitors (SSRIs) are commonly prescribed and can also cause dizziness.

F. **His only medications are aspirin, lisinopril, and atorvastatin, which he has been taking for many years. In the absence of an obvious medication side effect, what additional examination maneuver can further clarify the cause of continuous vertigo?**

Continue with the algorithm; many learners will not be familiar with the HINTS (Head Impulse, Nystagmus, Test of Skew) examination.

Teaching points

- HINTS is worth learning and practicing: a negative examination greatly decreases the risk of stroke (LR = 0.01, which virtually rules out the chance of stroke), more so than a normal diffusion weighted MRI (LR= 0.2, which corresponds to a decrease of 30%).
- The HINTS examination requires experience and practice. If you do not feel comfortable performing the HINTS examination, consider neuroimaging to evaluate for stroke and/or referral to a subspecialist

G. **How would you perform the HINTS examination on this patient?**

Write down the HINTS components and review the following video for demonstration of the HINTS maneuver: https://www.youtube.com/watch?v=1q-VTKPweuk

Teaching points

- <u>H</u>ead-<u>I</u>mpulse:
  - Have the patient sit with his head tilted slightly downward and focus on your nose.
  - Slowly move the patient's head back and forth between 10 and 20 degrees.
  - Briskly move the head to the center as you observe for catch-up saccade (rapid eye movement).
  - If any saccade is noted, repeat the examination to make sure it is reproducible.

- Nystagmus:
  - Instruct the patient to look straight ahead—observe for any abnormal eye movements.
  - Focusing on your finger, have the patient look laterally (about 20–30 degrees) and hold the gaze in this position—observe for nystagmus (defined as the direction of a fast beating eye movement).
  - Do not have the patient look in extreme lateral gaze or you may trigger a few beats of physiologic (normal) nystagmus that may be interpreted as a false positive.
  - Repeat in all directions (bilaterally, superiorly, inferiorly) and observe for unidirectional or bidirectional nystagmus.
- Test of Skew:
  - Instruct your patient to look straight ahead while you cover one eye at a time, back and forth, observing for vertical deviation of the eye that becomes uncovered

H. **Our patient has a saccade in both eyes with head movement, unilateral leftward horizontal nystagmus, and the absence of vertical eye deviation with cover–uncover testing. How do you interpret the HINTS examination? What findings suggest a peripheral etiology and what findings suggest a central etiology?**

Write down the findings for central and peripheral etiologies.

Teaching points

- The presence of saccade is reassuring and signifies a likely peripheral etiology.
- Nystagmus that is dominantly vertical or torsional or that changes direction with gaze (bidirectional) suggests a central etiology.
- Vertical deviation of the uncovered eye implies a central etiology.

I. **Depending on the results of the HINTS examination, what are some common causes of peripheral and central vertigo that this patient might have?**

Write down the main causes as shown in Fig. 43.1.

Our patient most likely has a benign peripheral etiology of vertigo. Since his symptoms are constant, he most likely has vestibular neuritis. If the HINTS examination demonstrates any of the signs suggestive of a central cause (absent saccade, bidirectional or vertical nystagmus, or vertical eye deviation) then the patient would require further investigation with neuroimaging and/or a subspecialist referral

Return to Objectives and Emphasize Key Points

1. Categorize vertigo as episodic or continuous and assess if it is triggered by head movement
   - The first step in the evaluation of vertigo is categorizing it as episodic (seconds to hours) or continuous (hours to days).
   - Remember that almost all vertigo is worsened by head movements and body positional changes; however, vertigo associated with BPPV is often triggered by such movements.
2. Understand how and when to perform the Dix-Hallpike examination to evaluate for benign paroxysmal positional vertigo
   - If the vertigo is positional, perform the Dix-Hallpike examination.
3. Introduce the HINTS examination and know how to interpret it to help differentiate peripheral from central etiologies of vertigo
   - Perform the HINTS examination when a patient has constant vertigo or enlist the help of an expert to perform the examination.
   - Vertical or bidirectional gaze nystagmus and vertical deviation during the cover test are worrisome examination findings for central causes of vertigo. The presence of saccade is reassuring and suggests a peripheral etiology.

Resources

1. Kerber KA, Newman-Toker DE. Misdiagnosing dizzy patients: common pitfalls in clinical practice. Neurol Clin. 2015;33(3):565–75.
2. Labuguen RH. Initial evaluation of vertigo. Am Fam Physician. 2006;73(2):244–51.
3. McGee S. Evidence based physical diagnosis. Philadelphia: Elsevier; 2012.
4. Muncie HL, Sirmans SM, Dizziness JE. Approach to evaluation and management. Am Fam Physician. 2017;95(3):154–62.
5. Newman-Toker DE, Edlow JA. TiTrATE: a novel, evidenced-based approach to diagnosing acute dizziness and vertigo. Neurol Clin. 2015;33(3):577–99.
6. Ji-Soo Kim MD, Zee DS. Benign paroxysmal positional vertigo. J Med. 2014;370:1138–47. https://www.youtube.com/watch?v=KLt2LtISPmQ.

Chapter 44
Approach to Intimate Partner Violence

Lindsay Gibbon and Nancy Sugg

Learning Objectives

1. Recognize clinical signs of physical, sexual, and/or psychological intimate partner violence (IPV).
2. Effectively screen for IPV and identify additional risk factors that suggest particular vulnerability to severe injury or death.
3. Utilize communication techniques to help patients appreciate the health consequences of IPV and assess individual psychosocial factors when creating a safety plan.
4. Formulate an appropriate and patient-centered safety plan for a patient experiencing intimate partner violence.

Clinical Vignette: Paula is a 46-year-old attorney with a history of type II diabetes, hypertension, and chronic neck pain who presents to primary care clinic with 3 months of atypical chest pain. Her vitals are BP 168/132, P 78, SpO2 97, and RR 16. An exercise treadmill test is negative and d-dimer is within normal limits. On a return visit, your patient shares that the chest pain is still bothersome despite a trial of omeprazole. She adds that she has been stressed out by some personal issues and has been drinking more alcohol to relax.

A. **As you reconsider your differential for Paula's chest pain, you note that intimate partner violence (IPV) could be one potential contributing factor. How is IPV defined?**

Write down the key features of IPV as shown in Fig. 44.1.

L. Gibbon (✉) · N. Sugg
Harborview Medical Center, Department of Medicine, Division of General Internal Medicine, University of Washington, Seattle, WA, USA
e-mail: lgibbon@uw.edu

S. Mookherjee et al. (eds.), *Chalk Talks in Internal Medicine*,
https://doi.org/10.1007/978-3-030-34814-4_44

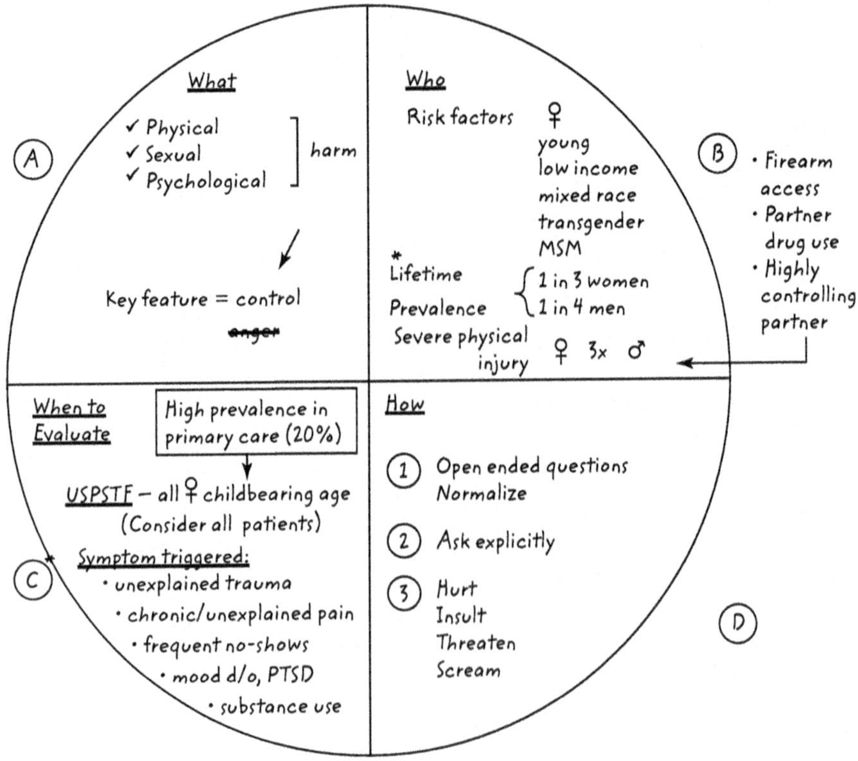

Fig. 44.1 (A–D) Approach to intimate partner violence

Teaching points

- IPV is physical, sexual, or psychological harm by a current or former intimate partner.
- Not driven by anger, but rather by a desire to control one's partner.
- Psychological abuse provides several key means of maintaining control and can often be the most distressing part of IPV:
  - Threats of harm to self, partner, or children unless certain conditions are met
  - Isolating partner by controlling movement, finances, social contacts, or access to information
  - Denying abuse or shifting responsibility for abuse

B. **What risk factors does the patient have for IPV?**

List correct risk factors as suggested by learners.

Teaching points

- Risk factors include female gender, young age, low income, mixed racial background, transgender status, and MSM.
- Absence of risk factors does *not* rule out IPV. IPV is highly prevalent in people of all age groups, genders, and sexual orientations.
  - More than one in three women and one in four men have experienced rape, physical violence, and/or stalking in their lifetime.
  - Studies in primary care clinics suggest that at any given time, up to one in five patients may be experiencing current IPV.
  - Women are three times more likely than men to suffer significant physical injury.
- Case–control studies suggest that female IPV patients with the following risk factors are at particularly high risk for death (OR 4–9):
  - Access to a firearm or previous threats with a weapon
  - Illicit drug use by abusive partner
  - Highly controlling abusive partner

C. **Should Paula be evaluated for IPV? Why?**

Write down indications under "when to evaluate" as shown in Fig. 44.1.

Teaching points

- Indications for routine screening:
  - The USPSTF recommends screening all women of childbearing age.
  - Since lifetime prevalence of IPV is high and the health consequences are serious, many experts and professional organizations suggest that all patients should be screened.

- Common “symptoms” of IPV that should trigger evaluation:
  - Frequent falls or unexplained traumatic injuries
  - Unexplained physical symptoms or chronic pain
  - Poorly controlled chronic medical problems, such as diabetes and hypertension
  - Frequent missed appointments or medication nonadherence
  - Symptoms of mood disorders or post traumatic stress disorder (PTSD)
  - Active substance use

D. **What questions should you ask the patient to evaluate for possible IPV?**

Ask learners to practice what questions they would ask and how they would ask them. Give feedback as needed.

Teaching points

- Start the conversation with open-ended questions. Normalize to help your patient feel more comfortable disclosing information: “Many of my patients tell me that their stress level has a big impact on their health. What sort of stresses are you dealing with in your personal life right now?”
- Ask explicitly about IPV: “Has anyone at home hit, hurt, or threatened you recently?”
- HITS (hurt, insult, threaten, scream) is another helpful screening tool for current IPV.

E. **You explicitly ask Paula about IPV. She shares that she and her boyfriend have been arguing more lately and sometimes it gets physical. What are concrete next steps you can take to help Paula?**

Continue with “Share provider concern” in Fig. 44.2.

Teaching points

- Share your concerns and medical expertise.
- Acknowledge IPV as a serious *health* issue: “I am concerned that these episodes of violence are having a serious impact on your health.”
- Educate about concrete changes in the patient’s health: “At your last few visits, I’ve noticed that your blood pressure and sugars have been much higher than in the past, and I’m concerned that this will have serious health consequences for you in the future.”

F. **After sharing your concerns the patient is quiet. How will you best determine her priorities?**

Ask learners to practice how they would evaluate patient priorities. Examples are given below.

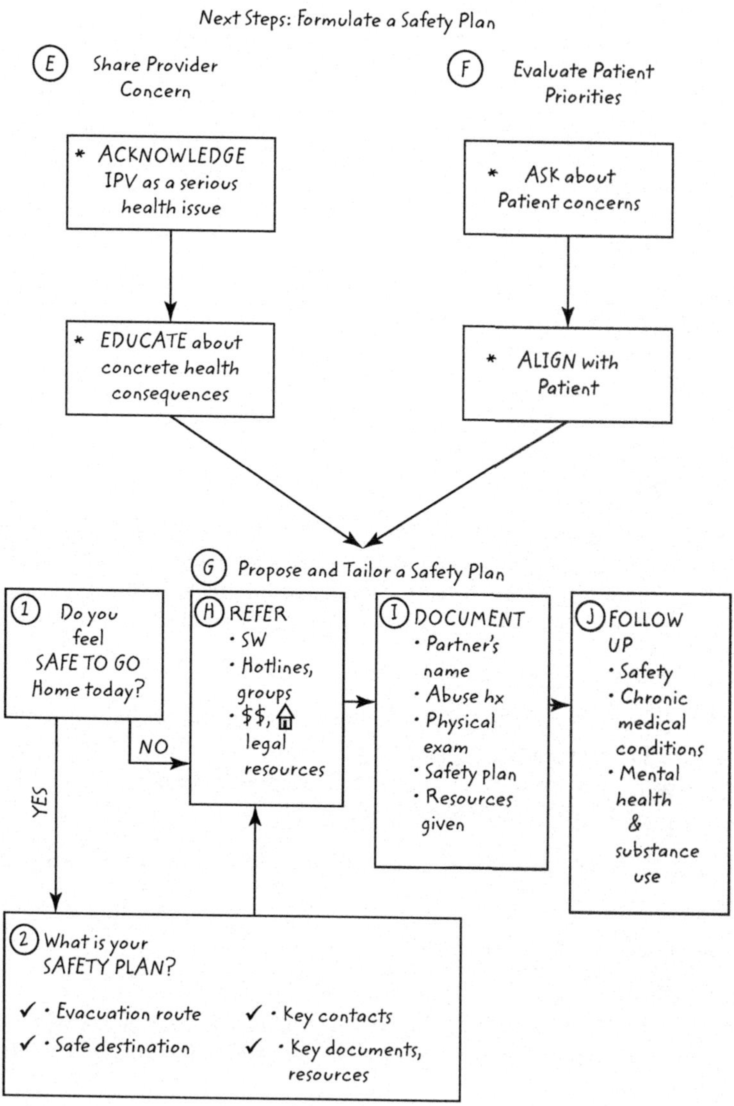

Fig. 44.2 (E–J) Approach to intimate partner violence

Teaching points

- Ask about *the patient's* biggest concerns
  - Provider: What's the most concerning part about this for you? (ASK)
  - Patient: Well, I've been really up tight lately and drinking a bottle of wine a night to get to sleep. Then at work, I'm sluggish and I can't concentrate the next day.
- Align with them.
  - Provider: *That sounds* exhausting. *It seems like* all the stress has really made it a struggle for you to function at work. (ALIGN)
  - Patient: Yes, exactly! I have some really big deadlines coming up. I can't keep going like this…

G. **After sharing your concerns and hearing the patient's priorities, you decide to help create a safety plan. What key questions should you ask her when creating a safety plan?**

Lead learners to the key steps: safety going home and safety plan.

Teaching points

- Do you feel safe to go home today?
  - If yes, reflect back what you have heard to help your patient think through her choice and ensure that you are both on the same page: "I'm hearing that you found a gun in your boyfriend's drawer last night and he has been escalating lately, but you feel pretty confident that you can handle the situation for now."
- What is your plan if you feel unsafe in the future?
  - Help patient identify a safe evacuation route, destination, and key contacts.
  - Assess financial and transportation resources.
  - Advise patient to make copies of important documents such as IDs, bank cards, and birth certificates.

H. **If the patient says she doesn't feel safe to go home, what resources can you offer?**

Continue the algorithm on Fig. 44.2 *as shown.*

Teaching points

- Your social worker can be very helpful in pointing out local resources.
- Ask about the possibility of staying with a friend/relative, or offer information about local shelters.
- Hotlines, support groups, financial/housing/legal resources.
- Pearl: Avoid giving your patient hard copies of support materials. These can be found by the abusive partner and may provoke escalating violence. Instead, consider conveying resources verbally or e-mailing written materials to a secure account.

I. **What information should be included in the patient's medical record?**

Continue the algorithm on Fig. 44.2 *as shown.*

Teaching points
- Name/relationship of alleged perpetrator
- History/physical exam pertaining to abuse
- Patient's safety plan and resources given

J. **When should we check in with Paula next?**

Continue the algorithm on Fig. 44.2 *as shown.*

Teaching points
- Weekly or biweekly appointments can be helpful for initial follow-up, since it can take multiple visits to build rapport, conduct motivational interviewing, arrange for social work resources, and re-establish care for poorly controlled chronic medical issues.
- Remember that patients can be adversely affected by mental and physical sequelae even after the abuse itself has ended.

Return to objectives and emphasize key points
1. Recognize clinical signs of physical, sexual, and/or psychological intimate partner violence (IPV)
   - Remember that the intimate partner engages in the abusive behaviors above due to a desire to control his/her partner, not because of anger.
   - Key clinical signs:
     - Unexplained trauma, falls, pain, or other symptoms
     - Frequent no-shows or nonadherence with medical therapy
     - Mood disorder or PTSD symptoms
     - Substance use
2. Effectively screen for IPV and identify additional risk factors that suggest particular vulnerability to severe injury or death.
   - Risk factors = female gender, young age, low income, mixed race, transgender, or MSM status.
   - Risk factors for severe physical harm = firearm access, partner substance use.
   - IPV is highly prevalent in primary care settings.
3. Utilize communication techniques to help patients appreciate the health consequences of IPV and assess individual psychosocial factors when creating a safety plan.
   - Use open ended questions and normalize patient's situation.
   - Ask explicitly about IPV.
   - HITS: Has anyone hurt, insulted, threatened, or screamed at you recently?

4. Formulate an appropriate and patient-centered safety plan.
   - Share your concern and educate about the health consequences of IPV.
   - Ask and align with patient concerns.
   - Propose and tailor a shared plan.
     - Do you feel safe to go home today?
     - Details include evacuation route/destination, key contacts, documents.
     - Refer to social worker, hotlines, groups, financial/housing/legal resources
     - Document carefully.
     - Arrange close follow-up.

Resources

1. Sugg N. Intimate partner violence. Med Clin North Am. 2015;99(3):629–49.
2. Rabin RF, Jennings JM, Campbell JC, Bair-Merritt MH. Intimate partner violence screening tools. Am J Prev Med. 2009;36(5):439–445.e4.
3. Campbell JC, Webster D, Koziol-McLain J, Block C, Campbell D, Curry MA, et al. Risk factors for femicide in abusive relationships: results from a multisite case control study. Am J Public Health. 2003;93(7):1089–97.
4. Novisky MA, Peralta RL. When women tell: intimate partner violence and the factors related to police notification. Violence Against Women. 2015;21(1):65–86.
5. Breiding M, Chen J, Black M. Intimate partner violence in the United States – 2010. Atlanta: National Center for Injury Prevention and Control, Centers for Disease Control and Prevention; 2014.

Chapter 45
Approach to Contraceptive Counseling

Ginger Evans and Stephanie Wheeler

Learning Objectives

1. Describe the various types of contraception: hormonal components, relative efficacy, major adverse effects.
2. Utilize resources for identifying contraindications to hormone-based contraception.
3. Manage minor side effects of all types of contraception.
4. Name an example of a recommended, first-line agent for combined oral contraception.

Clinical Vignette: A 35-year-old woman (G1P1) presents for contraceptive counseling. She is sexually active with men; she has had three different partners over the last year and was using condoms only. She wishes to discuss other contraception options.

A. **What forms of contraception might you discuss with the patient and which level of efficacy do they belong in?**

Draw the continuum of efficacy on the left side of the board, filling in number of pregnancies per 100 woman-years as shown in Fig. 45.1. *Add contraceptive methods as listed by learners at the appropriate place on the continuum. If learners use brand names, reorient them to the generic category. For example, write "copper intrauterine device (IUD)" instead of "ParaGard®."*

B. **What types of hormones are involved with each form of contraception?**

Ask learners if the contraceptives use estrogens, progestins, or neither, and fill out the chart as shown in Fig. 45.1.

G. Evans (✉) · S. Wheeler
VA Puget Sound Health Care System, Department of Medicine, Division of General Internal Medicine, University of Washington, Seattle, WA, USA
e-mail: gingere@uw.edu

S. Mookherjee et al. (eds.), *Chalk Talks in Internal Medicine*,
https://doi.org/10.1007/978-3-030-34814-4_45

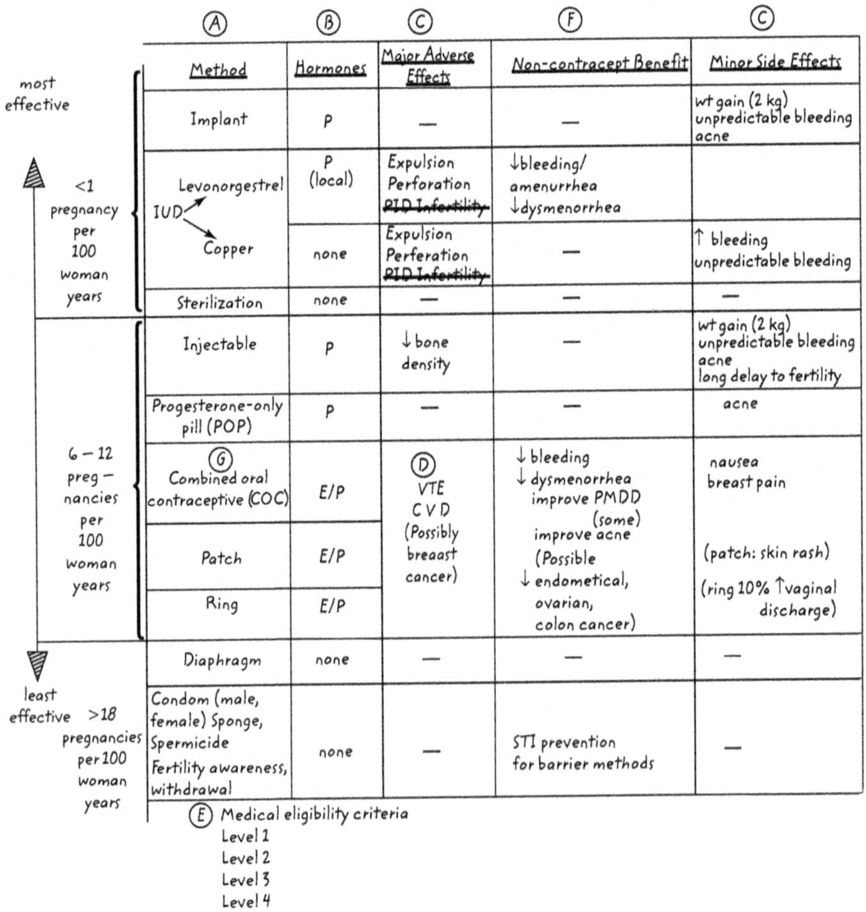

Fig. 45.1 (A–G) Approach to contraceptive counseling

Teaching points

- There are multiple types of estrogens (E) and progestins (P), but this need not be discussed unless learners inquire.
- Estrogen options include ethinyl estradiol (EE), estradiol valerate (EV), and mestranol.
- Progestin forms come in first, second, third, and fourth generation formulations.
- Commonly discussed options of progestin include levonorgestrel (LNG) which is a second generation formulation and recommended as first line progestin ingredient in a combined oral contraceptive by the Centers for Disease Control and Prevention (CDC).
- Drospirenone is a fourth generation formulation and a component of "Yaz®." The fourth generation progestins are the least androgenic and, therefore, in combination with estrogens in a combination oral contraceptive (COC) may be more effective against acne.
- The implant uses etonogestrel (third generation progestin) or LNG (second generation progestin).
- The IUD uses LNG.

C. **You elicit additional history that this patient has a remote history of gonorrhea and a current history of migraine without aura and hypertension. She has no significant family history and quit smoking at age 30. Her current BP is 150/94. Based on the type of device and the hormonal components, what are the major adverse effects we need to discuss with her?**

If learners name adverse effects that are not true, use that as a learning opportunity. Write them down and cross them off, for example, "pelvic inflammatory disease (PID)" and "Infertility" are crossed off under IUD because IUDs do not increase the risk of these. If the audience names minor risks, then add them to the final column and reorient learners back to major adverse effects.

Teaching points (references listed below under resources)

- Implant: Inserted on underside of upper arm, in groove between bicep and tricep. Can rarely migrate, but newest version (Nexplanon®) is now radioopaque.
- IUDs:
  - Risk of expulsion has been variably reported from 0% to 12% and there is mixed evidence about whether this is more common in younger women, but is likely not.
  - Risk of perforation is exceedingly low: </=0.1%.
  - No increased risk of pelvic inflammatory disease. In fact, although you should not place an IUD during an active cervical infection, patients with an IUD already in place who develop gonorrhea or chlamydia, can generally be treated without removing the IUD.
  - Fertility usually returns immediately upon removing the IUD.

- Injectable: possibly increased fracture risk.
- Combination hormonal contraception (CHC), includes COC, patch and ring:
  - Venous thromboembolic (VTE) risk: Baseline risk in users is about 0.2 per 1000 user-years. CHC use increases risk two to four times, which is still a low absolute risk.
  - Cardiovascular disease (CVD) risk: Baseline risk in users is about 0.1 per 1000 user-years. CHC use increases risk about one to two times.
  - The lower the estrogen dose, the less is the risk of VTE and CVD.
  - Cancer risk: Overall risk of cancer is decreased as a result of decrease colorectal, endometrial, and ovarian cancer. However, there may be a very slight increase risk in breast cancer (OR 1.08).

D. **What other risk factors could our patient have that would also increase her risk of VTE? What about additional risk factors she could have for CVD?**

Let the audience name various risk factors, but don't write them down (e.g., *inherited thrombophilia, family history of VTE, personal history of cancer, hypertension, diabetes, advanced age). Bring attention back to the vignette and ask which of these risk factors she has: migraine without aura, age, former smoker, elevated blood pressure, obesity.*

E. **How are you going to decide if any one of these risk factors that you named is a contraindication to adding on a COC, patch, or ring?**

Have learners download a "medical eligibility criteria" (MEC) app (search "Contraception"), bring a separate MEC printout, or search online at the time of the chalk-talk. Assign learners to look up each of the risk factors identified already in step D (hypertension, migraine, smoking, obesity) and have them report back what level of contraindication each is for different contraceptive methods.

Teaching points

- Risk levels aid in decision-making and in selecting a safe option.
- Level 1 = no restriction for use of this contraceptive method.
- Level 2 = advantages generally outweigh theoretical or proven risks.
- Level 3 = theoretical or proven risks generally outweigh advantages.
- Level 4 = unacceptable health risk if this method is used.

F. **Now that you have decided what the range of safe options are for this patient, you can choose between them based on her preferences, including concerns about noncontraceptive benefits and minor side effects. On further questioning, this patient shares that she has regular cycles q28 days, bleeds for 5 days, and is not bothered by heavy bleeding or cramps. She does not wish to be pregnant again now but may want to in the next 1–2 years. What potential benefits of various contraceptive methods should you discuss with the patient?**

Fill in the column for noncontraceptive benefits and complete the column for any minor side effects not previously mentioned.

Teaching points

- Minor side effect often can be dealt with, tips for dealing with them are given below:
  - For nausea, suggest taking it at night or decreasing the estrogen dose.
  - For breast tenderness, suggest the lowest estrogen dose or a progesterone-only option.
  - For rash, suggest rotating the site.
  - For breakthrough bleeding, counsel her that it will improve over first 3 months, but you can also increase estrogen dose if it is intolerable.
- Weight gain is not typical. When objectively studied, weight gain is nonexistent (comparable to placebo) or is very minimal (less than 2 kg in a year).
- Acne decreases with any estrogen-containing option because the estrogen effects outweigh the androgen effects of the progesterone. The fourth generation progestins are more anti-androgenic, so *might* be slightly better than other CHCs at reducing acne.

G. **Now, let's pretend for a minute that she didn't have any contraindications and you had jointly chosen a COC—how would you decide which one to prescribe?**

Ask learners how they would choose.

Teaching points

- Include patient preference or experiences.
- Generic formulations cost less.
- Monophasic preparations should be first line.
- Of the available options, LNG with EE at either 20 μg or 30 μg have the smallest increase in the risk of VTE. Either of these two are a good first-line choice.

Return to Objectives and Key Points

1. Describe the various types of contraception: hormonal components, relative efficacy, major adverse effects:
   - Hormonal options include combination estrogens and progestins or progesterone-only
   - Effectiveness:
     - Most effective (<1 pregnancy/100 women-years): Implant, IUD, sterilization
     - Medium effectiveness (6–12 pregnancies/100 women-years): injectable or oral progesterone, combination oral contraceptives, patch, and ring
     - Least effective (>18 pregnancies/100 women-years): condoms, fertility awareness ("rhythm"), withdrawal method
   - Major adverse effects:
     - IUD: expulsion, perforation (rare)
     - CHC: VTE, CVD

2. Utilize resources for identifying contraindications to hormone-based contraception:
    - Medical eligibility criteria.
    - Risk stratify patients who are considering CHC based on patient-specific factors including age, smoking status, comorbidities, and family history.
3. Manage minor side effects of all types of contraception.
    - For nausea, suggest taking it at night or decreasing the estrogen dose.
    - For breast tenderness, suggest the lowest estrogen dose or a progesterone-only option.
    - For breakthrough bleeding, counsel her that it will improve over first 3 months, but you can also increase estrogen dose if it is intolerable.
    - Weight gain is not typical and when it does occur is very minimal.
    - Acne decreases with any estrogen-containing option because the estrogen effects outweigh the androgen effects of the progesterone.
4. Name an example of a recommended, first-line agent for combined oral contraception.
    - Ethinyl estradiol 20 mg + levonorgestrel

Resources

1. Jutalia TC, Riley HE, Curtis KM. The safety of intrauterine devices among young women: a systematic review. Contraception. 2017;95(1):13–9.
2. Lopez LM, Chen M, Mullins Long S, Curtis KM, Helmerhorst FM. Steroidal contraceptives and bone fractures in women: evidence from observational studies. Cochrane Database Syst Rev. 2015(7):CD009849. https://doi.org/10.1002/14651858.CD009849.pub3.
3. Tricotel A, Raguideau F, Collin C, Zureik M. Estimate of venous thromboembolism and related-deaths attributable to the use of combined oral contraceptives in France. PLoS One. 2014;9(4):e93792. https://doi.org/10.1371/journal.pone.0093792.
4. Lidegaard O, Lokkegaard E, Jensen A, Skovelund CW, Keiding N. Thrombotic stroke and myocardial infarction with hormonal contraception. New Engl J Med. 2012;366(24):2257–66.
5. Hannaford PC, Selvaraj S, Elliot AM, Angus V, Iversen L, Lee AJ. Cancer risk among users of oral contraceptives: cohort data from the Royal College of General Practitioner's oral contraception study. BMJ. 2007;335(7621):651.
6. Van Vliet HAAM, Grimes DA, Lopez LM, Schulz KF, Helmerhorst FM. Triphasic versus monophasic oral contraceptives for contraception. Cochrane Database Syst Rev. 2011(11): CD003553. https://doi.org/10.1002/14651858.CD003553.pub3.
7. de Bastos M, Stegeman BH, Rosendaal FR, Van Hylckama Vlieg A, Helmerhorst FM, Stijnen T, et al. Combined oral contraceptives: venous thrombosis. Cochrane Database Syst Rev. 2014(3):CD010813. https://doi.org/10.1002/14651858.CD010813.pub2.
8. Evans GE, Sutton EL. Oral contraception. Med Clin N Am. 2015;99(3):479–503.

Chapter 46
Approach to Secondary Amenorrhea

Adelaide McClintock and Catherine P. Kaminetzky

Learning Objectives
1. Define secondary amenorrhea.
2. Build a differential for a patient with secondary amenorrhea based on knowledge of the hypothalamic–pituitary–ovarian (HPO) axis.
3. Design and interpret an appropriate workup.

Clinical Vignette: A 27-year-old woman presents for evaluation of irregular periods. She has experienced unpredictable bleeding and spotting x3 years. Her last period was 4 months ago. Past medical history is significant for bipolar disorder and she takes lithium and risperidone. She is sexually active with one, monogamous male partner, and they use condoms irregularly. On exam, vitals are normal, she has a BMI of 32, and the rest of her exam is normal.

A. **Does this patient have primary or secondary amenorrhea?**

Write the definitions on the whiteboard as shown in Fig. 46.1.

Teaching points
- **Primary amenorrhea**: No menses by age 15. Not discussed in this chalk talk (or addressed in the diagram). Can be anatomical, endocrine, or developmental. Rarely evaluated primarily by general internists (usually pediatrics or gynecology). This is an appropriate referral to a gynecologist.

A. McClintock (✉)
University of Washington Medical Center, Department of Medicine, Division of General Internal Medicine, University of Washington, Seattle, WA, USA
e-mail: ahearst@uw.edu

C. P. Kaminetzky
VA Puget Sound Health Care System, Department of Medicine, Division of General Internal Medicine, University of Washington, Seattle, WA, USA

S. Mookherjee et al. (eds.), *Chalk Talks in Internal Medicine*,
https://doi.org/10.1007/978-3-030-34814-4_46

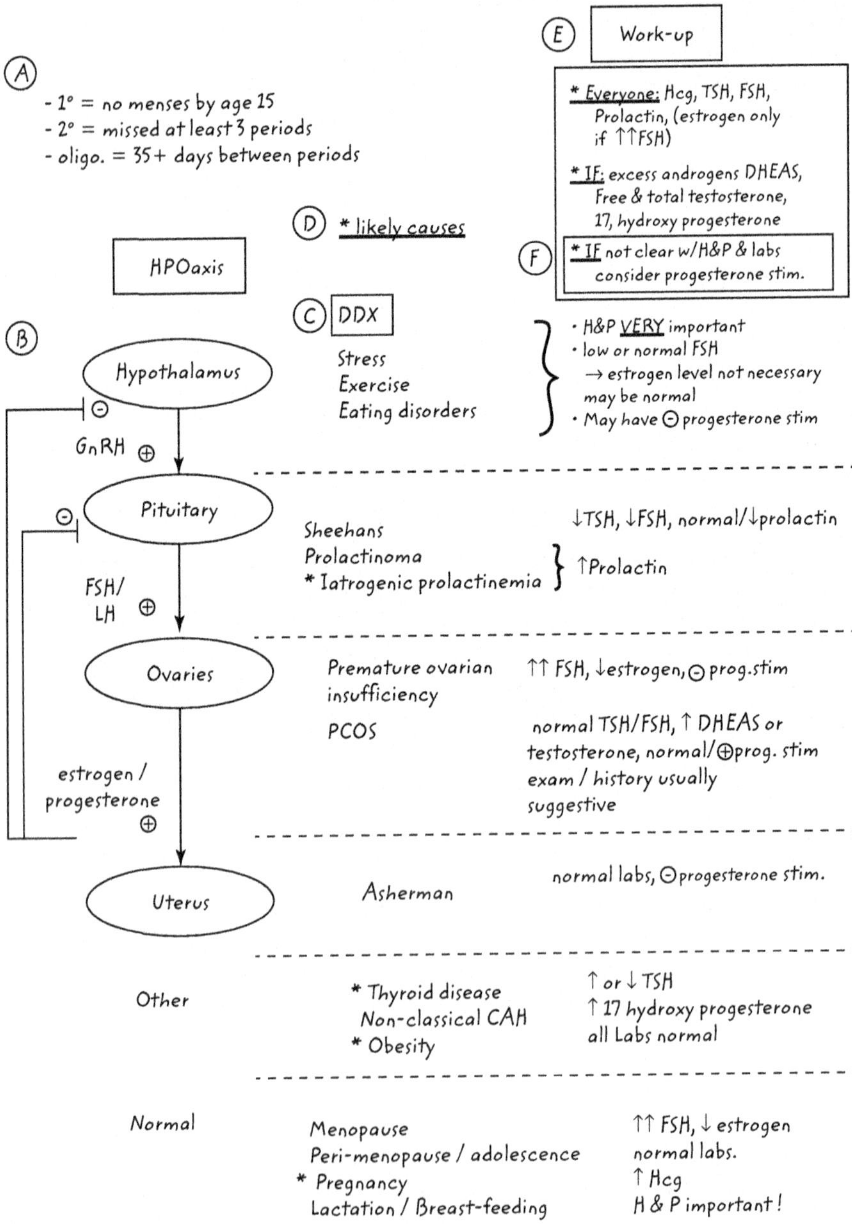

Fig. 46.1 (A–F) Approach to secondary amenorrhea

- **Secondary amenorrhea**: Women who have missed at least three menstrual periods in a row have secondary amenorrhea. This is the focus of this chalk talk.
- **Oligomenorrhea**: Women who regularly go more than 35 days without menstruating.

B. **What are the four possible locations in the hypothalamic–pituitary–ovarian (HPO) hormonal pathway that could be causing this patient's amenorrhea?**

Draw the HPO axis as shown in Fig. 46.1., *including the hormone signaling involved in each step of the axis, including negative feedback loops.*

C. **Based on the HPO axis, what possible disorders could cause secondary amenorrhea?**

Use the HPO axis to structure the differential, organizing by broad categories (hypothalamic, pituitary, ovarian, uterine). List potential causes based on the location of the primary insult. Have people name one to two items per anatomic location/cause, and fill in what isn't named. Add "other" and "normal" categories to complete the differential.

D. **What causes are most likely in our patient?**

Read the case presentation again and ask learners to identify clues for potential causes. Add asterisks for likely causes of amenorrhea in this patient.

Teaching points

- Pregnancy (most common cause of secondary amenorrhea)
- Hypothyroid (lithium-induced)
- Hyperprolactinemia (risperidone side effect)
- Obesity
- Learners might suggest polycystic ovarian syndrome (PCOS), but the case does not support this diagnosis as written, as there is no suggestion of hyperandrogenism:
  - Insulin resistance
  - Hirsutism
  - Acanthosis nigricans
  - Acne

E. **Looking at our diagram and differential, which labs should we order to investigate this patient's amenorrhea?**

Write in labs and studies in a second column alongside the differential. Note the labs that all patients should have at the top.

Teaching points

- All patients should have:
  - Pregnancy test (human chorionic gonadotropin, Hcg) → pregnancy
  - Thyroid stimulating hormone (TSH) → hypothyroidism
  - Prolactin → hyperprolactinemia
  - Follicle stimulating hormone (FSH) → primary ovarian insufficiency
- Don't need estradiol level unless you suspect ovarian insufficiency or want to confirm menopause. Estradiol is typically only useful in the event of a high FSH.
- In women who have physical evidence of excess androgens (hirsutism, hair thinning, mandibular acne, virilization) consider androgen testing:
  - Testosterone (free and total)
  - Dehydroepiandrosterone sulfate, aka DHEAS (PCOS)
  - 17-Hydroxyprogesterone (nonclassic congenital adrenal hyperplasia, which can be misdiagnosed as PCOS)
- Note that each of these labs correspond roughly to some key points along the HPO axis, as well as other endocrine disorders.

F. **What if your lab workup is negative and you still don't have a diagnosis based on history, physical, and labs?**

Add "progesterone stimulation" as shown in Fig. 46.1.

Teaching points

- Consider progesterone stimulation (5–10 days of progesterone).
- Bleeding after progesterone stimulation suggests adequate estrogen and normal genital tract. Therefore, the patient has anovulatory cycles.
- If no bleeding following progesterone stimulation can try estrogen stimulation followed by progesterone. If bleeding occurs following estrogen and progesterone administration, the patient likely has low estrogen (usually hypothalamic cause or ovarian failure).
- If still no bleeding after estrogen stimulation and progesterone challenge, cause may be structural (for example, Asherman's syndrome/scarring).

The patient's labs show an elevated prolactin and a slightly elevated TSH. This patient likely has hypothyroidism from her lithium and elevated prolactin from her risperidone. She has both hypothyroidism and iatrogenic hyperprolactinemia. Both of these meds need to be changed in discussion with her mental health provider. If she does not desire pregnancy, more consistent condom use +/– another form of contraception should be discussed with her.

Return to Objectives and Emphasize Key Points

1. Secondary amenorrhea is defined as three or more missed menstrual periods in a row; and oligomenorrhea is defined as cycles regularly lasting more than 35 days.
2. Every patient with secondary amenorrhea should have a pregnancy test, as well as TSH, prolactin and FSH, at a minimum.

3. Further testing can be done, including estradiol levels if FSH is abnormal, or testosterone, DHEAS, and 17-hydroxyprogesterone if there is evidence of excess androgens.
4. Treat underlying endocrine disorders directly. Assess patient's fertility goals, tailoring treatment to patient needs, and prevent downstream effects of endocrine abnormalities (osteoporosis or endometrial cancers, for example).

Resources

1. American College of Obstetricians and Gynecologists. Primary ovarian insufficiency in adolescents and young women. Committee Opinion No. 605. Obstet Gynecol. 2014;124:193–7.
2. Klein D, Poth MA. An approach to diagnosis and management. Am Fam Physician. 2013;87(11):781–8.
3. Speiser PW. 2001. Congenital adrenal hyperplasia owing to 21-hydroxylase deficiency. Endocrinol Metab Clin N Am. 2001;30(1):31.

Chapter 47
Approach to Abnormal Uterine Bleeding

Jocelyn James and Alexandra Molnar

Learning Objectives

1. Define abnormal uterine bleeding (AUB) and provide a differential diagnosis of other sources of bleeding.
2. Classify AUB.
3. Distinguish features that might indicate structural or nonstructural causes of bleeding and choose diagnostic tests accordingly.
4. Recognize indications for endometrial biopsy in the evaluation of abnormal uterine bleeding.

Clinical Vignette: A 44-year-old woman who presents to establish care complains of painful, heavy periods ever since menarche at age 14. She reports increased fatigue and bleeding over the last several years. Her periods have always been regular.

A. **Does this patient have AUB?**

Write the characteristics of AUB as shown in Fig. 47.1.

Teaching points

- AUB is menstrual bleeding of abnormal quantity, duration, or schedule (normal bleeding lasts up to 8 days and occurs every 24–38 days).
- Determination of excessive bleeding should be based on patient's perception.

B. **According to this definition, this patient appears to have AUB. When should uterine bleeding be considered an emergency?**

Continue with the algorithm as shown in Fig. 47.1.

J. James (✉) · A. Molnar
Harborview Medical Center, Department of Medicine, Division of General Internal Medicine, University of Washington, Seattle, WA, USA
e-mail: jorose@uw.edu

S. Mookherjee et al. (eds.), *Chalk Talks in Internal Medicine*,
https://doi.org/10.1007/978-3-030-34814-4_47

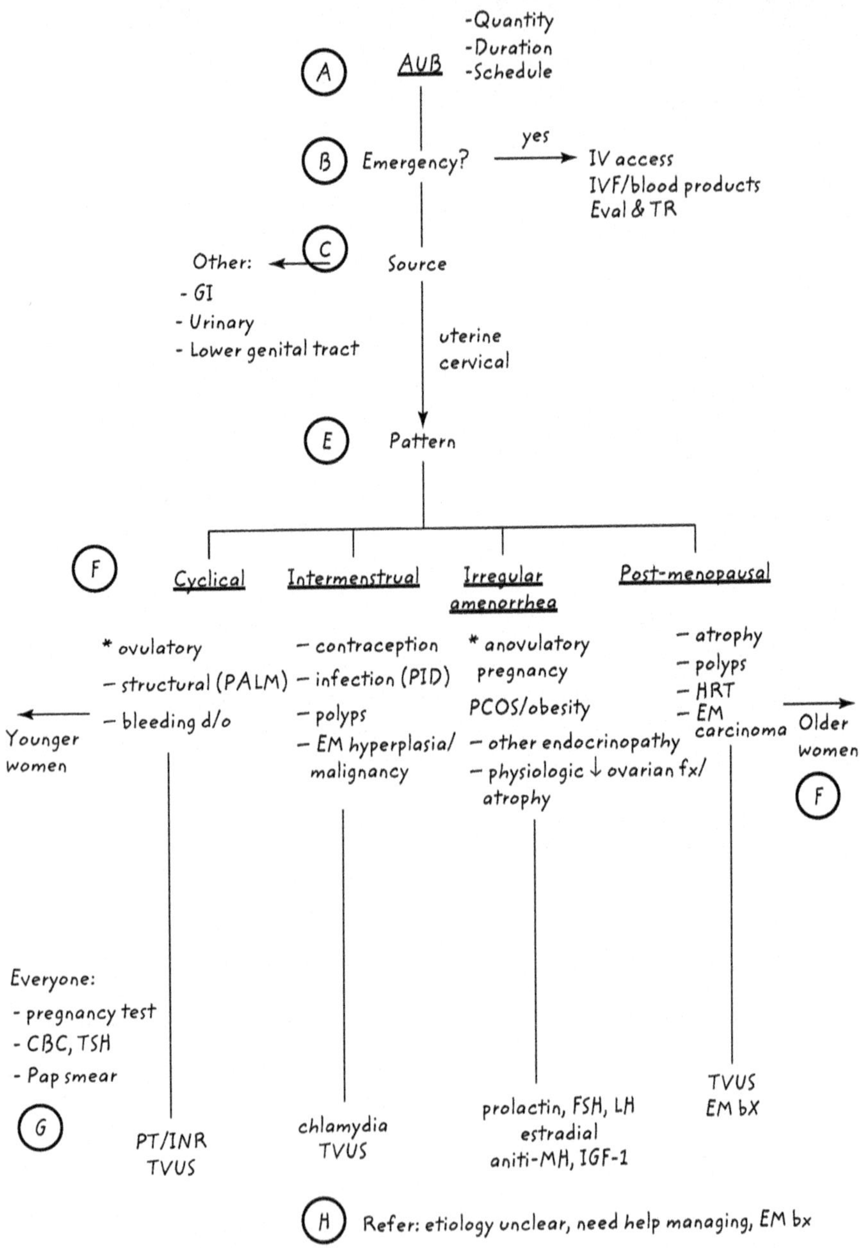

Fig. 47.1 (A–H) Approach to abnormal bleeding

Teaching points

- AUB is an emergency when signs of hypovolemia or hemodynamic instability are present.
- Emergent bleeding should be promptly identified and treated by obtaining IV access, administering IVF or blood products, and evaluating and treating the source of bleeding.

C. **What external sources of blood loss should be considered in a woman with suspected AUB?**

Draw potential external sources of blood loss as shown in Fig. 47.2.

Teaching points

- It is critical to evaluate the most likely etiology of bleeding so that appropriate treatment can be provided.
- The external genitalia should be examined for rash, fissures, or lesions.
- A speculum exam should be performed to evaluate the cervix for friability or bleeding from the os.

D. **What internal sources of blood loss should be considered in a woman with suspected AUB?**

Draw an outline of the uterus and ovaries as shown in Fig. 47.2. *Label structural etiologies as suggested by learners, and list nonstructural etiologies on the side.*

Teaching points

- PALM is the mnemonic used for these **structural etiologies:**
  - **P**olyp
  - **A**denomyosis
  - **L**eiomyoma (fibroids)
  - **M**alignancy/hyperplasia
- COE is the mnemonic for **nonstructural etiologies:**
  - **C**oagulopathy
  - **O**vulatory dysfunction—pregnancy, hormonal contraception, PCOS, obesity, age-related decline in ovarian function, stress-related hypothalamic hypogonadism, pituitary disorder
  - **E**ndometrial atrophy

E. **Returning to our patient, how do we classify her pattern of bleeding?**

Return to Fig. 47.1 *to show the four patterns of AUB.*

Teaching points

- Cyclical (heavy or prolonged) menses suggests ovulatory bleeding.
  - More common than anovulatory AUB

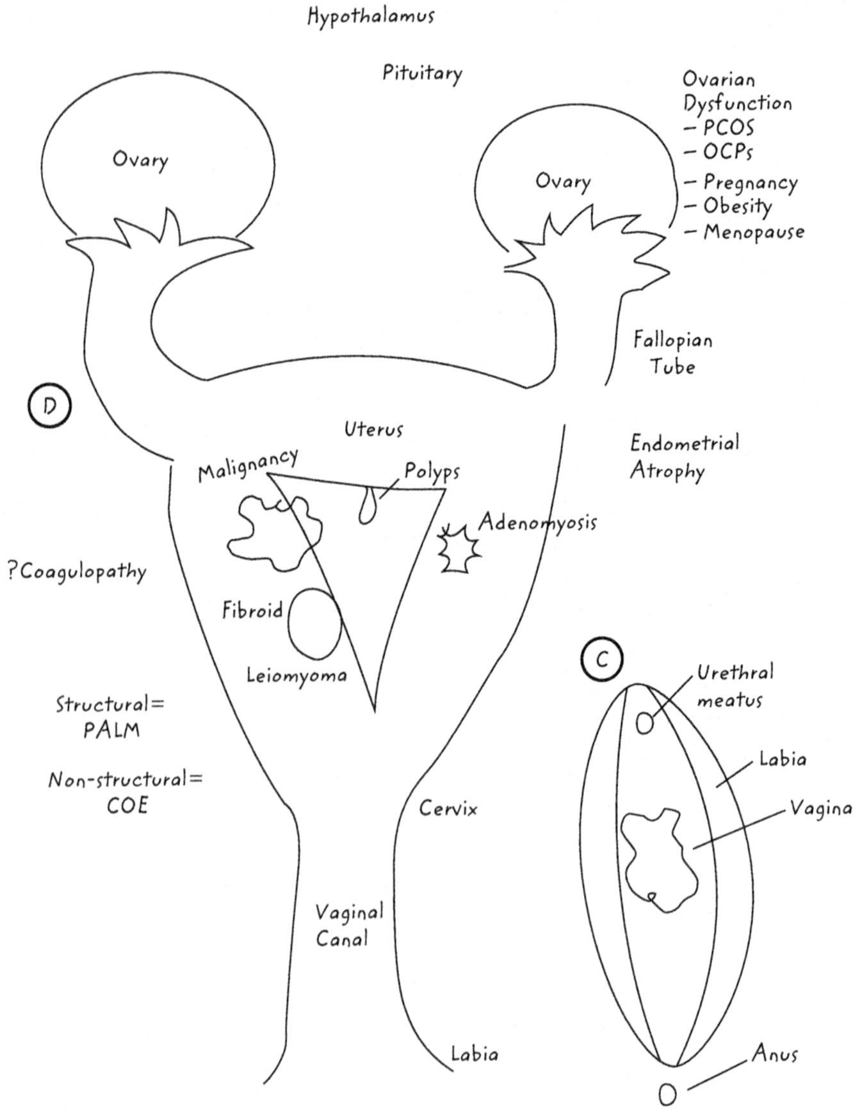

Fig. 47.2 (C and D) Approach to abnormal uterine bleeding

- Leiomyoma, adenomyosis, cesarean scar defects, bleeding disorders, idiopathic
- Heavy menses since menarche-> evaluate for bleeding disorder

• Intermenstrual bleeding or bleeding between regular cycles.

- Contraception, infection (pelvic inflammatory disease (PID)), structural (polyps, endometrial hyperplasia/malignancy)

• Irregular menses or amenorrhea suggests anovulatory bleeding, typically associated with an endocrinopathy (see Chap. 46).

- Pregnancy, polycystic ovarian syndrome (PCOS), obesity, other endocrinopathy, physiologic decline in ovarian function/atrophy

• Postmenopausal bleeding.

- Endometrial carcinoma, vaginal atrophy, polyps, hormone replacement therapy

F. **Recall that our patient is 44 years old. What etiologies of AUB are more likely in women aged 40 through menopause, and what etiologies more commonly present in younger women?**

Draw arrows indicating typical etiologies for older and younger woman as shown in the figure.

Teaching points

• Generally, etiologies toward the left are more common in younger women and those on the right are more common in older women.

- Age 19–39: pregnancy, hormonal contraception, endocrinopathy
- Age 40–menopause: physiologic anovulatory bleeding (declining ovarian function), endometrial atrophy, endometrial carcinoma

• Note that fibroids and endometrial hyperplasia are common in both groups.

G. **Due to the heavy but regular periods, we suspect a structural problem or perhaps a bleeding disorder explains the bleeding in this patient. Which diagnostic procedures are indicated? Which are indicated in other patterns of bleeding?**

Write out appropriate diagnostics as suggested by learners.

Teaching points

• Indicated regardless of bleeding pattern:

- Pregnancy test
- Complete blood count (CBC), thyroid stimulating hormone (TSH)
- Cervical cancer screening

- Cyclical bleeding:
  - Coagulopathy evaluation with prothrombin time (PT/INR), partial thromboplastin time
  - Transvaginal ultrasound (TVUS) or sonohysterography to assess for a structural problem
- Intermenstrual bleeding:
  - Chlamydia testing if risk factors for sexually transmitted infection
  - TVUS
- Irregular bleeding or amenorrhea:
  - Other pituitary/ovarian hormones: prolactin, follicle-stimulating hormone (FSH), luteinizing hormone (LH), estradiol, occasionally anti-Mullerian hormone (anti-MH) or insulin-like growth factor-1 (IGF-1)
- Postmenopausal bleeding:
  - TVUS
  - Endometrial (EM) biopsy

H. **When should patients with AUB be referred to gynecology?**

Write out reasons to refer.

Return to objectives and emphasize key points

1. Define abnormal uterine bleeding (AUB) and provide a differential diagnosis of other sources of bleeding.
   - Menstrual bleeding of abnormal quantity, duration, or schedule
   - Exclude GI, urinary or lower urinary tract sources with careful exam
2. Classify AUB.
   - Cyclical
   - Intermenstrual
   - Irregular/amenorrhea
   - Postmenopausal
3. Distinguish features that might indicate structural or nonstructural causes of bleeding and choose diagnostic tests accordingly.
   - All patients require pregnancy testing, CBC, TSH, and cervical cancer screening.
   - Additional testing should be directed at specific classification of bleeding.
     - Cyclical—PT/INR, TVUS
     - Intermenstrual—chlamydia testing, TVUS
     - Irregular/amenorrhea—prolactin, FSH/LH, estradiol, etc.
     - Postmenopausal—TVUS, endometrial biopsy

4. Recognize indications for referral to gynecology in the evaluation of abnormal uterine bleeding.
    - Unclear etiology
    - Endometrial biopsy

Resources

1. Bradley LD, Gueye NA. The medical management of abnormal uterine bleeding in reproductive-aged women. Am J Obstet Gynecol. 2016;214(1):31–44. https://doi.org/10.1016/j.ajog.2015.07.044. Epub 2015 Aug 5. Review. PubMed [citation] PMID:26254516.
2. American College of Obstetricians and Gynecologists. ACOG committee opinion no. 557: management of acute abnormal uterine bleeding in nonpregnant reproductive-aged women. Obstet Gynecol. 2013;121(4):891–6. https://doi.org/10.1097/01.AOG.0000428646.67925.9a. PubMed [citation] PMID: 23635706.
3. Committee on Practice Bulletins—Gynecology. Practice bulletin no. 128: diagnosis of abnormal uterine bleeding in reproductive-aged women. Obstet Gynecol. 2012;120(1):197–206. https://doi.org/10.1097/AOG.0b013e318262e320. No abstract available. PubMed [citation] PMID: 22914421.
4. Munro MG, Critchley HO, Broder MS, Fraser IS, FIGO Working Group on Menstrual Disorders. FIGO classification system (PALM-COEIN) for causes of abnormal uterine bleeding in nongravid women of reproductive age. Int J Gynaecol Obstet. 2011;113(1):3–13. https://doi.org/10.1016/j.ijgo.2010.11.011. Epub 2011 Feb 22. PubMed [citation] PMID: 21345435.
5. Bayer SR, DeCherney AH. Clinical manifestations and treatment of dysfunctional uterine bleeding. JAMA. 1993;269(14):1823–8. Review. PubMed [citation] PMID: 8459515.
6. Bacon JL. Abnormal uterine bleeding: current classification and clinical management. Obstet Gynecol Clin North Am. 2017;44(2):179–93.

Chapter 48
Approach to Transgender Health

Tyra Fainstad and Kamala B. Jain

Learning Objectives

1. Use the correct terminology regarding the transgender population.
2. Describe indications, contraindications, and effects of masculinizing/feminizing hormone therapy.
3. Initiate and follow patients on masculinizing/feminizing hormone therapy.

Clinical Vignette: Brian is a 31-year-old transman who is seeing you in clinic. He identifies as male and has female anatomy. He hopes to begin masculinizing hormone therapy.

A. **What are the best ways to refer to the patient in person and in your documentation?**

Ask learners for their ideas and emphasize that it is best to ask the patient.

Teaching points

- Always ask your patients how they identify and which pronouns and names they prefer. If you have not met them yet, gender neutral pronouns are: they/their/them.
- Gender identity does not refer to sexual orientation. Gender identity refers to the innate, deep-seated knowledge of one's own gender, which may or may not match biological sex assigned at birth.
- Sexual orientation refers to whom the person is attracted.

T. Fainstad (✉)
University of Washington Medical Center, Department of Medicine, Division of General Internal Medicine, University of Washington, Seattle, WA, USA
e-mail: tyrat@uw.edu

K. B. Jain
VA Puget Sound Health Care System, Department of Medicine, Division of General Internal Medicine, University of Washington, Seattle, WA, USA

S. Mookherjee et al. (eds.), *Chalk Talks in Internal Medicine*,
https://doi.org/10.1007/978-3-030-34814-4_48

B. **What are the more accurate and respectful terms to use when referring to the patient?**

Elicit terms from learners and list them under "best" as shown in Fig. 48.1.

- Trans: umbrella for nonbinary gender or gender nonconforming identity
- Transgender: gender identity does not equal sex that they were born with (as opposed to cisgender)
- Gender dysphoria: *DSM-5* diagnosis referring to distress about one's gender identity and natal sex (note: not all transpatients are uncomfortable with their body)

C. **What terms should you definitely avoid when referring to the patient?**

Elicit terms from learners and list them under "avoid" as shown in Fig. 48.1.

- "Transgendered" (implies that something happened)
- "F->M, M->F" (better to say transman/masculine or transwoman/feminine)
- "Transsexual" (this is confusing since "trans" has nothing to do with sexuality)
- "Transvestite" (considered pejorative, use "crossdresser" instead)

D. **What are some gender affirming interventions for trans patients such as Brian?**

Continue with "therapy initiation" as shown in Fig. 48.1.

Teaching points
- Hormones, surgery, hair removal, speech intervention, behavioral (genital tucking/packing, chest binding)

E. **Is there any specific testing needed to determine if Brian is a candidate for masculinizing hormone treatment?**

Continue Fig. 48.1 *as shown.*

Teaching points
- No special testing needed other than a good history, physical exam and capacity determination
- WPATH (World Professional Association for Transgender Health) uses four criteria for hormone therapy:

    1. Persistent, well-documented gender dysphoria
    2. Capacity to make an informed decision and consent to treatment (see Chap. 50)
    3. >18 years old
    4. If significant medical or mental health concerns: must be reasonably well-controlled

- If he does not meet all criteria, consider referring to mental health or endocrine for help.

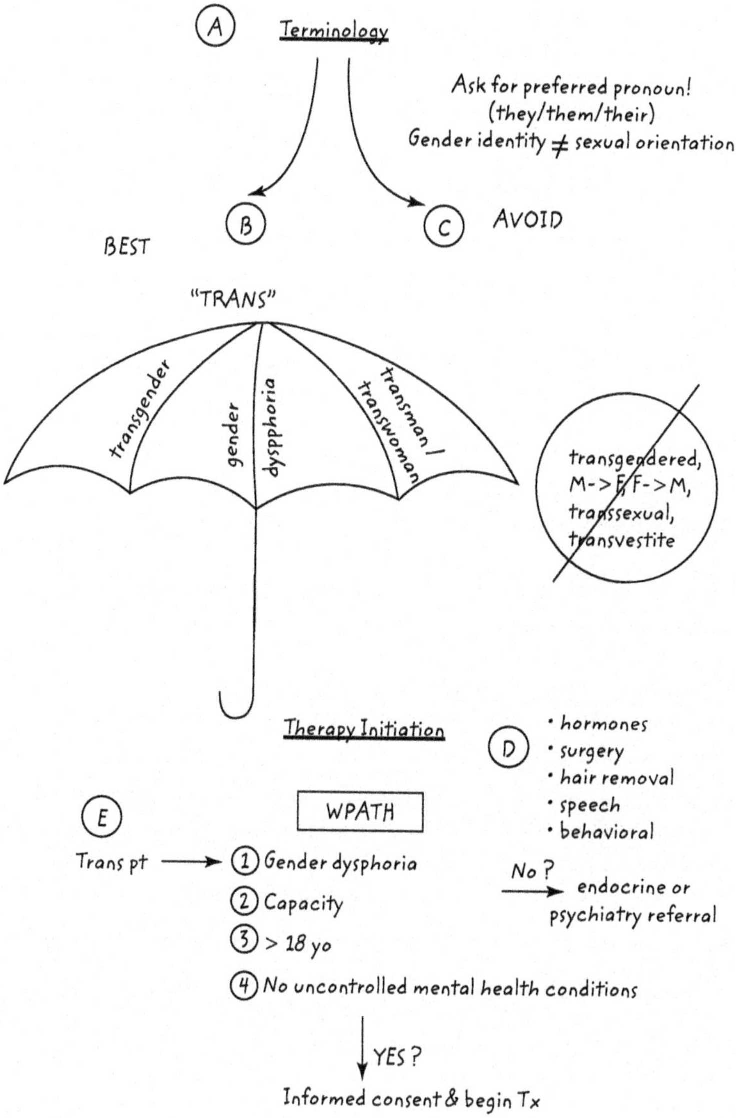

Fig. 48.1 (A–E) Approach to transgender health

- If he does, initiate informed consent: a discussion about risks/benefits/alternatives. PCP does a "psychosocial assessment" (get a sense of support, work life, risks if/when they come out). Can refer to mental health for help with this.
- Historically, WPATH recommended a psychologist letter and 3–6 months of living as the opposite gender first, *but* many studies actually found this was harmful prior to receiving hormonal Tx.
- Now most major guidelines support the Informed Consent for Access to Transgender Health (ICATH) model, i.e., *informed consent only as the basis for treatment.*

F. **What is the goal of gender affirming hormone therapy?**

Write down the goal as shown at the top of Fig. 48.2.

G. **What will you tell Brian about expected changes with masculinizing hormones?**

Write down desired and undesired effects as suggested by learners.

Teaching points

- Desired effects
  - Permanent facial hair (won't resolve if Tx stopped!)
  - Male pattern baldness
  - Acne
  - Permanent deepening of voice (won't resolve if Tx stopped!)
  - Increased muscle mass
  - Increased body hair
  - Shifts body fat towards midline
  - Enlarged clitoris, cessation of menses (possible permanent infertility, but NOT a reliable birth control!)
- Undesired effects: Possible polycythemia, adverse lipids effects, mood changes/irritability, liver function test (LFT) abnormalities, atrophic vaginitis (spotting)
- Note: Can't pick and choose effects (i.e., "you may want a beard, but you'll also go bald. You may want a deep voice, but you'll also get acne")

H. **What are the expected changes with feminizing hormone therapy?**

Write down the desired and undesired effects as suggested by learners.

Teaching points

- Reduce male pattern baldness
- Skin softening

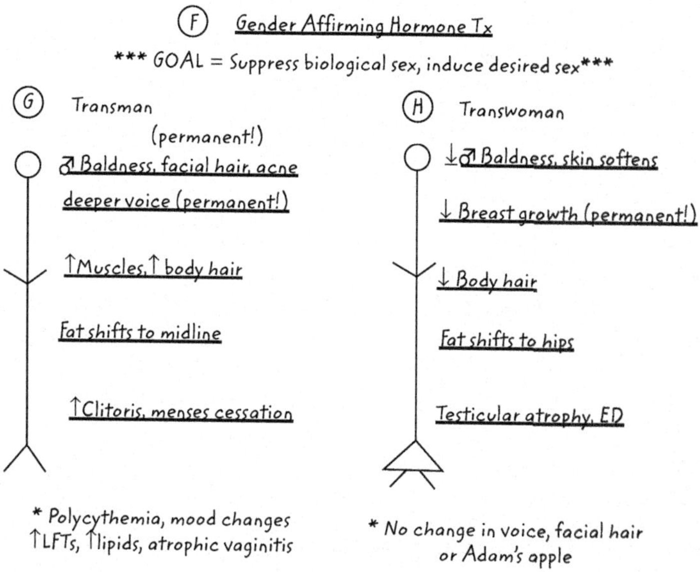

(I)

Drug	Contraindications
Testosterone (IM, SQ, gel)	active testosterone responsive cancer (i.e. prostate)

(J)

Drug	Contraindications
Estradiol	active estrogen responsive cancer or active VTE relative: CAD, migraine + aura, prolactinoma
Spirondactone	renal dysfunction, hyperkalemia
Finasteride	none

Fig. 48.2 (F–J) Approach to transgender health

- Permanent breast growth (won't resolve if Tx stopped!)
- Decreased body hair
- Fat redistribution
- Testicular atrophy
- Erectile dysfunction (ED), infertility (recommend sperm banking)
- Note: Will NOT change: voice, facial hair, or Adam's apple

I. **How do you initiate masculinizing hormone therapy for Brian? What drugs are available and what are the contraindications?**

Write down the drug and contraindications as shown in Fig. 48.2.

Teaching points
- Main drug is testosterone. Choose formulation based on preferences/need/cost. Most common are injections (more peak/trough effect) and gel (may be more expensive, but avoids peak/trough).
- Note: Increases should be based on patient response and/or monitored hormone levels. Once within the normal male range, higher doses/levels don't necessarily result in more virilization.
- Monitor labs (can look up specifics when needed) and see patient Q3 months for first year, then yearly thereafter.
- An absolute contraindication to testosterone use is active hormone responsive malignancy, i.e., prostate cancer.

J. **How would you initiate feminizing hormone therapy and what are the contraindications?**

Write down the drugs and contraindications as shown in Fig. 48.2.

- There are many estrogen formulations, estradiol is most widely used.
- Monitor estradiol, sex binding hormone globulin (SBHG), and testosterone every 3 months × 1 year then yearly. Ok to look this up as needed!
- Spironolactone and finasteride are androgen suppressing and may be used to reduce male secondary sexual characteristics and allow for lower dose of estrogen. Monitor basic metabolic panel (BMP) yearly for spironolactone, and prostate specific antigen (PSA) yearly for finasteride.
- Contraindications to feminizing hormone therapy include:
  - Active estrogen responsive cancer or active venous thromboembolism (VTE) for estrogen
  - Use estrogen with caution in coronary artery disease (CAD), migraine w/ aura, Hx of VTE, or prolactinoma
  - Renal dysfunction or hyperkalemia with spironolactone
  - No contraindications to finasteride, but remember it reduces PSA levels by 50%, so your cut off for cancer workup is a PSA of ~2

Return to Objectives and Emphasize Key Points
1. Use the correct terminology regarding the transgender population.

- Gender identity does NOT refer to sexual orientation.
- Avoid using F->M or M->F, better to use transman/transwoman. Also avoid transsexual/transvestite.
- Ask the patient about preferred pronouns.

2. Describe indications and effects of masculinizing/feminizing hormone therapy.

- WPATH guidelines for indications: Informed Consent is all that is needed to start therapy.
- Review effects of gender affirming hormonal therapy—circle main points on stick figures.

3. Initiate and monitor patients on masculinizing/feminizing hormone therapy.

- Three feminizing drugs: estradiol, spironolactone, and finasteride. One masculinizing drug: testosterone.
- Need to see patient (to evaluate response) and monitor labs every 3 months for the first year in everyone.
- Only absolute contraindication to hormone therapy is active hormone-responsive malignancy (for both) or active VTE (for estrogen).
- Increase hormones based on response/satisfaction and/or levels. Higher doses are not always move effective.

Resources

1. Spack NP. Management of transgenderism. JAMA. 2013;309(5):478–84.
2. Albert J, et al. Gender identity and the management of the transgender patient: a guide for non-specialists. J R Soc Med. 2017;110(4):144–52.
3. ICATH: www.icath.org
4. UCSF Center for Transgender Excellence: www.transhealth.ucsf.edu
5. Fenway Guidelines for Transgender Care: fenwayhealth.org/care/medical/transgender-health

Chapter 49
Inpatient Treatment of Opioid Withdrawal

David S. Levitt and Alexandra Moretti Morrison

Learning Objectives
1. Articulate the importance of addressing acute opioid withdrawal in hospitalized patients.
2. Strengthen the therapeutic alliance with patients by acknowledging the discomfort of withdrawal, expressing provider support, and discussing a plan for medication to address withdrawal symptoms.
3. Assess symptoms of acute opioid withdrawal.
4. Use methadone appropriately to safely mitigate withdrawal symptoms.

Clinical Vignette: A 22-year-old woman with 2 weeks of subjective fevers and chills is admitted for treatment of endocarditis after a bedside ultrasound revealed a mobile mitral valve mass. She has been injecting heroin daily for the last 6 months, but prior to that she had no medical problems. She has had no complications from her drug use until now. She agreed to be admitted, but you have just received a page from her nurse stating that she is getting anxious about how long she will need to be hospitalized because she is experiencing opioid cravings and withdrawal symptoms.

A. **Does this patient meet the criteria for the opioid use disorder (OUD)?**

Draw the "time" and "condition" axes as shown in Fig. 49.1. *Fill out the labels: "withdrawal," "normal," "euphoria," "acute use," and "chronic use." Draw the curved line indicating episodes of opioid use with decreasing euphoria and increasing withdrawal over time. Do not draw the curve for initiation of medications for OUD yet. Highlight the key features of OUD: impairment/distress.*

D. S. Levitt (✉) · A. M. Morrison
Harborview Medical Center, Department of Medicine, Division of General Internal Medicine, University of Washington, Seattle, WA, USA
e-mail: figment@uw.edu

S. Mookherjee et al. (eds.), *Chalk Talks in Internal Medicine*,
https://doi.org/10.1007/978-3-030-34814-4_49

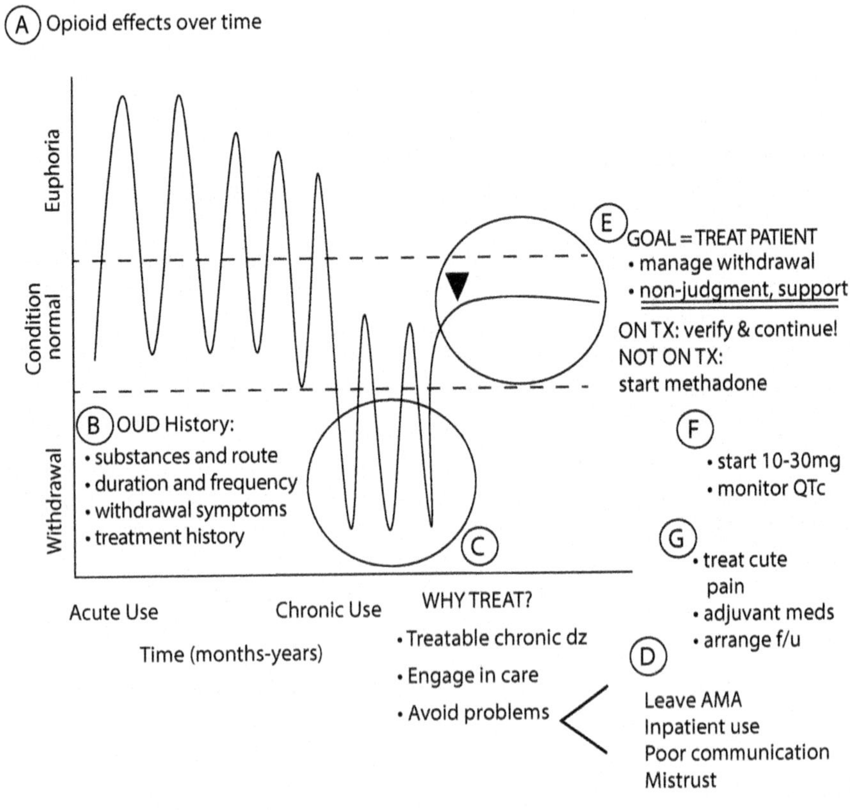

Fig. 49.1 Management of opioid withdrawal, A–G

Teaching points

- OUD is defined by *DSM-5* as a problematic pattern of opioid use leading to clinically significant impairment/distress, including at least two of the following criteria in a 12-month period:

Opioids are often taken in larger amounts or over a longer period than was intended.
There is a persistent desire or unsuccessful efforts to cut down or control opioid use.
A great deal of time is spent in activities necessary to obtain the opioid, use the opioid, or recover from its effects.
Craving, or a strong desire or urge to use opioids.
Recurrent opioid use resulting in a failure to fulfill major role obligations at work, school, or home.
Continued opioid use despite having persistent or recurrent social or interpersonal problems caused or exacerbated by the effects of opioids.
Important social, occupational, or recreational activities are given up or reduced because of opioid use.
Recurrent opioid use in situations in which it is physically hazardous.
Continued opioid use despite knowledge of having a persistent or recurrent physical or psychological problem that is likely to have been caused or exacerbated by the substance.
Exhibits tolerance.
Exhibits withdrawal.

- With acute use, patients experience euphoria with each episode. Over time (months-years, depending on intensity of use) patients experience dysphoria/withdrawal between episodes of use. This is a major driver of continued opioid use.

B. **A detailed history is essential for developing a treatment plan. What information should you gather about the patient's opioid use?**

Add the key history components as suggested by learners.

Teaching points

- Are they now in outpatient treatment?
- What opioids do they use and how often?
- What withdrawal symptoms do they feel if they don't use?
- Consider assessment for objective signs of withdrawal using the Clinical Opioid Withdrawal Score (COWS) scale.
- Quantifying precisely how much they use isn't as helpful as determining if they experience withdrawal symptoms when they don't use.

C. **Why is it important to address withdrawal symptoms in addition to treating her primary reason for admission?**

Circle the withdrawal curves on the diagram; add the key points for why to treat withdrawal.

Teaching points

- OUD, like emphysema and diabetes, is a medical illness and should not be treated as a moral failure or dismissed as a consequence of lifestyle choices.
- We have safe and effective medications for treating opioid withdrawal.
- Treating acute withdrawal can open the door for discussion about outpatient medication treatment and harm-reduction strategies.

D. **If this patient's concerns about withdrawal go unaddressed, what challenges might arise in treating her acute medical condition?**

Add challenges as suggested by learner.

Teaching points

- Leaving against medical advice (AMA), or threatening to do so.
- Illicit drug use in the hospital.
- Obscured diagnostic information because of vital sign abnormalities and inhibited communication with the patient.
- Decreased trust in her health care providers and the health care system.

E. **Our patient reports injecting heroin two to three times daily for the last 6 months. She is not currently in treatment. How will you establish a therapeutic relationship with this patient? What expectations will you set before initiating treatment?**

Fill in the remainder of Fig. 49.1 *with a horizontal line extending to the right past the upside-down triangle indicating initiation of medication treatment.*

Teaching points

- Primary goal of treatment is to stabilize withdrawal symptoms and facilitate management of acute medical or surgical conditions.
- As such, it is essential to provide reassurance (early and often) that you will aggressively treat withdrawal.
  - Recognize that psychological factors play a major role in opioid withdrawal syndrome.
  - Nonjudgmental, supportive, and clear communication is essential.
  - Medication alone is unlikely to address the distress of anticipating withdrawal.
- If currently receiving methadone, verify dose with the opioid treatment program. If on buprenorphine, verify dose by checking your state's Prescription Monitoring Program (PMP) or clinic notes.
- If NOT currently receiving treatment, start methadone with or without short-acting opioids as discussed below.

F. **She expresses understanding and agreement starting methadone. What features of methadone make it ideal for treating opioid withdrawal in the inpatient setting?**

Write out methadone treatment pearls as shown in Fig. 49.1.

- Long half-life provides consistent control of symptoms.
- Co-administration with short-acting opiates allows the provider to safely titrate to effect.
- Dosing recommendations:
  - Start with up to 30 mg methadone ×1.
  - For patients with limited prior opioid use, mild withdrawal symptoms, active benzodiazepine use, or baseline neurologic compromise, consider starting with as little as 10 mg of methadone for the first dose.
  - Peak initial dose effect occurs around 4 h, so at that time, reassess and give an additional one-time dose of 5–10 mg if they are still in active withdrawal.
  - Total daily dose should not exceed 40 mg when starting methadone.
- Low risk of overdose and respiratory depression when appropriately dosed.
- QTc prolongation:
  - Use caution and monitor if QTc is above 500 ms.
  - A stable QTc is the goal, so repeating electrocardiograms (ECGs) is warranted when the initial QTc is prolonged or with dose increases to ensure that the QTc is rising.

G. **The patient initially endorses some improvement in severe withdrawal symptoms within a few hours of receiving methadone 30 mg, but on hospital day 4 she wants to leave against medical advice. What will you discuss with her on discharge?**

Write down key points as suggested by learners.

Teaching points

- Offer emotional support and avoid judgement!
- Acknowledge that a safe dose of methadone may not completely suppress cravings, but should prevent uncomfortable withdrawal symptoms.
- Treat acute pain with short-acting opioids.
- Consider using adjuvant medications:
  - Gabapentin, antihistamines, antiemetics, antidiarrheals, and melatonin.
  - A2-agonists (e.g. clonidine or lofexidine) can mitigate symptoms as well, but watch for hypotension.
- Can continue methadone on discharge at a methadone clinic if this can be arranged, OR discontinue on discharge if not possible or the patient is not interested in continuing methadone.
- Do not prescribe methadone for treatment of OUD at discharge.
- Harm reduction:

– Information about needle exchanges, outpatient treatment resources.
– Naloxone prescription for overdose prevention.

Return to Objectives and Emphasize Key Points

1. Articulate the importance of addressing acute opioid withdrawal in hospitalized patients:
   - Treating withdrawal helps prevent complications and disruptions of care for acute medical problems.
   - Potential to engage patients in ongoing addiction treatment.
2. Strengthen the therapeutic alliance with patients by acknowledging the discomfort of withdrawal, expressing provider support and discussing a plan for medication to address withdrawal symptoms.
3. Assess symptoms of acute opioid withdrawal:
   - Ask patients about their typical experience.
   - Look for objective signs (mydriasis, diaphoresis, piloerection, etc.).
   - Consider checking COWS score.
4. Use methadone appropriately to safely mitigate withdrawal symptoms:
   - Start with up to 30 mg of methadone, with a one-time dose of 5–10 mg after 4 h if still in active withdrawal, but don't go above 40 mg/day in the first 4 days.
   - Use scheduled short-acting oral opioids to fill the gaps until methadone dose levels out.
   - Engagement with outpatient treatment is Not a pre-requisite for management of withdrawal with methadone during an inpatient admission.

Resources

1. American Psychiatric Association. Diagnostic and statistical manual of mental disorders. 5th ed. Arlington: American Psychiatric Association; 2013.
2. Phillips GT, Gossop M, Bradley B. The influence of psychological factors on the opiate withdrawal syndrome. Br J Psychiatry. 1986;149:235–8.
3. Cohen AJ, Klett CJ, Ling W. Patient perspectives of opiate withdrawal. Drug Alcohol Depend. 1983;12(2):167–72.
4. Elkader AK, Brands B, Callaghan R, Sproule BA. Exploring the relationship between perceived inter-dose opioid withdrawal and patient characteristics in methadone maintenance treatment. Drug Alcohol Depend. 2009;105(3):209–14. https://doi.org/10.1016/j.drugalcdep.2009.07.003.
5. Fanucchi L, Lofwall MR. Putting parity into practice — integrating opioid-use disorder treatment into the hospital setting. New Engl J Med. 2016;375(9):811–3.
6. Donroe JH, Holt SR, Tetrault JM. Caring for patients with opioid use disorder in the hospital. CMAJ. 2016;188(17–18):1232–9.

7. Noska A, Mohan A, Wakeman S, Rich J, Boutwell A. Managing opioid use disorder during and after acute hospitalization: a case-based review clarifying methadone regulation for acute care settings. J Addict Behav Ther Rehabil. 2015;4(2):1000138.
8. Nielsen S, Larance B, Lintzeris N. Opioid agonist treatment for patients with dependence on prescription opioids. JAMA. 2017;317(9):967–8.
9. Clinical Opiate Withdrawal Scale (COWS) https://www.drugabuse.gov/sites/default/files/files/ClinicalOpiateWithdrawalScale.pdf
10. American Society of Addiction Medicine (ASAM) National Practice Guideline for the Use of Medications in the Treatment of Addiction Involving Opioid Use https://www.asam.org/docs/default-source/practice-support/guidelines-and-consensus-docs/asam-national-practice-guideline-supplement.pdf

Chapter 50
Approach to Determination of Decision-Making Capacity

Jessica Woan and Kara Mitchell

Learning Objectives
1. Define the terms informed consent, medical decision-making capacity, competence.
2. Recognize when a formal capacity evaluation is necessary.
3. Evaluate a patient to determine his or her medical decision-making capacity.
4. Identify factors that may influence a patient's medical decision-making capacity, including "pseudo-incapacity."

Clinical Vignette: Ms. C. is a 70-year-old woman with history of diabetes, heart disease, and chronic obstructive pulmonary disease (COPD). Her daughter brings her to the emergency room because of 2 days of worsening right upper quadrant pain, fevers, and chills. Imaging demonstrates a stone in the common bile duct and urgent decompression with endoscopic retrograde cholangiopancreatography (ERCP) is recommended. She receives IV morphine, fluids, and antibiotics, and feels better. You must consent her for the procedure.

A. **What are the components of informed consent to consider when discussing ERCP with this patient?**

Write down the three key components as shown in Fig. 50.1.

J. Woan (✉)
VA Puget Sound Health Care System, Department of Medicine, Division of General Internal Medicine, University of Washington, Seattle, WA, USA
e-mail: Jessica.Woan@va.gov

K. Mitchell
University of Washington Medical Center, Department of Medicine, Division of General Internal Medicine, University of Washington, Seattle, WA, USA
e-mail: karajo@uw.edu

S. Mookherjee et al. (eds.), *Chalk Talks in Internal Medicine*,
https://doi.org/10.1007/978-3-030-34814-4_50

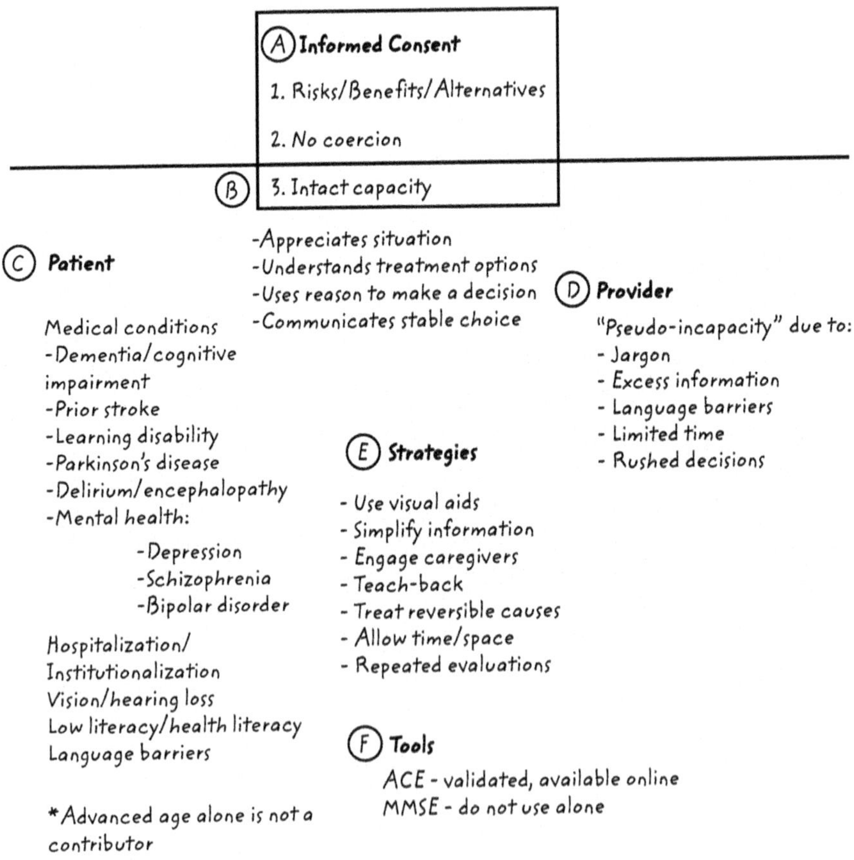

Fig. 50.1 Approach to determination of decision-making capacity: A–F

Teaching points

- Criteria for valid consent to medical treatment vary from state to state but are based on the following three elements:
  - The patient must be given adequate information regarding and demonstrate understanding of the nature and purpose of the proposed treatment, the risks and benefits of treatment, and alternatives to treatment, including no treatment.
  - The patient must be free from coercion.
  - The patient must have medical decision-making capacity.

B. **She declines to have the ERCP and wants to go home. You wonder if she has decision-making capacity. How will you assess her decision-making capacity?**

Ask learner how they would assess her decision-making capacity: Draw a line between "No coercion" and "Intact capacity," then write down the key elements as shown in Fig. 50.1.

Teaching points

- Medical decision-making capacity (MDMC) is the ability to understand and appreciate the nature and consequences of health care treatment decisions. Its determination is based on the patient's decision-making process rather than the final decision itself. Any licensed physician can make a determination of capacity.
- Patients are presumed to have decision-making capacity unless a clinical evaluation suggests that it is lacking. Studies suggest, however, that clinicians frequently fail to recognize when patients lack MDMC.
- In most United States jurisdictions, the patient is required to demonstrate four abilities to have capacity. The patient should be able to:
  - Appreciate his or her situation (including underlying values and current medical situation)
  - Understand the relevant information about proposed diagnostic tests or treatment
  - Use reason to make a decision
  - Communicate a choice (that is durable over time)
- A decision that is a result of a patient's consideration of his or her individual medical situation and treatment options in the context of his or her values demonstrates the patient's ability to reason effectively. There is no "right" or "wrong" decision against which the patient's decision should be judged.
- Capacity is situational and temporal.
- Because of this, evaluation of MDMC should occur in the context of specific medical decisions.

C. **On questioning, Ms. C states that she knows she has a severe infection, but does not believe she needs the ERCP. "I'm feeling better already." She is not sure what the alternatives to treatment are despite your counseling earlier.**

She states, "I don't believe in surgery" but cannot articulate reasons for this. She states she wants to live longer, but isn't sure what would happen if she refused the ERCP. When told again she could develop a life-threatening infection, she responds, "Well, it really wouldn't matter anyway." When asked the meaning behind this response, she states, "I've lived long enough already. I've suffered so much." The provider probes further, but the patient states, "I'm tired of all this talking. Can you stop asking so many questions?" Does our patient have medical decision-making capacity? What patient factors increase risk for incapacity?

Ask learners for their assessment, and then share that the patient does not demonstrate decision-making capacity. List patient factors that increase risk for incapacity.

Teaching points

- The patient does not demonstrate intact medical decision-making capacity. She seems to appreciate that she has a severe infection, but does not show a clear understanding of the risks and benefits of her treatment options. She seems to believe that because she feels improved, the ERCP is unnecessary. She does not clearly understand the potential complications of not removing the stone.
- Many factors may influence a patient's ability to make medical decisions. For example, certain diagnoses such as dementia, schizophrenia, or hospitalization for medical illness correlate with a higher prevalence of incapacity. A significant proportion of these patients, however, will possess intact MDMC.
- Of note, advanced age does not carry increased likelihood of decisional incapacity.

D. **What are some provider-related factors that might contribute to an inappropriate capacity determination?**

Write down causes of "pseudo-incapacity" as shown in Fig. 50.1.

E. **What factors are influencing the patient's current lack of capacity? What strategies could you use to increase the chances that Ms. C has decision-making capacity around the ERCP?**

Ask for specific strategies that could be used to address the factors negatively effecting the patient's MDMC and write then down as shown in Fig. 50.1.

Teaching points

- Factors that may be contributing to our patient's lack of capacity are her current illness, effects of morphine, and possible hypoxemia from COPD and/or heart failure, undiagnosed hearing loss, depression, delirium, or dementia.

- It is also possible her provider used excessive jargon or may not have given enough time for decision-making. In addition, she hasn't stated why she is making a choice to refuse, and has asked the provider to stop the assessment.
- Provider strategies to optimize potential for improving capacity are as follows:
  - Use visuals.
  - Shorten or simplify information.
  - Engage family members and caregivers.
  - Acknowledge that fear, anxiety, and the illness itself can affect capacity.
  - Collateral information can be helpful in making determinations regarding capacity.
  - Use teach-back methods.
  - Address reversible causes: pain, fever, hypoxemia, uremia, sedation, delirium, psychosis, undiagnosed depression.
  - Optimize potential to improve thought processing and communication.
  - Allow sufficient time and space for discussion, questions, and decision-making.
  - Repeat the evaluation.

F. **What formal tools are available to help screen for incapacity?**

Write down Aid to Capacity Evaluation (ACE) and Mini-Mental State Examination (MMSE) as shown in Fig. 50.1.

- The Aid to Capacity Evaluation (ACE) is a semistructured evaluation of the participant's ability to understand relevant information and appreciate reasonably foreseeable consequences with regard to the specific treatment decision. This specific capacity assessment can be performed within 30 minutes and has been validated against a clinical gold standard, has a reasonable level of evidence to support its use, and is available online for free.
- The Mini-Mental State Examination (MMSE) is a good screening tool for cognitive impairment, but do not use it as a capacity assessment by itself. It can, however, help you decide if a formal evaluation is needed:
  - Scores <20 had an increased likelihood of incapacity (LR = 6.3).
  - Scores >24 had significantly lowered likelihood of incapacity (LR = 0.14).
  - Scores 21–24 do not change the pretest probability for MDMC.

G. **We've talked about several different aspects about medical decision-making capacity—time to put it together. What would your first step be?**

Walk through the flowsheet in Fig. 50.2 *with Ms. C in mind.*

Teaching points

- It is usually accepted that competence is a legal term by which courts of law deem a patient unable to make decisions for him or herself. In cases where the courts deem a patient legally incompetent, there may be rare situations in which

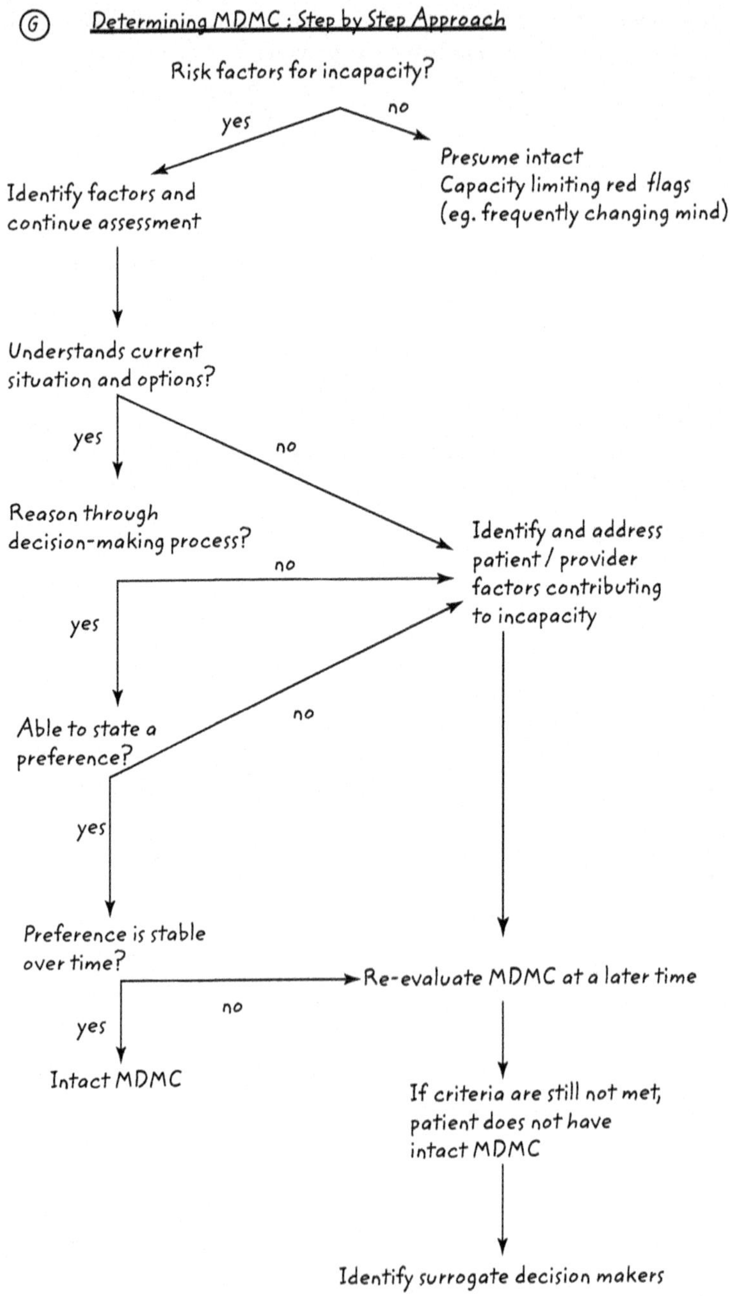

Fig. 50.2 Approach to determination of decision-making capacity: G

a patient does exhibit MDMC. If this is the case, an ethics committee consultation will be helpful.

- Because she is clinically stable, you've decided to evaluate for and treat potentially reversible causes and to reevaluate her decision-making capacity for ERCP at a later time.
- It would be also helpful to ascertain if her daughter is an appropriate surrogate for medical decision-making.

Return to Objectives and Emphasize Key Points

1. MDMC is usually presumed to be intact, but incapacity is frequently missed.
2. Patient and provider factors can influence capacity.
3. MDMC is specific to time and place. To have intact capacity, a patient must be able to:

   - Appreciate his or her situation (including underlying values and current medical situation).
   - Understand the relevant information about proposed diagnostic tests or treatment.
   - Use reason to make a decision.
   - Communicate a choice (that is durable over time).

Resources

1. Applebaum PS. Assessment of patients' competence to consent to treatment. N Engl J Med. 2007;357:1834–40.
2. Etchells E, Darzins P, Silberfeld M, et al. Assessment of patient capacity to consent to treatment. J Gen Intern Med. 1999;14(1):27–34. https://doi.org/10.1046/j.1525-1497.1999.00277.x.
3. Fields LM, Calvert JD. Informed consent procedures with cognitively impaired patients: a review of ethics and best practices. Psychiatry Clin Neurosci. 2015;69:462–71. https://doi.org/10.1111/pcn.12289.
4. Merel SE, Murray SB. Decisional capacity. In: Scheurer D, editors. Hosp Med Clin. 2013;2:e263–73. https://doi.org/10.1016/j.ehmc.2012.10.002.
5. Mitchell KJ. Chapter 34: decision-making capacity. In: Wong CJ, Hamlin NP, editors. The perioperative medicine consult handbook. New York: Springer Science + Business Media; 2013. https://doi.org/10.1007/978-1-4614-3220-3_34.
6. Sessums LL, Zembrzuska H, Jackson JL. Does this patient have medical decision-making capacity? JAMA. 2011;306:420–7.
7. Community tools: Aid to capacity evaluation (ACE). University of Toronto Joint Centre for Bioethics. Available at http://jcb.utoronto.ca/tools/ace.shtml.

Chapter 51
Management of Pharmacotherapy for Depression

Nicole Chow Ahrenholz and Amy Baernstein

Learning Objective
1. Choose an antidepressant suitable for a patient.
2. Be aware of psychiatric and medical comorbidities that affect medication choice.
3. Monitor response to a medication and adjust when needed.
4. Develop an approach to discontinuing antidepressants.

Clinical Vignette: A 46-year-old woman describes feelings of depressed mood, anxiety, insomnia, and tearfulness. She is no longer enjoying teaching kindergarten or attending her middle school children's activities. Her patient health questionnaire-9 (PHQ-9) score is 18 (moderately severe depression). These symptoms have persisted for several months and she is ready to "do something about it." Together you decide to start an antidepressant medication.

A. **What comorbidities are important to explore in this patient?**

List the categories "psychiatric symptoms," "medical mimics," "impacts dosing," and "conditions that exclude certain meds," as shown in Fig. 51.1.

Teaching points
- Consider psychiatric consultation before starting an antidepressant when there is a history of mania, psychosis, actively suicidal, substance use disorders.
- Medical conditions may mimic depression including hypothyroidism, sleep apnea.

N. C. Ahrenholz (✉)
Harborview Medical Center, Department of Medicine, Division of General Internal Medicine, University of Washington, Seattle, WA, USA
e-mail: ncahren@uw.edu

A. Baernstein
University of Washington Medical Center, Department of Medicine, Division of General Internal Medicine, University of Washington, Seattle, WA, USA

S. Mookherjee et al. (eds.), *Chalk Talks in Internal Medicine*,
https://doi.org/10.1007/978-3-030-34814-4_51

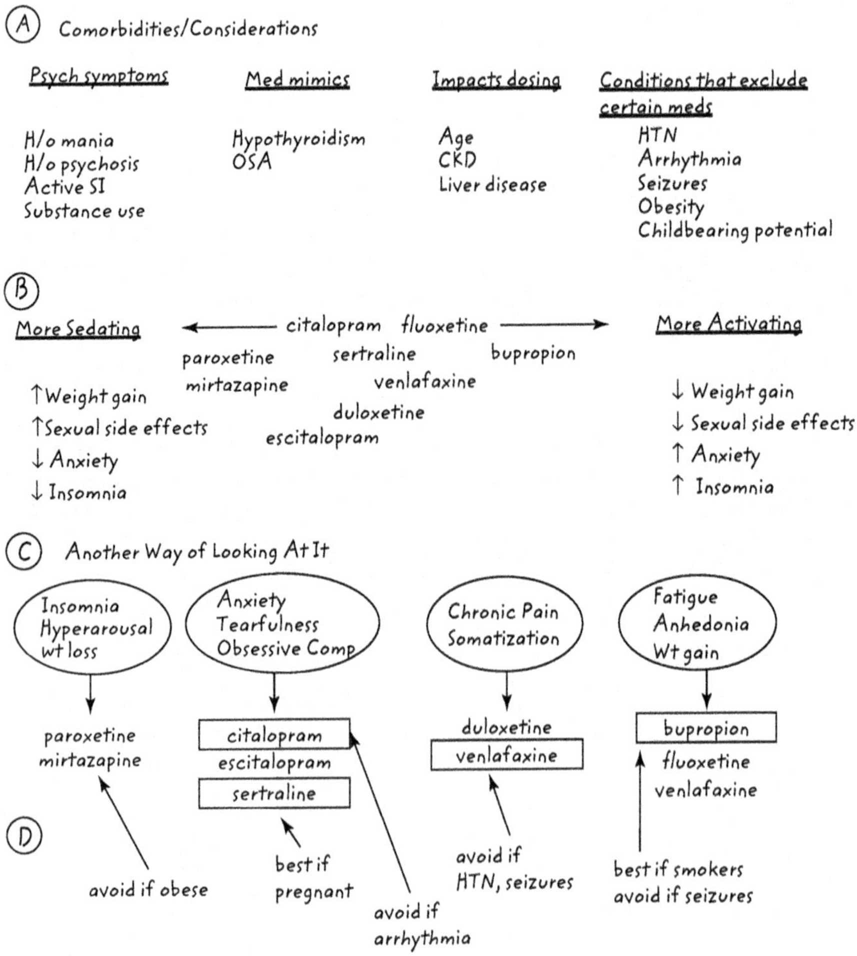

Fig. 51.1 Management of pharmacotherapy for depression, A–D

- Conditions that may impact dosing: age, chronic kidney disease (CKD), and liver disease.
- Conditions that might exclude certain agents: hypertension (HTN), arrhythmia, seizures, obesity, childbearing potential.

B. **The patient is most bothered by her insomnia and is concerned that medications might cause her to gain weight. What medication would you recommend for her?**

Draw out the continuum between "more sedating" and "more activating" as shown in Fig. 51.1. *Name common antidepressants and add them to the appropriate place as shown in* Fig. 51.1.

Teaching points
- First-line treatment is a second-generation antidepressant (not a tricyclic antidepressant (TCA) or monoamine oxidase inhibitor (MAOI)).
- Drug choice can be tailored to the patient's predominant symptoms, though there is not strong evidence for this approach.
- Citalopram or sertraline are reasonable initial choices for most patients; escitalopram, paroxetine, and fluoxetine are other first-line agents.

C. **If the patient had a history of chronic pain, how would that change your recommendation for initial medication?**

Write out the four groups of symptom complexes under "another way of looking at it." Ask learners which medications fall under each column.

D. **If the patient had a history of arrhythmia, how would that change your recommendation?**

Indicate the preferred and contraindicated medications as shown in Fig. 51.1.

E. **You decide to start citalopram 20 mg daily. When would you see her back?**

Start the algorithm in Fig. 51.2.

Teaching points
- Return to the clinic within 1–2 weeks to assess adherence, side effects, suicidal ideation (SI).
- Consider seeing younger patients (<25 years old) weekly for the first month due to higher suicide risk.

F. **After 2 weeks, she still feels depressed and has been having nausea and headaches. You encourage her to persist through her side effects and at 4 weeks she feels significantly less depressed, though not back to her usual self. PHQ-9 is down to 15. Side effects have resolved. What should you do now?**

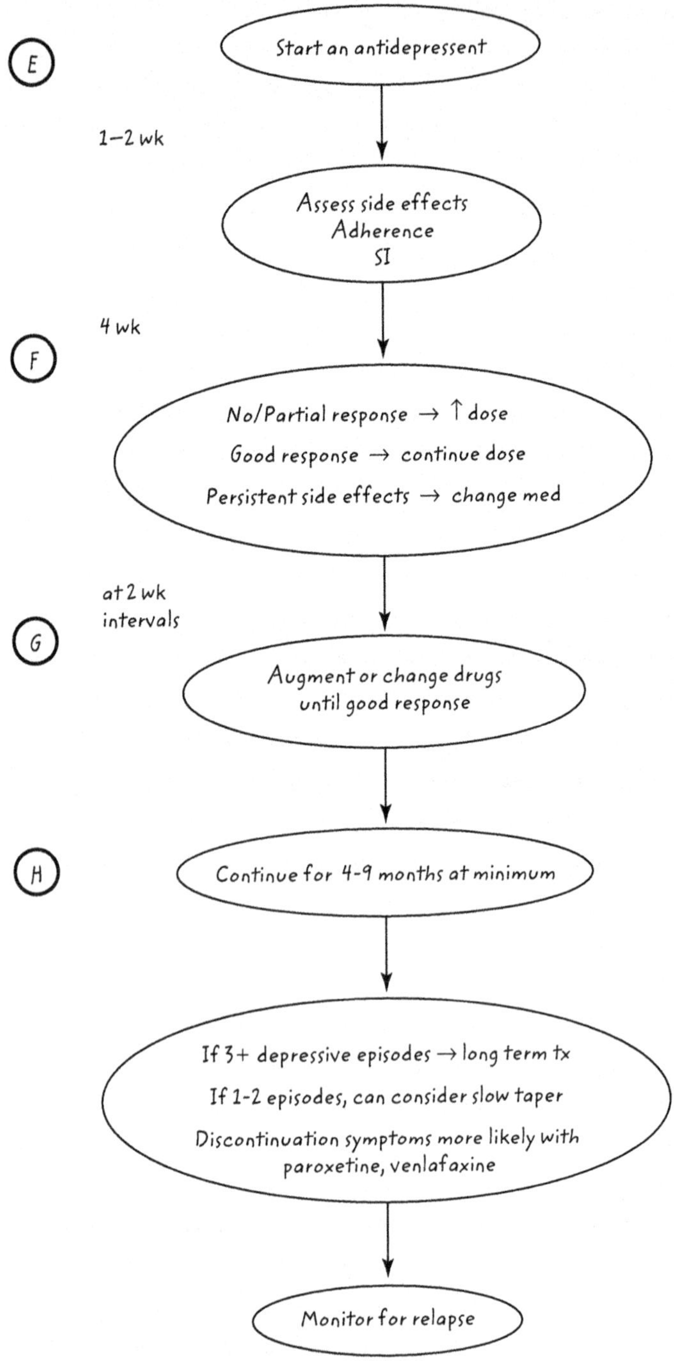

Fig. 51.2 Management of pharmacotherapy for depression, E–H

Continue the algorithm in Fig. 51.2.

Teaching points

- Remind patients that side effects tend to wane after 2 weeks, whereas mood improvement does not start until at least 2 weeks and takes at least 6 weeks for maximal effect.
- For no or partial response, increase the dose of citalopram.
- For full response, continue same dose.
- If side effects are persistent and bothersome, change medication.

G. **She's been on the maximum dose of citalopram for 12 weeks and still feels depressed but not as bad as before the medication. PHQ-9 is down to 10. What should you do now?**

Continue the algorithm in Fig. 51.2.

Teaching points

- For partial response, augment with bupropion (more activating) or buspirone (better relief from anxiety).
- If no response, switch to another second-generation antidepressant, either from the same class or from a different class.
- Have patient at a maximum dose for 8 weeks before deeming that drug a failure.

H. **You see her 4 months later and she has been feeling normal on citalopram and bupropion. Is it advisable to discontinue? If so, how?**

Continue the algorithm in Fig. 51.2.

Teaching points

- Antidepressants should be continued at least 4–9 months to reduce risk of relapse.
- Many patients self-discontinue.
- Long-term maintenance is necessary for patients with three or more episodes of depression and may be helpful in other settings.
- Tapering SSRIs mitigates the unpleasant (though not dangerous) discontinuation symptoms
  - Abdominal pain
  - Sleep disturbance
  - Neurologic symptoms (dizziness, tremor, paresthesias)
- Discontinuation symptoms are more likely with some medications (venlafaxine, paroxetine) than others (fluoxetine). A tapering plan can be tailored to the anticipated degree of symptoms.

Return to Objectives and Emphasize Key Points

1. Choose an antidepressant suitable for a patient
   - Start a second-generation antidepressant.

- Consider tailoring medication choice to a patient's predominant symptom (anxiety, insomnia, fatigue, chronic pain).
- Citalopram 20 mg daily is a reasonable initial choice for most depressed patients.

2. Be aware of psychiatric and medical comorbidities that affect medication choice

   - Mania, psychosis, suicidality, substance use, HTN, arrhythmia, seizures, obesity, childbearing potential

3. Monitor response to a medication and adjust when needed

   - Return in 1–2 weeks to assess adherence, side effects, suicidal ideation.
   - Return in 4 weeks to assess response, and consider increasing dose.
   - Return in 2 weeks intervals to assess response. For partial response, consider augmenting with bupropion or buspirone. For no response, switch to another second-generation antidepressant (can be from the same class or a different class).

4. Develop an approach to discontinuing antidepressants

   - Advise continuing for at least 4–9 months after remission to prevent relapse.
   - Advise patients to taper gradually to avoid discontinuation symptoms.

Resources

1. McCarron RM, Vanderlip ER, Rado J. In the clinic. Depression. Ann Intern Med. 2016;165(7):ITC49–64.
2. Lin SY, Stevens MB. The symptom cluster-based approach to individualize patient-centered treatment for major depression. J Am Board Fam Med. 2014;27(1):151–9.
3. Sinyor M, Shaffer A, Levitt A. The sequenced treatment alternatives to relieve depression (STAR*D) trial: a review. Can J Psychiatr. 2010;55(3):126–35.
4. American Psychiatric Association: Practice Guideline for the Treatment of Patients with Major Depressive Disorder, 3rd ed., 2010. http://psychiatryonline.org/guidelines.aspx. Accessed 25 May 2017.

Chapter 52
Approach to Pharmacotherapy for Alcohol Withdrawal

Albert Ackil and Genevieve L. Pagalilauan

Learning Objective

1. Review the basic physiology of alcohol intoxication, tolerance, and withdrawal.
2. Determine appropriate treatment setting for managing acute alcohol withdrawal.
3. Apply a symptom-triggered benzodiazepine treatment plan for alcohol withdrawal.
4. Become familiar with the three main medications used to support long-term recovery from alcohol use disorder.

Clinical Vignette: A 65-year-old man presents to the emergency department (ED) complaining of severe anxiety, nausea, and palpitations. He has a history of severe alcohol withdrawal, including seizures and alcoholic hallucinosis. He normally drinks 12 to 18 beers a day. Last drink was ~12 h ago and he says he tried to "quit cold turkey." He denies suicidal ideation. Vitals include mild tachycardia and hypertension but are otherwise stable. His examination is notable for anxious mood, diaphoresis, and diffuse fine tremor but normal orientation and sensorium. Initial Clinical Institute Withdrawal Assessment (CIWA) score is 14.

A. **Should this patient be managed in the hospital or referred to outpatient detox treatment? What are the three factors that should go into making the decision?**

Draw the three boxes for "CIWA score," "Clinical factors," and "Local resources" as shown in Fig. 52.1. *Lead learners through the algorithm.*

A. Ackil (✉)
University of Colorado Hospital, Department of Medicine, Division of Hospital Medicine, University of Colorado, Denver, CO, USA

G. L. Pagalilauan
University of Washington Medical Center, Department of Medicine, Division of General Internal Medicine, University of Washington, Seattle, WA, USA

S. Mookherjee et al. (eds.), *Chalk Talks in Internal Medicine*,
https://doi.org/10.1007/978-3-030-34814-4_52

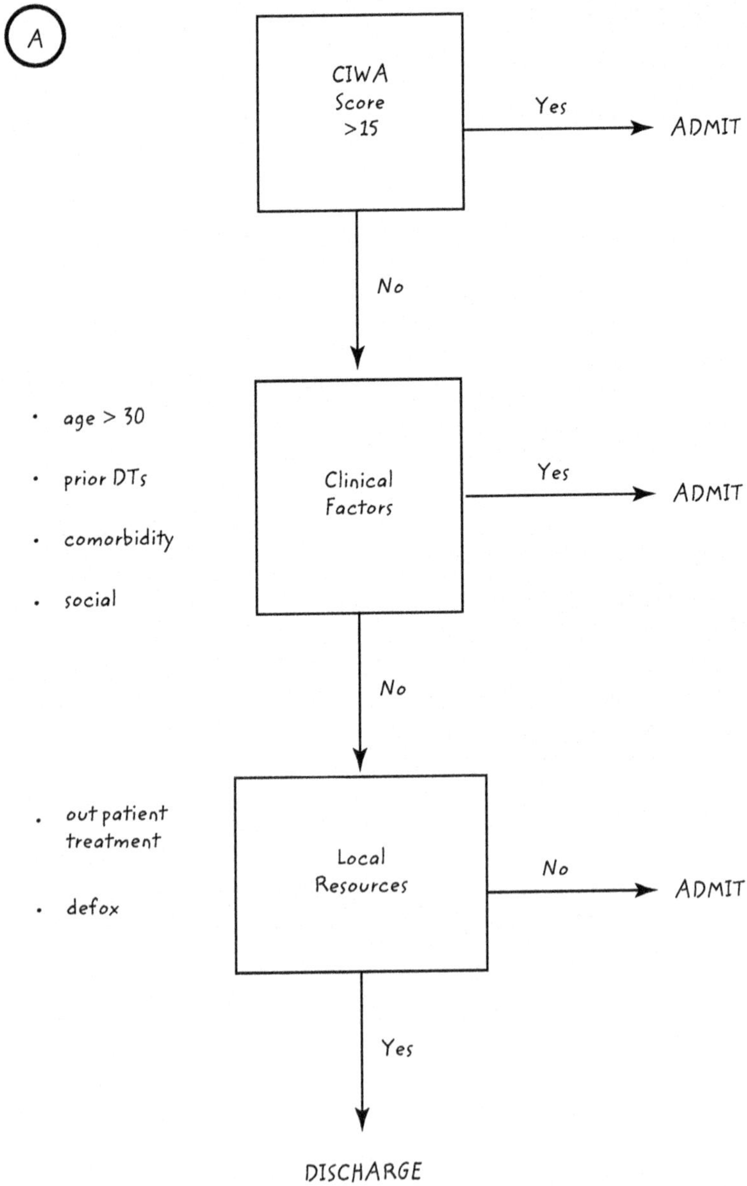

Fig. 52.1 Approach to pharmacotherapy for alcohol withdrawal, A

Teaching points

- The triage decision of outpatient versus inpatient treatment of alcohol withdrawal should take into consideration the initial CIWA scores, clinical factors, and local resources.
- Initial CIWA score.
  - Strong predictor of overall withdrawal episode severity (must wait for blood alcohol level (BAL) to drop <0.02 g/dL before assessing).
  - Well-validated assessment scale of alcohol withdrawal severity. Includes 10 domains of subjective (headache, nausea, anxiety, hallucinations) and objective (tremor, diaphoresis, orientation) findings associated with withdrawal, each domain is scored 0–7 based on severity. Usually nursing task. There can be high intraoperator variability.
  - <8—very mild withdrawal. No need for medication, low risk for progression to severe withdrawal.
  - 8–15—mild withdrawal, clinical decision for admission versus output treatment based on clinical factors.
  - >15—moderate withdrawal, generally needs admission to hospital.
  - >20—severe withdrawal, usually needs intensive care unit (ICU) level care.
- Clinical factors associated with more severe withdrawal episodes include:
  - Age >30 years
  - Alcohol-specific factors—history of prior delirium tremens (DTs) or seizures, longer history of heavy drinking
  - Active comorbid conditions—acute kidney injury, electrolyte derangements, infection, unstable mental illness, or cognitive impairment
  - Psychosocial—stable housing, family support, ability to return to daily outpatient appointments, prior unsuccessful treatment
- Local resources—what are the limitations of local outpatient programs? Is there a medical detox facility available?

B. **What is the mechanism of alcohol's effect to create intoxication, tolerance, and withdrawal states in the central nervous system (CNS)?**

Draw the four see-saws as shown in Fig. 52.2*, leaving the circles containing "GABA" and "GLUT" unlabeled. Title each see-saw as "normal," "alcohol intoxication," "alcohol tolerance," and "alcohol withdrawal." Ask learners to indicate the GABA/GLUT balance in each case.*

Teaching points

- Normal balance of excitatory glutamate (GLUT)/N-methyl-D-aspartate (NMDA) and inhibitory gamma-aminobutyric acid (GABA) neurotransmitter tone in the CNS maintains alertness and normal brain function.

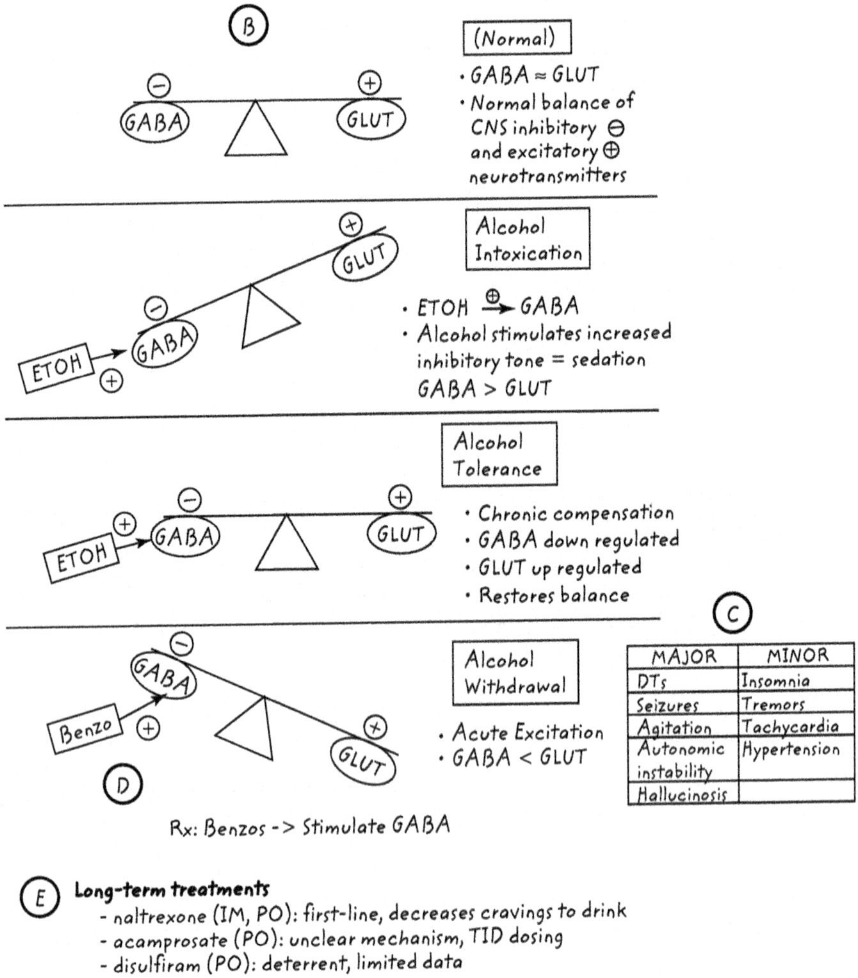

Fig. 52.2 Approach to pharmacotherapy for alcohol withdrawal, B–E

- With alcohol intoxication, GABA receptors are disproportionately activated, leading to sedation.
- Tolerance represents a state of chronic compensation with downregulation of GABA receptors and upregulation of glutamate receptors.
- Alcohol withdrawal occurs when there is removal of GABA activation, leading to inappropriate overstimulation of excitatory glutamate receptors.
- Patients first need to develop tolerance before withdrawal can occur.
- Even 1 week of heavy steady drinking can lead to minor withdrawal.
- Need >1 month of steady use to develop moderate/severe withdrawal.

C. **What are some major and minor alcohol withdrawal symptoms and complications?**

Label two columns "major" and "minor" and add symptoms and complications as listed by learners.

Teaching points

- Major—delirium tremens, seizures, alcoholic hallucinosis (not to be confused with DTs), severe agitation, autonomic instability
- Minor—insomnia, tremors, anxiety, nausea, anorexia, headache, hypertension, tachycardia, palpitations
- Other—hypovolemia, electrolyte derangements, gastrointestinal bleeding, malnutrition

D. **You admit the patient to your medicine service. He receives a "banana bag," an intravenous infusion of isotonic fluids, electrolytes, and vitamins including thiamine. What other treatments are commonly used for acute alcohol withdrawal?**

Draw an arrow showing how benzodiazepines stimulate GABA release.

Teaching points

- Benzodiazepines (Benzos)!—Enhance GABA release and receptor binding.
- No one benzodiazepine shown to work better than others—choice determined by half-life and local pharmacy availability.
  - Lorazepam, oxazepam—short half-life, 4–6 h
  - Chlordiazepoxide, diazepam—longer half-life, can be >20 h
- Evidence favors using a symptom-triggered strategy versus fixed dose taper, incorporating CIWA scoring as a method of determining timing of doses.

- Phenobarbital—used as adjunct for refractory withdrawal or DTs—works synergistically with benzodiazepines by increasing duration of GABA receptor channel opening.
- Supportive care also very important—IV fluids, antiemetics, electrolyte repletion, nutritional support.

E. **Over the next 72 h, your patient's acute withdrawal symptoms improve with benzodiazepine treatment. You discuss his last period of sobriety, which was about 3 years ago and lasted for 18 months. This was managed through an outpatient addiction clinic and he formerly used naltrexone depot injections to help maintain sobriety. He is motivated to change his drinking and wants to restart naltrexone. What are the commonly used medications to treat alcohol use disorder?**

List medications as suggested by learners.

Teaching points
- Naltrexone—mu-opioid receptor antagonist, oral (PO) or depot intramuscular (IM) injection available.
- Acamprosate—mechanism of action not well understood, possible glutamate modulation, dosed three times per day (TID).
- Disulfiram—blocks aldehyde dehydrogenase causing buildup of toxic acetaldehyde levels.
- Medications need to be combined with psychosocial interventions—motivational interviewing, group therapy, cognitive behavioral therapy (CBT)—often delivered by specialty addictions clinic.
- The goal is "bridge to maintenance" strategy at discharge with referral to outpatient addiction treatment clinic or inpatient rehabilitation facility.

Return to Objectives
1. Review the basic physiology of alcohol intoxication, tolerance, and withdrawal
   - Balance of inhibitory (GABA) and excitatory (glutamate) neurotransmitters.
2. Determine appropriate treatment setting for managing acute alcohol withdrawal
   - Use CIWA score, clinical factors, and available local resources to determine safety of discharge versus inpatient observation.
3. Apply a symptom-triggered benzodiazepine treatment plan for alcohol withdrawal
   - Short-acting agents are cornerstone of this treatment strategy.
   - CIWA scores determine need for medication dosing.
4. Become familiar with the three main medications used to support long-term recovery from alcohol use disorder.
   - Naltrexone, acamprosate, and disulfiram.

Resources

1. Perry E. Inpatient management of acute alcohol withdrawal syndrome. CNS Drugs. 2014;28(5):401–10.
2. Gortney J, Raub J, Patel P, Kokoska L, Hannawa M, Argyris A. Alcohol withdrawal syndrome in medical patients. Cleve Clin J Med. 2016;83(1):67–79.
3. Mayo-Smith M. Pharmacological management of alcohol withdrawal. A meta-analysis and evidence-based practice guideline. American Society of Addiction Medicine Working Group on Pharmacological Management of Alcohol Withdrawal. JAMA. 1997;278(2):144–51.
4. Schuckit M. Recognition and management of withdrawal delirium (delirium tremens). N Engl J Med. 2014;371(22):2109–13.
5. Muncie H, Yasinian Y, Oge' L. Outpatient management of alcohol withdrawal syndrome. Am Fam Physician. 2013;88(9):589–95.

Index

S. Mookherjee et al. (eds.), *Chalk Talks in Internal Medicine*,
https://doi.org/10.1007/978-3-030-34814-4

V

W

X

The manufacturer's authorised representative in the EU is Springer Nature Customer Service Centre GmbH, Europaplatz 3, 69115 Heidelberg, Germany. If you have any concerns regarding our products, please contact ProductSafety@springernature.com

Printed and bound by CPI Group (UK) Ltd, Croydon, CR0 4YY
22/09/2026
02220957-0006